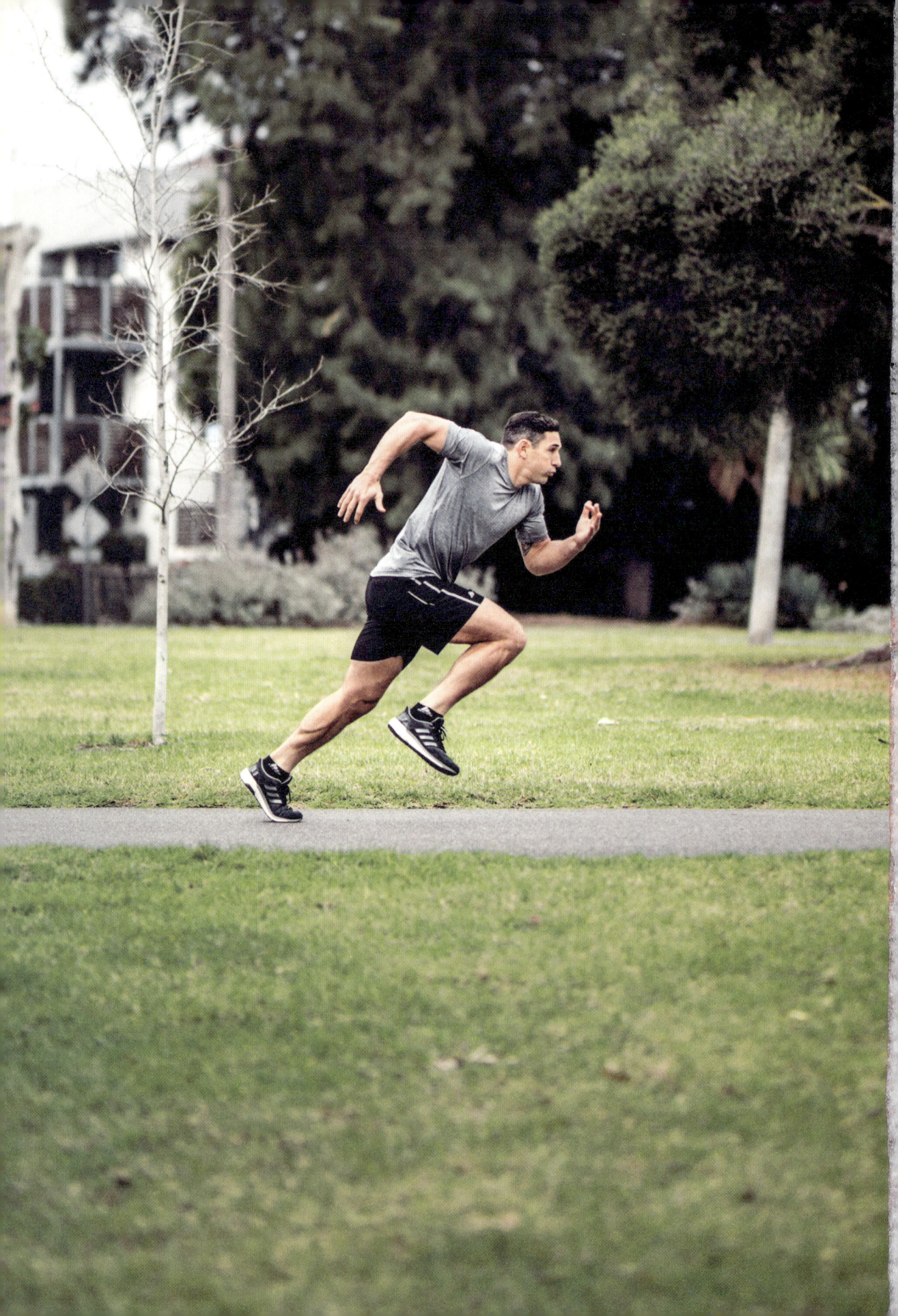

MOVE
WITH
BILLY SLATER
AND COACH MICHAEL CHAPMAN

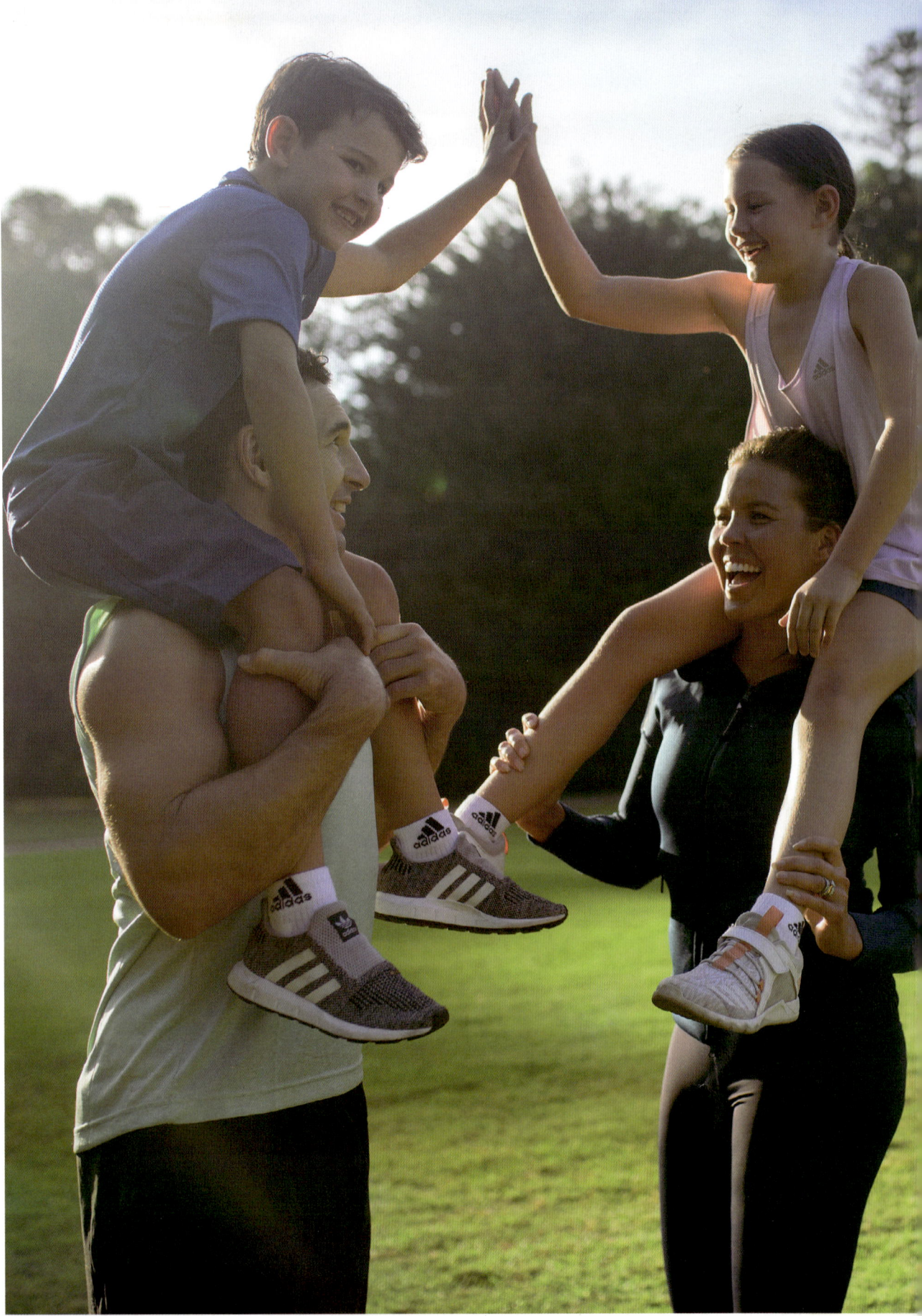

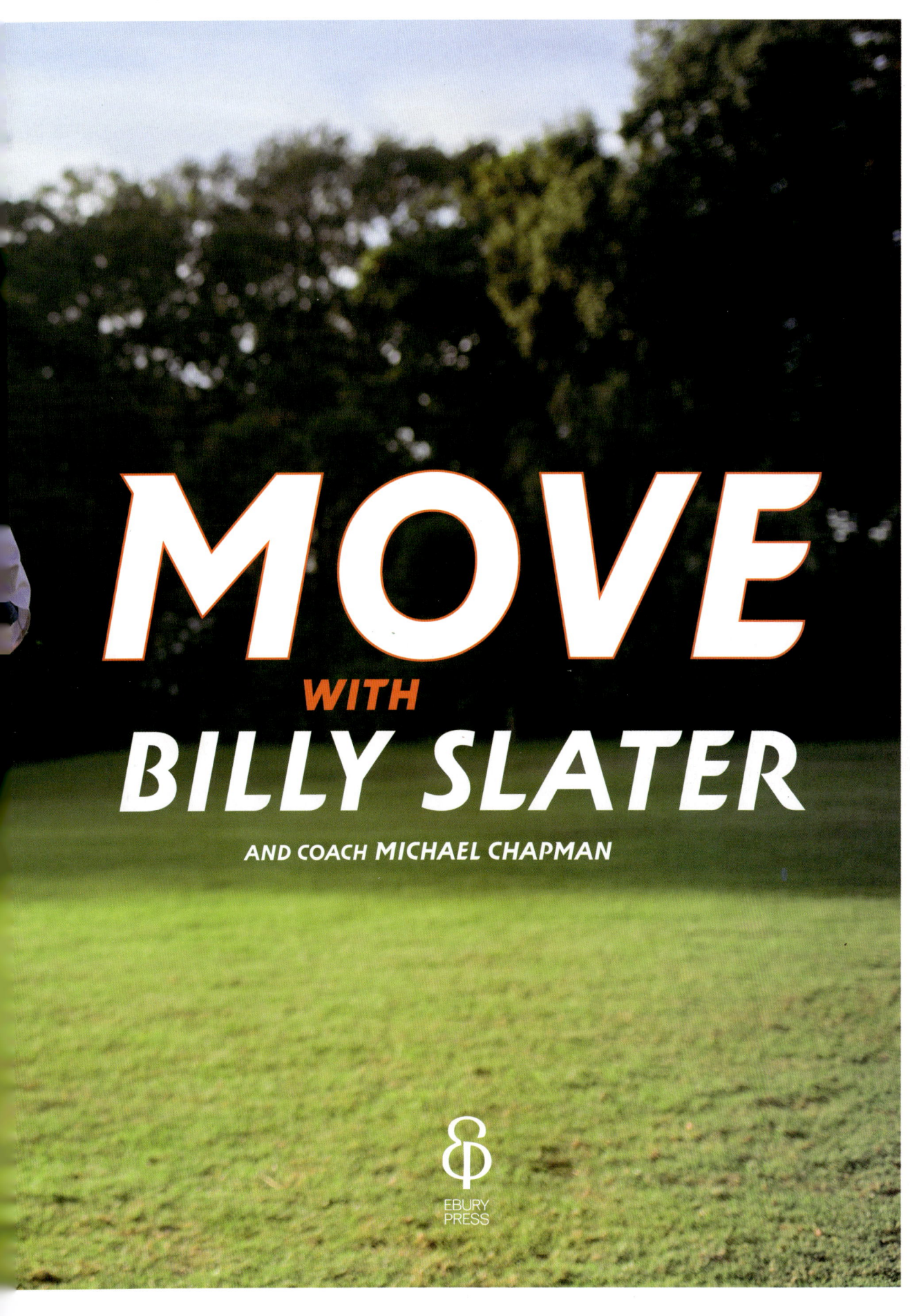

MOVE
WITH
BILLY SLATER
AND COACH MICHAEL CHAPMAN

EBURY PRESS

This book is not intended as a substitute for professional medical advice. The reader should regularly consult a physician in matters relating to his/her health, particularly with respect to any symptoms that may require diagnosis or medical attention, and must obtain their own professional medical advice before relying on or otherwise making use of the dietary and exercise information in this book.

An Ebury Press book

UK | USA | Canada | Ireland | Australia
India | New Zealand | South Africa | China

Penguin Books is part of the Penguin Random House group of companies whose addresses can be found at global.penguinrandomhouse.com.

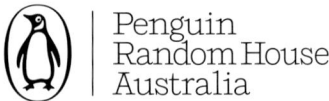

First published by Penguin Random House Australia Pty Ltd 2018

Text copyright © Billy Slater 2018
Photography copyright © Daily Press 2018

The moral right of the author has been asserted.

All rights reserved. Without limiting the rights under copyright reserved above, no part of this publication may be reproduced, stored in or introduced into a retrieval system, or transmitted, in any form or by any means (electronic, mechanical, photocopying, recording or otherwise), without the prior written permission of both the copyright owner and the above publisher of this book.

Text and cover design by Nada Backovic © Penguin Random House Australia Pty Ltd
Internal and cover photography by Daily Press
Typeset in Joanna Sans Nova by Post Pre-Press Group, Brisbane, Queensland
Colour separation by Splitting Image Colour Studio, Clayton, Victoria
Printed and bound in China by RR Donnelley

 A catalogue record for this book is available from the National Library of Australia

ISBN 978 0 14379 320 5

penguin.com.au

Contents

FOREWORD – VII

INTRODUCTION – VIII

MEET THE SLATERS – 3

FUELLING YOUR MOVEMENT – 4

PREPPING FOR EXERCISE – 6

HOW TO USE THIS BOOK – 10

BLOCK 1: WESTERN AUSTRALIA – 13

    ADVICE FOR BEGINNERS – 39

BLOCK 2: NEW SOUTH WALES – 41

    GETTING THE KIDS FIRED UP – 65

BLOCK 3: QUEENSLAND – 67

    FINDING YOUR MOTIVATION – 93

BLOCK 4: SOUTH AUSTRALIA – 95

    HALF-TIME COACH'S PEP TALK – 121

BLOCK 5: AUSTRALIAN CAPITAL TERRITORY – 123

    STAYING IN THE HABIT – 149

BLOCK 6: VICTORIA – 151

    EXERCISING THROUGH INJURY – 175

BLOCK 7: TASMANIA – 177

    KEEPING IT UP IN SCHOOL HOLIDAYS – 203

BLOCK 8: NEW ZEALAND – 205

ACKNOWLEDGEMENTS – 231

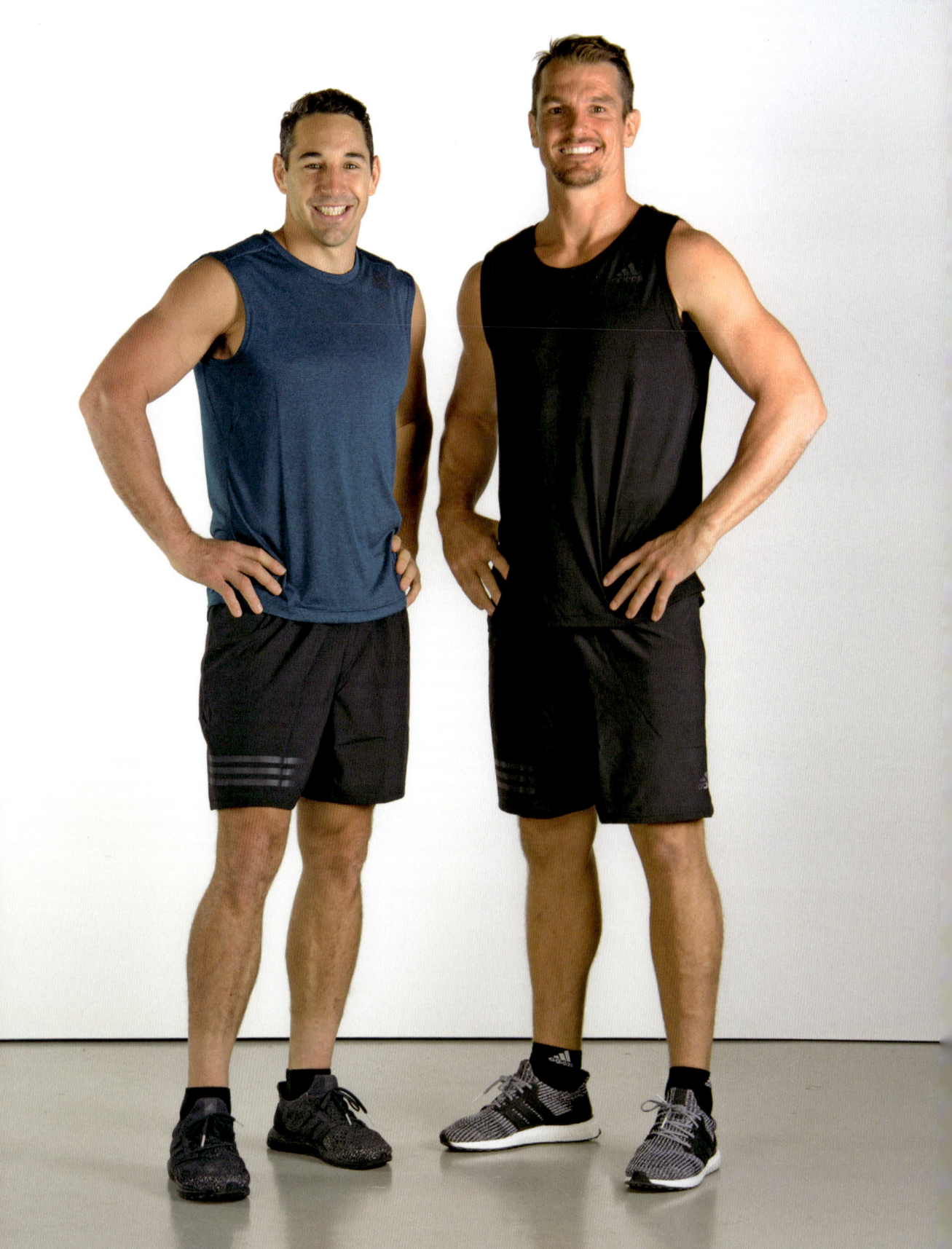

Foreword

Hi Team Move,

I have spent a large part of my life using regular and active functional movements to build and maintain a healthy outlook. Cornerstone to this: your body is the greatest fitness tool you can use.

I'm thrilled to be able to share some of the fantastic bodyweight workouts and functional movements that I incorporate into my daily personal training sessions. These movements will increase your cardio work rates and endurance, and help you lose weight while building core body strength. Importantly, they can be undertaken by anyone of any fitness level because they solely rely on your own body at your own level of intensity.

Billy and I have worked together to create these workouts so they're ideal for you and your family. Your training goals are probably different from those of other members of your family (or friends), but the key is to keep your focus and aim to achieve your best.

You can build your fitness in as little as 10 minutes for a workout. The range of motions included within this practical guide will provide you with a solid understanding of how to correctly perform specific movements. It will also, in combination with a balanced diet and positive mindset, improve your overall body health.

The workouts and movements are designed so you can MOVE at home, MOVE in a hotel room, MOVE at work or MOVE in the backyard. In fact, you can MOVE anywhere! You don't need equipment to get healthy.

It might sound a little bit on the serious side here, guys, but that's about as serious as we get. Have fun with your workouts. Get your friends involved, to help get to the better you. Exercising should be done with a smile, as well as a bit of sweat, with the aiming of improving your goals!

If you want to lose some weight, get rid of the dad bod, get your pre-baby body back, develop your summer shape or just get fitter, stronger and healthier, we're here to get this sorted for you.

Have fun and train well.

Cheers,

Coach Mike

> Mike is an internationally trained and accredited expert bodyweight trainer. A former professional athlete himself, on a daily basis he trains all manner of people looking to achieve their health and wellness goals, including elite athletes.

Introduction

Hi guys,

We're really excited to be able to share some of our fitness tips and exercises with you.

We've tried to keep a lot of these movements and exercises so that they are not only achievable but also enjoyable for you (and your family) to do. Over time, you should see an increase in your fitness levels, enjoyment of exercise and ability to do those movements you may have thought were not for you.

As you can appreciate, I do a lot of training, both for personal fitness and for the big game each weekend. What I know to be true is that you have to get the basics right. We've included basics that focus on core muscle groups and are created to help you become fitter.

We've had a heap of fun putting this book together. My family – wife Nicole, daughter Tyla and son Jake – have not stopped laughing, jumping, squatting, rolling around and smiling, as we've done these exercises as a family.

We love being a healthy family. I know that it might sound easy coming from me, but anyone can do it, anywhere and anytime.

You don't have to be a fitness guru or even a full-time athlete. All you have to do is to want to be a better, healthier and fitter version of yourself. Only you can make this happen, so what are you waiting for?

It's really quite simple to do. In just 10 minutes for a workout, you can get moving. You don't need to spend money on gym memberships or fancy equipment. Everything that you need is either in your home, in the yard or at the park. Your body is made for exercising. Sometimes, all it needs is a little helping hand to remind it that nature intended us to MOVE.

You feel better when you MOVE.
Your mind is clearer when you MOVE.
Your heart is healthier when you MOVE.
Your outlook on life is more positive when you MOVE.

Let's get moving together and kick your goals!

Cheers,

Billy

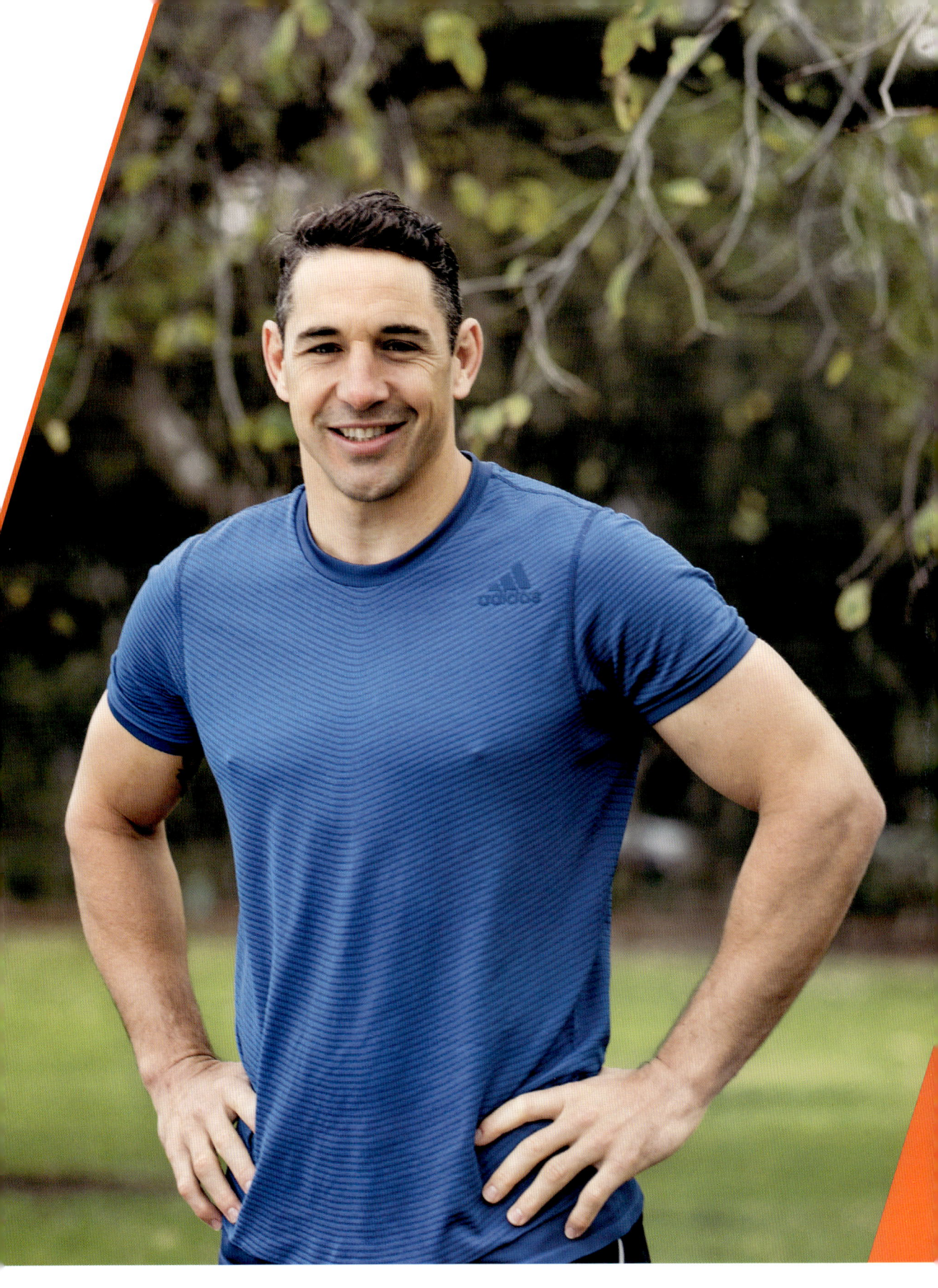

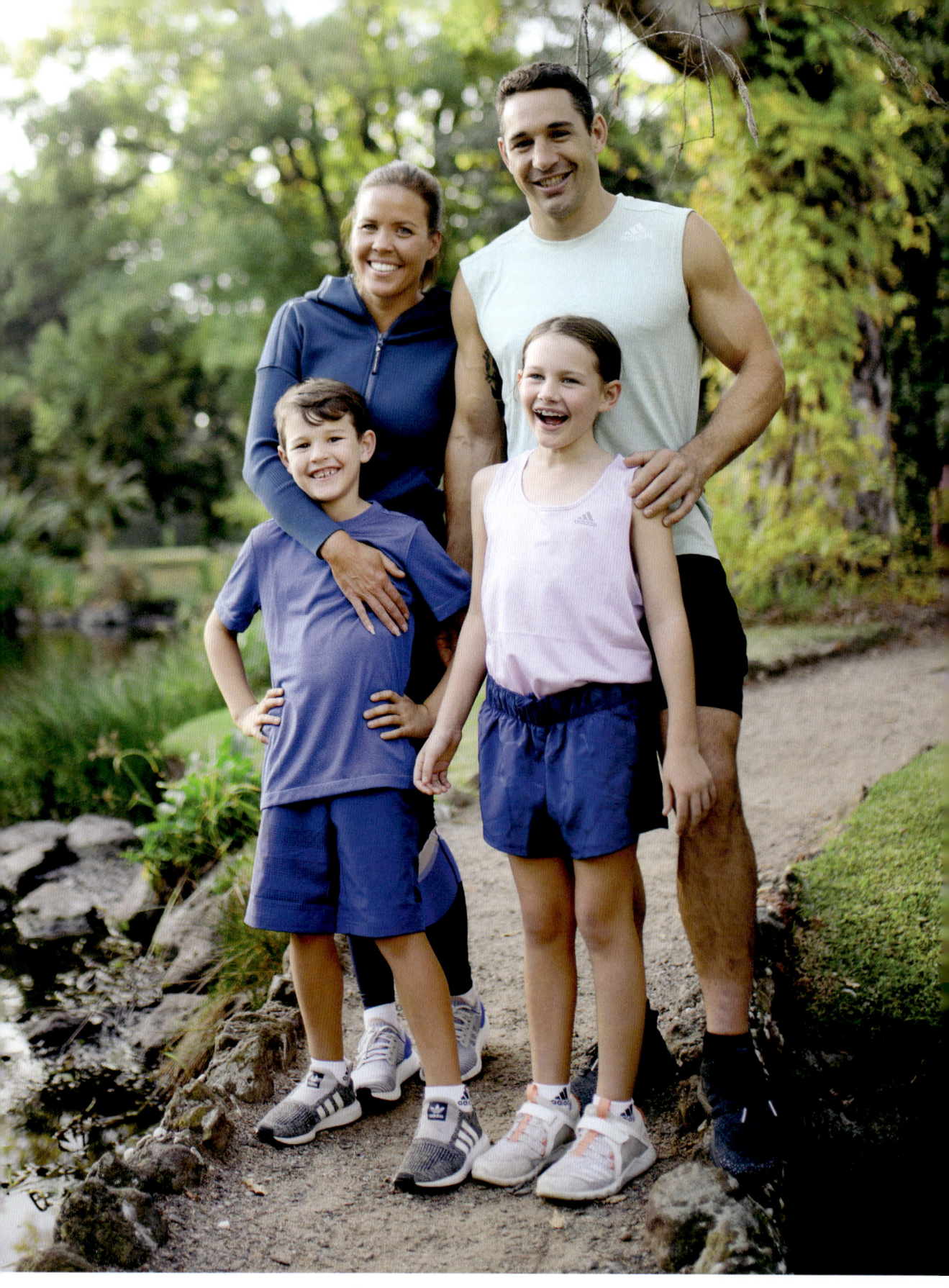

Meet the Slaters

Billy
One of the most recognisable athletes in Australian sport. In a rugby league career spanning more than 15 years and 300 top-level NRL games, Billy has achieved everything that has been put in front of him and more. He's a future immortal of the game. He has also won the coveted title of Australia's greatest athlete on two occasions, a testament to his all-round health and fitness approach to everyday living. Billy is a family man, husband to Nicole and father to Tyla and Jake.

Nicole
Well-regarded self-taught artist and loving mother of two. Nicole is focused on raising the two kids to be respectful, healthy and well-rounded people. Her passion for horses and the outdoors provides her with a strong sense of identity and appreciation for nature. Nicole is an active mother who loves playing with her kids and doing outdoor activities with the family. She is also passionate about her training with her girlfriends.

Tyla
Ten years old. Tyla has a beautiful outlook on life which is highlighted by her love of play, exercise and being active. She enjoys playing and running around the park with her friends. The ideal day for Tyla would be waking up, having bacon, eggs and avocado for breakfast, and listening to her fave music while dancing in the kitchen. She has a passion for animals, with her horses being number one.

Jake
Eight years old. Fun-loving young boy who enjoys being outdoors, whether this is running around with Buddy (the family dog) or out on the footy field. Constantly has a big smile on his face and is a really positive boy. If Jake had to pick which one he'd prefer, study or sneakers, there's little doubt that he'd grab his sneakers and head out the door!

Fuelling Your Movement

The whole philosophy around what you eat and when you eat it has changed from when Billy first started playing rugby league. Back then it was all carbs for your energy, whereas now it's good fats, avocados, nuts, bacon, eggs – that sort of stuff. He tries to stay relatively light leading into physical activity, just bananas or sometimes even just Vegemite sandwiches, so he doesn't feel too heavy or full.

There's a lot of information available about healthy eating and positive food habits, and it's good to be mindful of what you eat if you are exercising for a goal. One of the most important things to keep in mind is balance.

By balance, we mean you should try to eat fruit and vegetables every day. The benefits they bring are fantastic. There are many essential vitamins and nutrients within fruit and veggies that give us the energy to exercise, the resources to think and the ability to achieve our goals.

While we may have defined nutritional and supplement plans as a part of our professional training programs, we still enjoy eating a balanced diet. In combination with fruit and vegetables, we recommend eating legumes (nuts and beans), protein (eggs, chicken, red meats, pork, fish and turkey) and carbs (think wholegrain bread, pasta, cereals and brown rice).

Supplements are also a useful way to top up on your balanced eating approach. Remember, these supplements, whether they be multivitamins, protein shakes or meal-replacement drinks, should not form the foundation of your dietary needs. Use them in addition to the fruits, vegetables, grains, legumes, carbs and proteins that will make your body feel great.

With all of these foods to choose from to help you feel and become fitter, try to change up your weekly meals so you enjoy these nutritious ingredients in a variety of ways. For example, if you like chicken, make a chicken stir-fry one week, a lightly crumbed chicken schnitzel the next and perhaps a poached chicken salad for dinner the week after.

Don't forget to keep hydrated throughout the day, not just when you're training. Drinking water is a great way to keep your body ready to combat any toxins, improve your skin complexion, relieve fatigue and increase your energy levels.

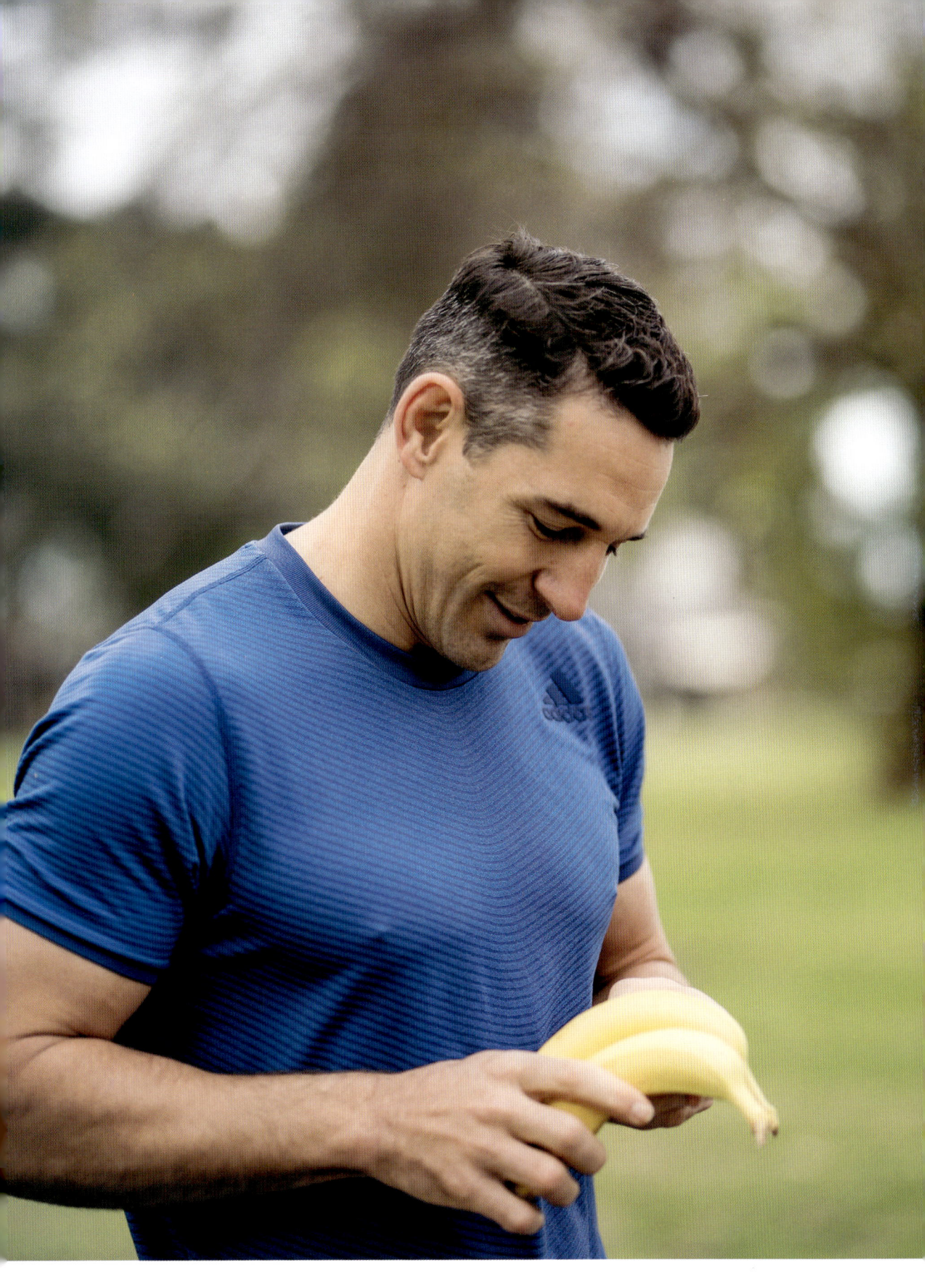

Prepping for Exercise

Before you're ready for your workout, you'll need to do some stretching. The whole point here is to let your body know there's going to be some action soon. Really good stretches help your muscles and joints prepare for the higher-impact fun to come. With any pre- and post-workout stretching, remember not to overdo it. There's no medal for the world's best workout stretching champion! Listen to your body, guys – it will tell you when it's ready to move on.

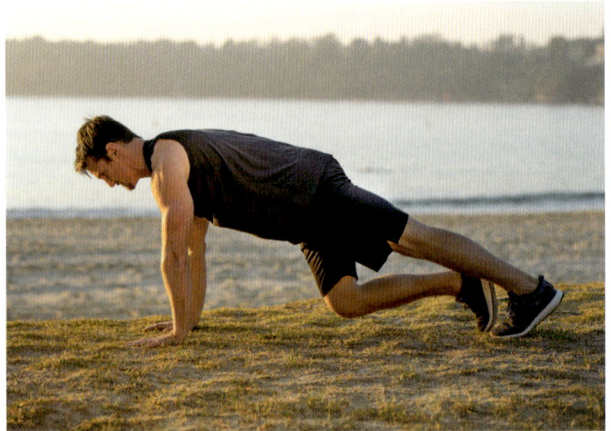

Calf stretch

Start in a high plank position, with your feet and hands both flat on the ground. From here, slowly transfer your weight onto one foot by releasing the heel of the other. Move backwards and forwards for 10 seconds. Repeat 3 times.

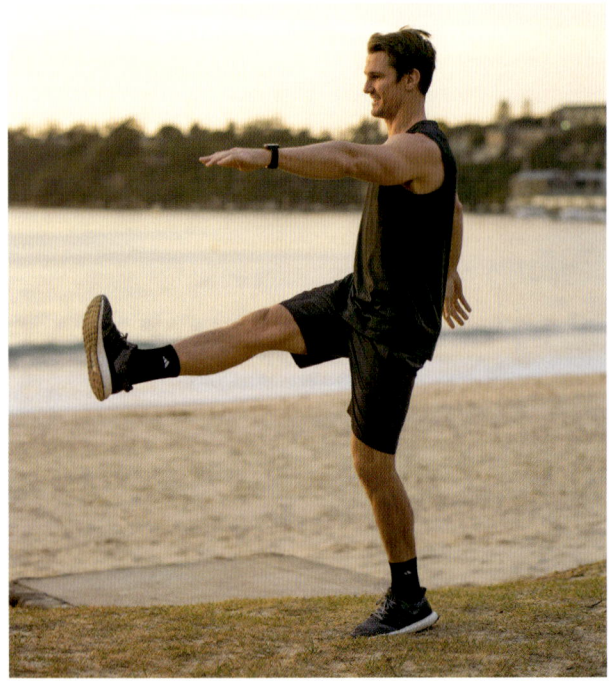

Leg swing

Swing your leg backwards and forwards, repeating this motion 10 times for each leg. (If you have trouble balancing, hold a wall or chair for stability.)

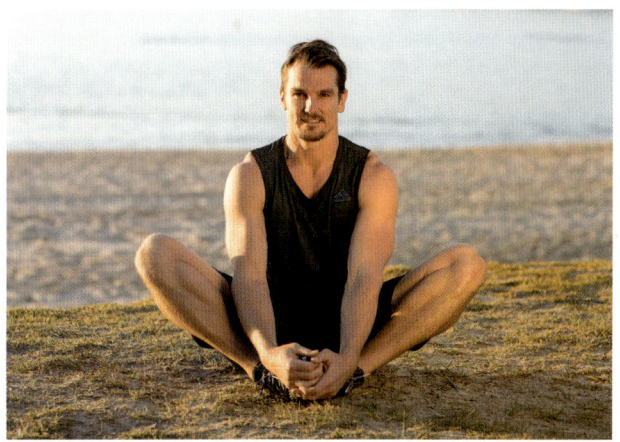

Adductor stretch
Sitting down with the soles of your feet together, grab your ankles and slowly push down your legs with your elbows until you feel a stretch in your adductors/groin. Hold this stretch for 20 seconds.

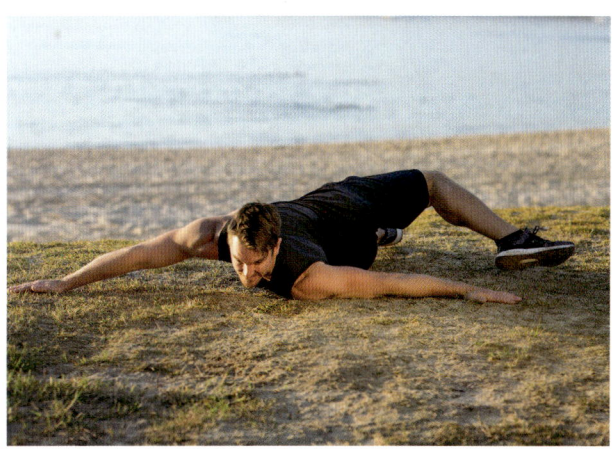

Scorpion stretch
Start facedown on the floor with your arms fully outstretched to the sides. Lift one leg off the floor, cross it over the body and touch the floor on the other side. Return your leg to the starting position and repeat on the other side.

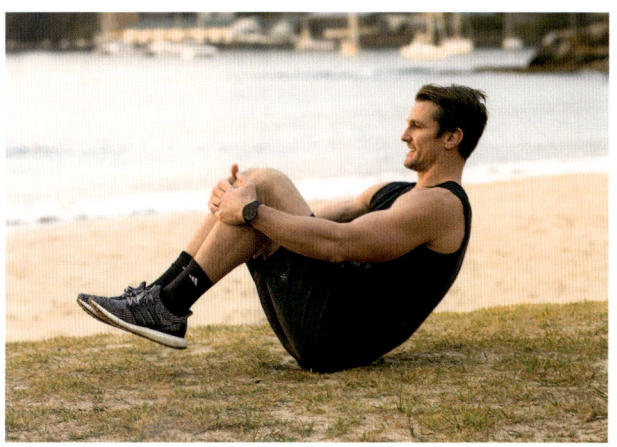

Back roll
Sitting on the floor, bring your knees towards your chest. Put your hands on your knees. From here, slowly rock backwards and forwards, repeating 10 times.

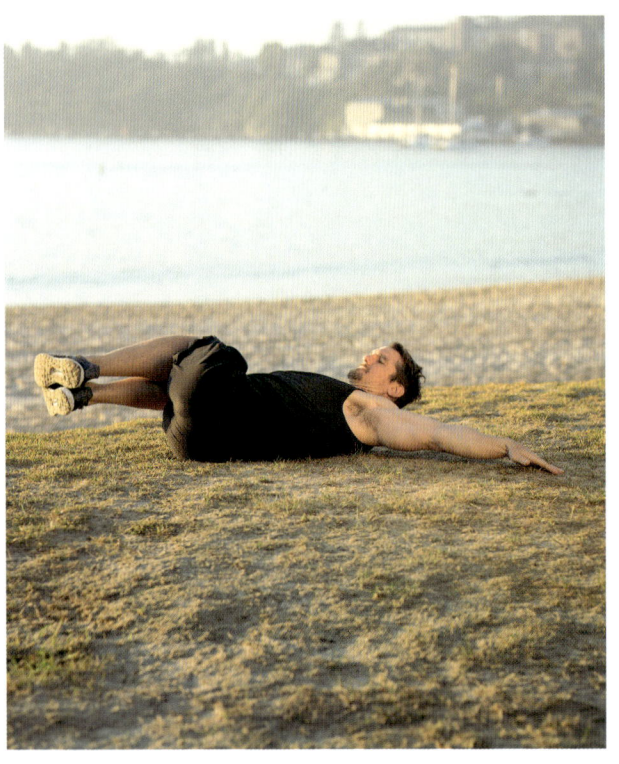

Knee drop

Start by lying on your back with your knees bent on a 90-degree angle and your arms spread out to your sides. Keeping your back firmly against the ground, move your knees to the side until your bottom leg is about to touch the ground. Lift your legs back up to the starting position and repeat on the other side.

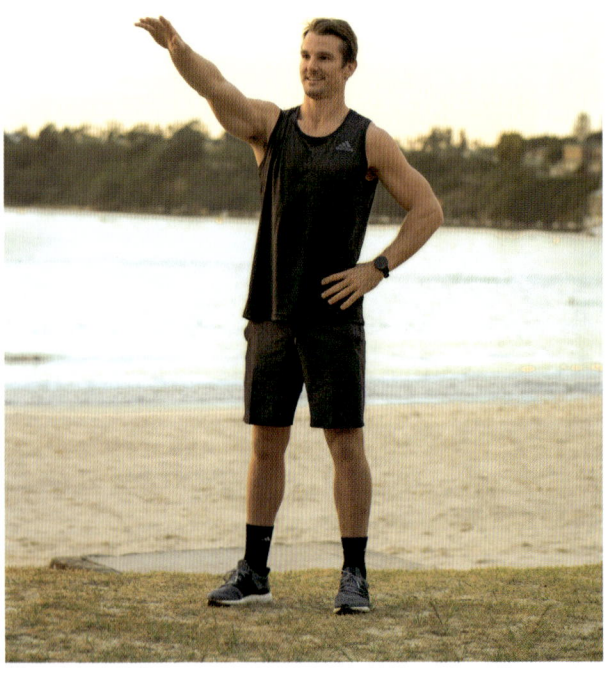

Upper body windmill

Place one hand on your hip. Lift your opposite arm straight out in front of you, then swing it down and back behind you then forward over your head in a circle motion. Swing forwards this way 5 times then reverse the motion backwards for 5 swings. Change arms and repeat.

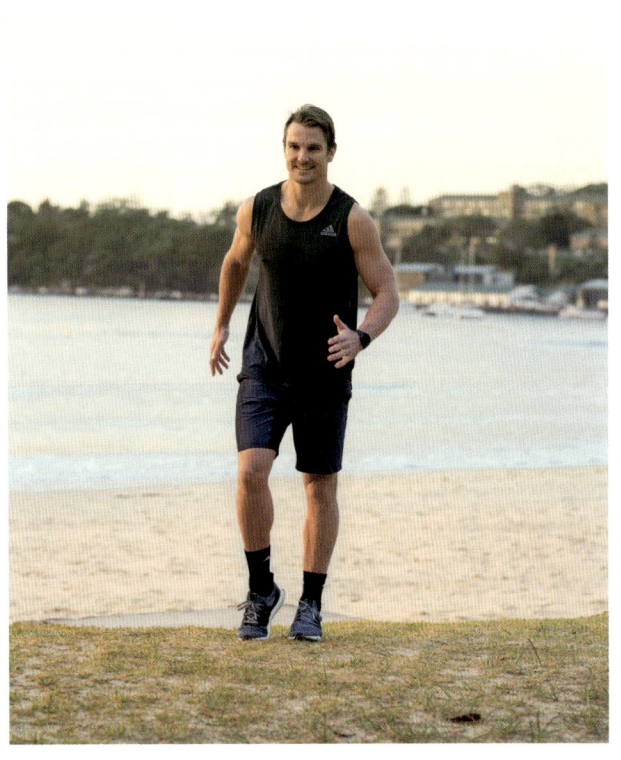

Tempo fast feet
Standing on the spot, sprint for 10 seconds at full speed then 5 seconds slow. Repeat 3 times.

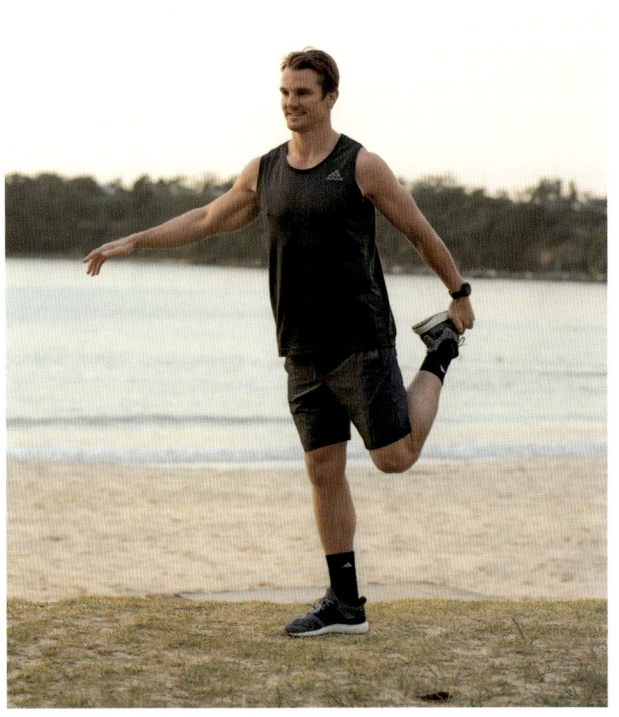

Quad stretch
Stand on one leg. Grab your other leg with one hand and pull towards your butt. Keep your chest out proud and hold for 20 seconds. Repeat on other leg. (If you have trouble balancing, hold a wall or chair for stability.)

How to Use This Book

Our book is designed to help you achieve your fitness goals. The exercises and body movements can be done inside at home, in the backyard, at the park – pretty much anywhere.

Each of the eight blocks are designed to take you through the week – four days of varied workouts, with a rest day in the middle.

We will give you the tools so that you feel confident in doing these exercises. Some of them may be new to you, while others you will be familiar with. We will give you the tips on not only how to perform these exercises properly, but also how they affect different body parts.

The workouts that we have created are set out to suit your fitness level or available time, so you can either train for a quick 10-minute burst, 20 minutes or a full half-hour. In some cases there's a special workout for the longer sessions – in the others, simply do two or three reps of the 10-minute option.

If you want to train for longer to challenge yourself further, fantastic. Remember, listen to your body. It's usually a great judge on how much training you should do! With a good training intensity, a 10-minute workout will burn calories and improve your overall fitness, so there's no need to overdo it.

By following our workout plan, you will be varying the exercises you do each week and adding some new movements to your fitness program to keep you progressing. This also keeps things fresh so that you can always enjoy your exercise.

As you MOVE through the book, you'll see we've included some of Nicole and Billy's Best scores. For example, Billy's best 10-second score = 18 for push-ups, which means he did 18 push-ups in 10 seconds. This is by no means designed to push you to achieve this number . . . but well done if you do! It's rather a guide for how Billy went. In the same way, consider keeping a diary of your personal bests for each exercise. Once you see the improvement in your scores, it's a great motivator to keep going.

In addition, you'll notice the letters 'BPT' at the beginning of each workout. That stands for 'Body Parts Targeted', so you know which parts of you are going to feel a bit sore tomorrow! Use this as a guide for tailoring workouts to you and your family's needs, or work through the book from cover to cover. We've designed MOVE as an overall fitness program.

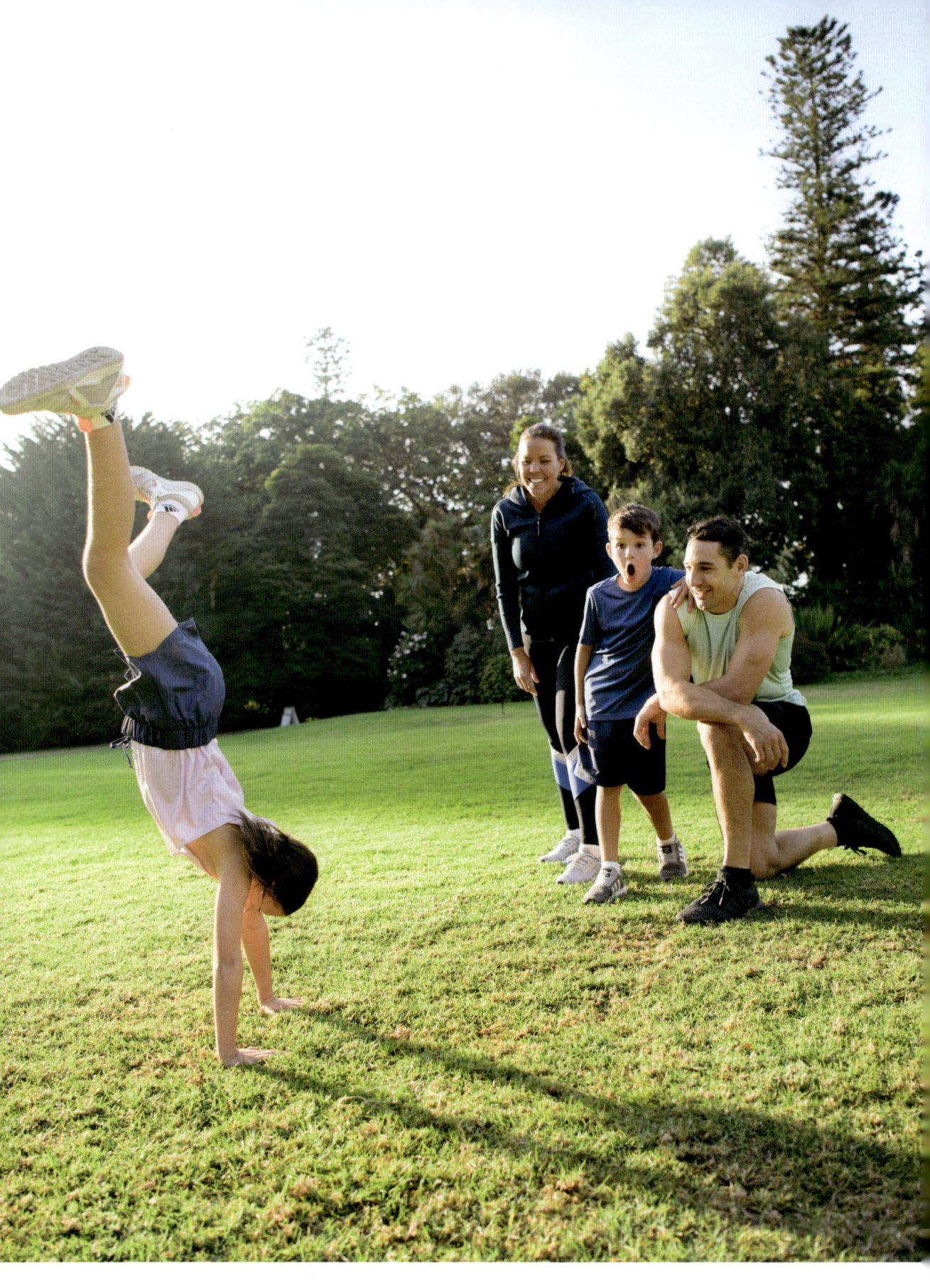

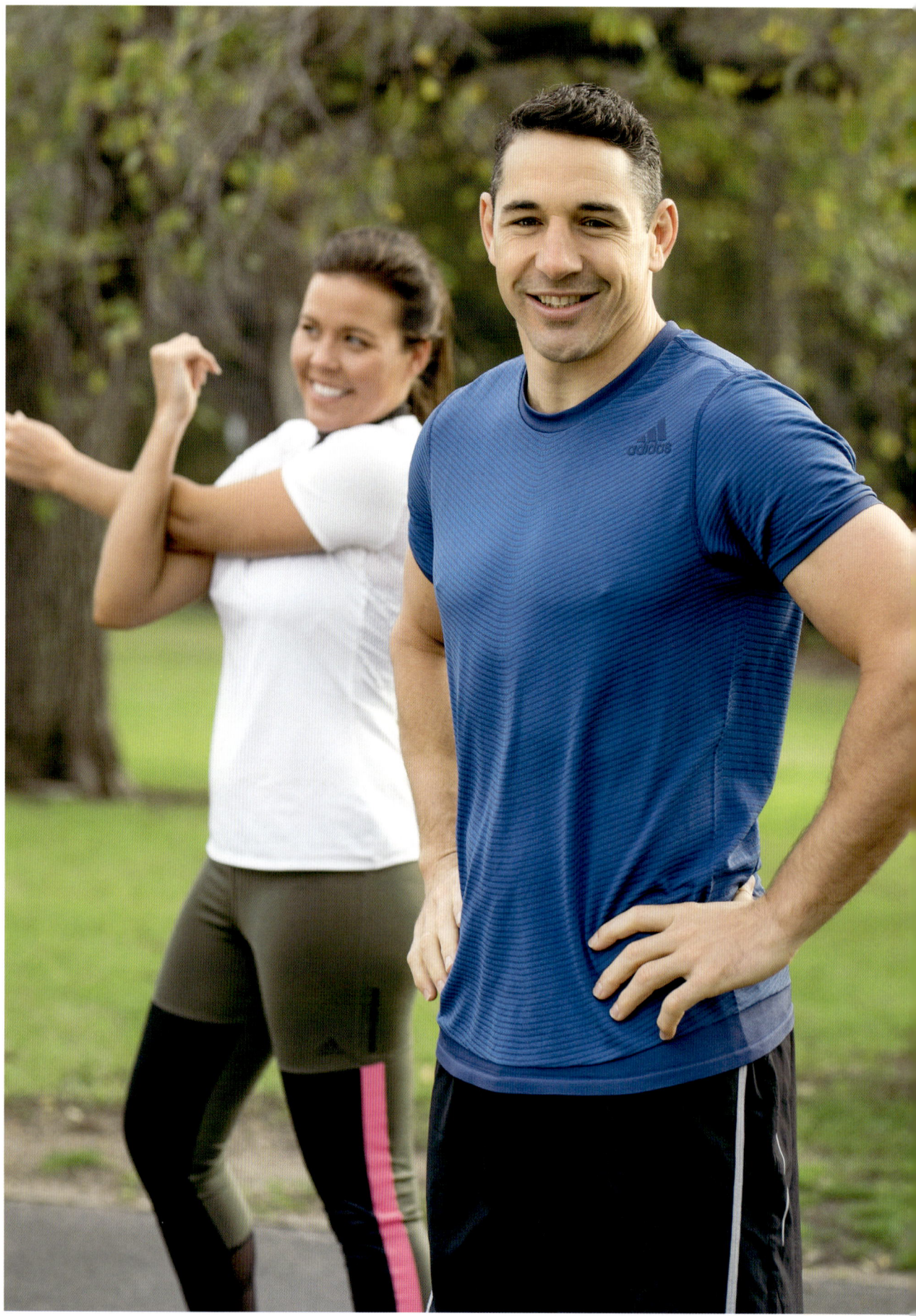

BLOCK 1: WESTERN AUSTRALIA

'The trips to WA are always memorable. I played a World Cup Test Match there a few years back. While I don't get across as often as I would like, the backdrops that Perth and its surrounds offer make moving around outside a treat.'

Billy

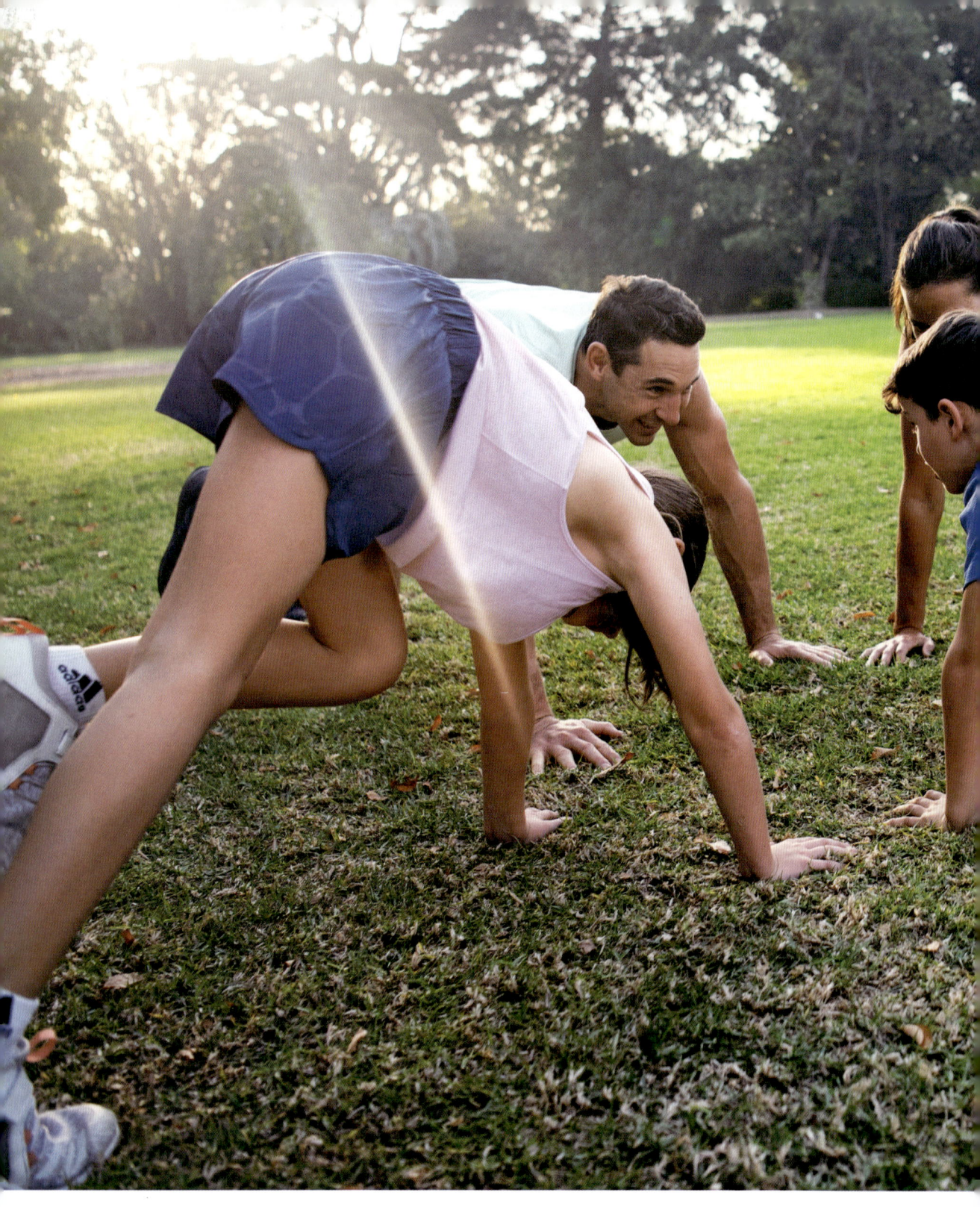

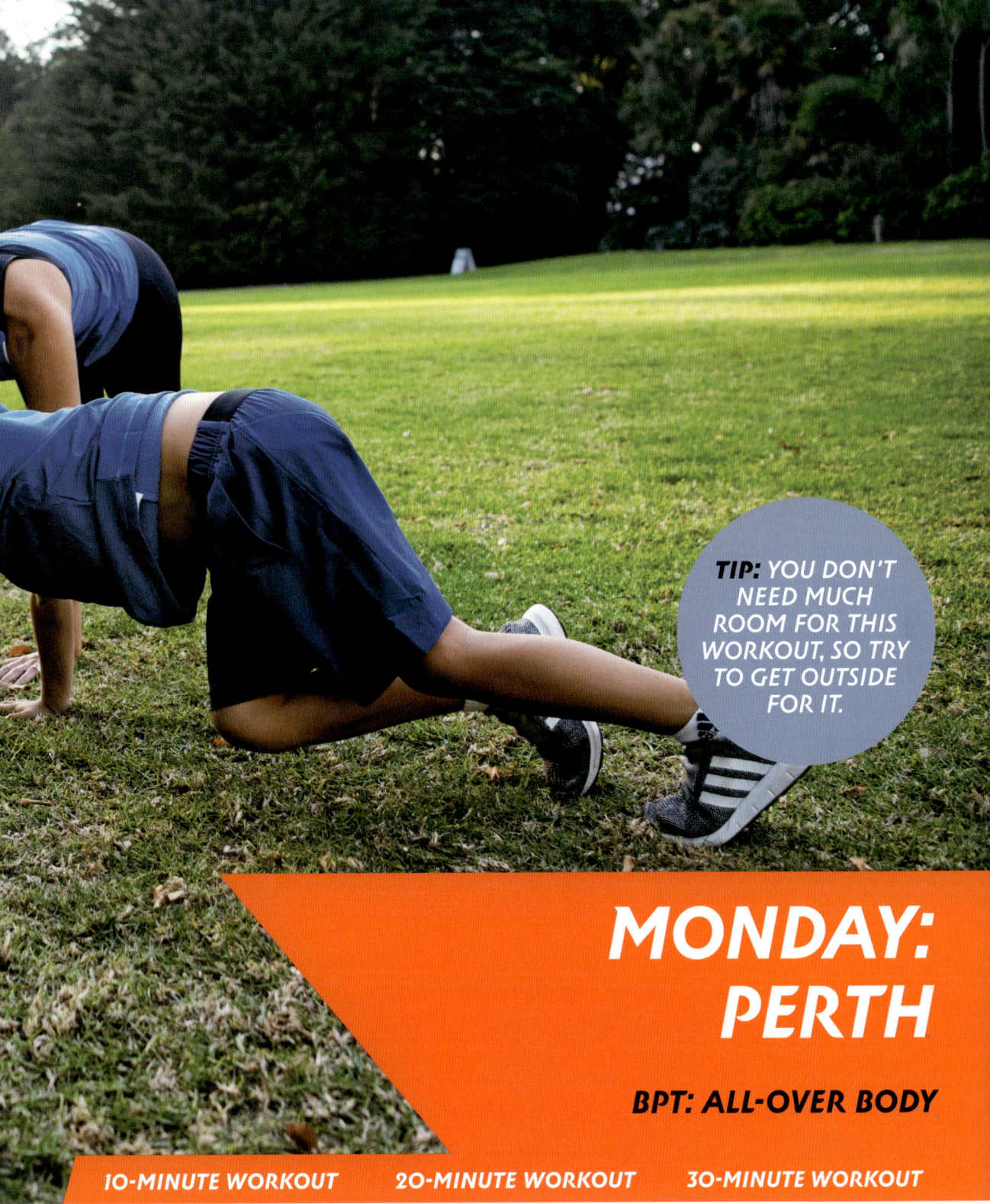

TIP: YOU DON'T NEED MUCH ROOM FOR THIS WORKOUT, SO TRY TO GET OUTSIDE FOR IT.

MONDAY: PERTH

BPT: ALL-OVER BODY

10-MINUTE WORKOUT	20-MINUTE WORKOUT	30-MINUTE WORKOUT
20 seconds movement / 10 seconds rest 2 sets of each exercise (one lap)	20 seconds movement / 10 seconds rest 2 sets of each exercise (two laps)	20 seconds movement / 10 seconds rest 2 sets of each exercise (three laps)

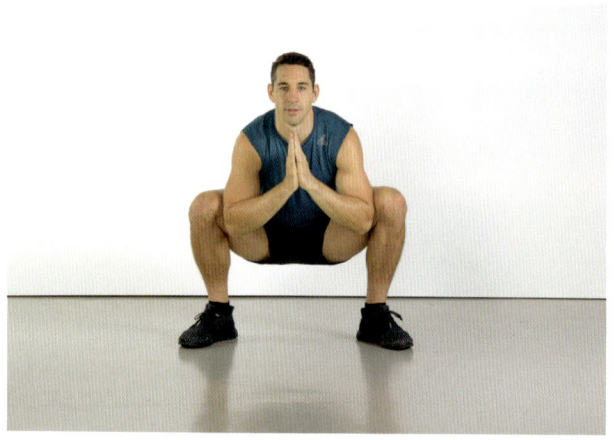

1 **Frog squats**

Stand with your feet shoulder-width apart and your feet slightly tracked out. Bend down to full squat position with your elbows tucked inside your legs. This is the starting position. From here, raise your hips and then lower them back to the starting position.

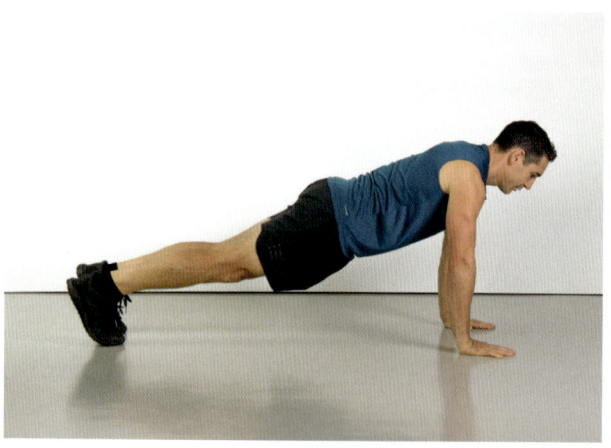

2 **Push-ups**

2.1 Get into high plank position with your hands shoulder-width apart, your shoulders over your wrists and your feet elevated on your toes. This is the starting position. Now lower yourself down to transfer all your weight into your shoulders and back. Press back up to the starting position.

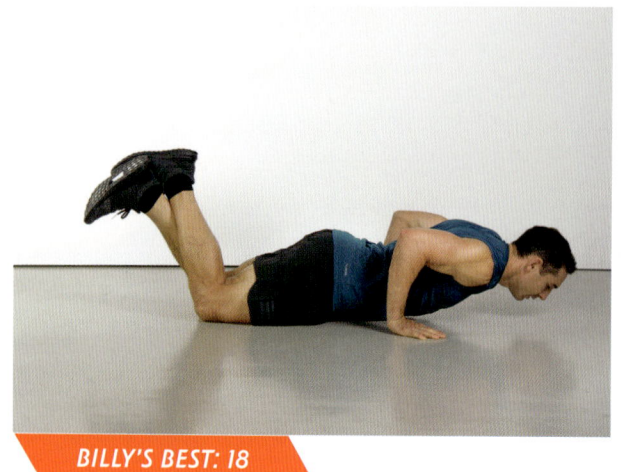

2.2 Alternatively, place one ankle over the other while your knees are on the floor in the starting position. Now lift yourself up so your shoulders are over your wrists. Lower yourself down to the ground and then press back up to the starting position.

BILLY'S BEST: 18

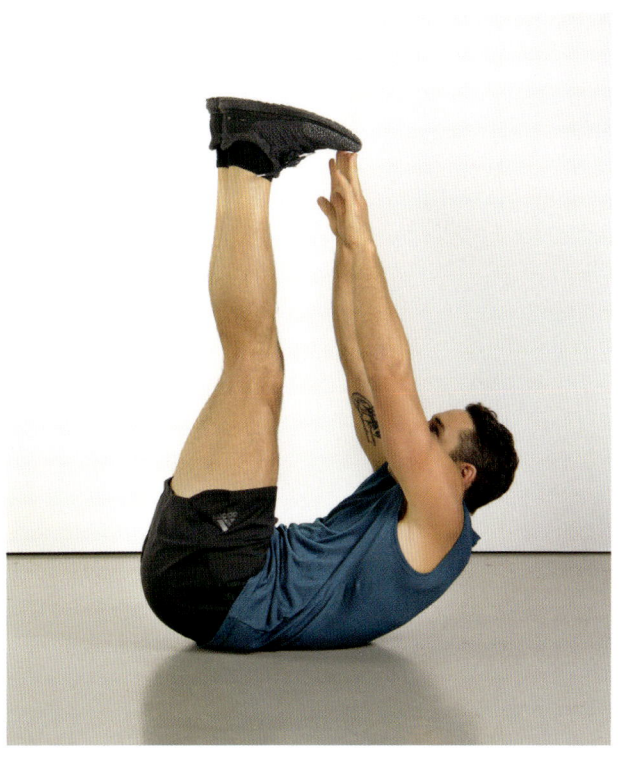

3 **Sit-up toe touches**
Sitting up, bring both legs up and touch the toes with your hands. Lie back down and repeat.

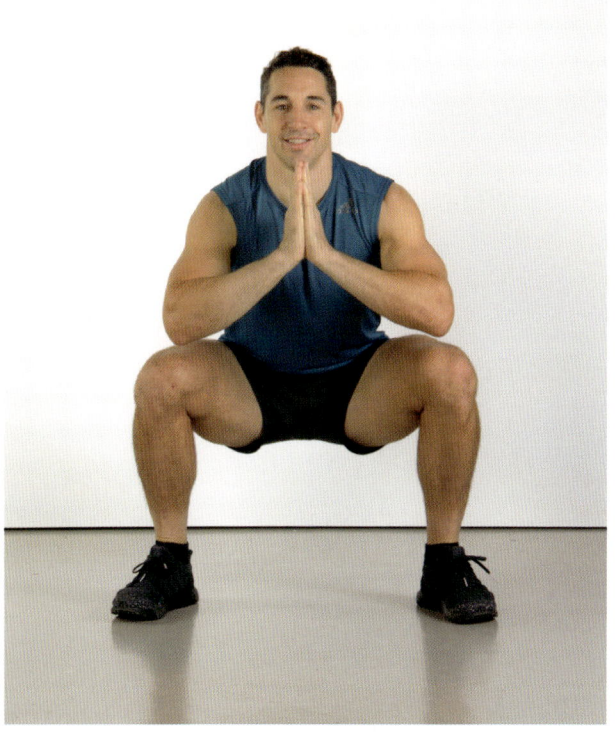

4 **Pulse squats**
Stand with your feet just past shoulder-width apart and slightly tracked out. Squat with your hips back and your legs at a 90-degree angle, then pulse up and down.

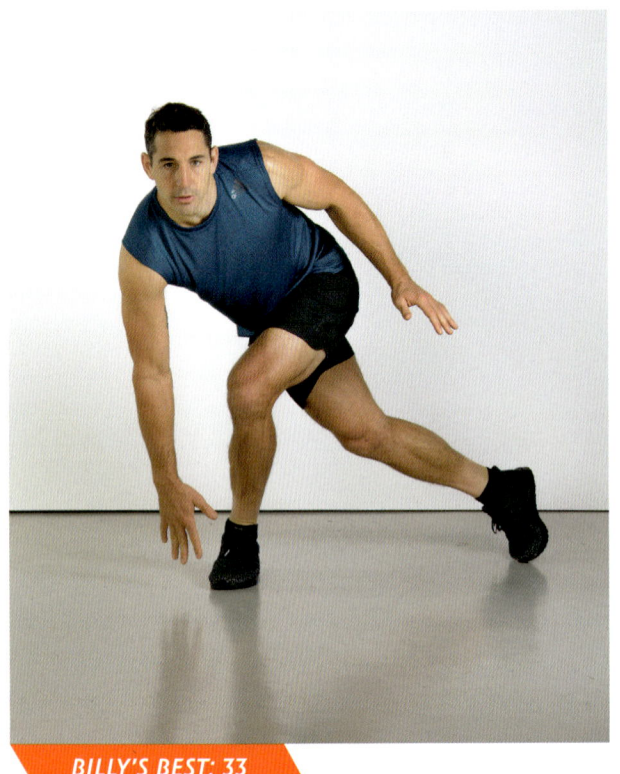

BILLY'S BEST: 33

5 **Ice skaters**

Start with your feet shoulder-width apart. Take a step to your left, swing your right leg behind your left leg, and with your right hand touch your left toe. From here, step to your right, swing your left leg behind your right leg, and with your left hand touch your right toe.

6 **Shoulder taps**

Starting in plank position and engaging your core, transfer your weight into your right arm, and with your left hand touch your right shoulder. Return to the starting position and repeat on the left side.

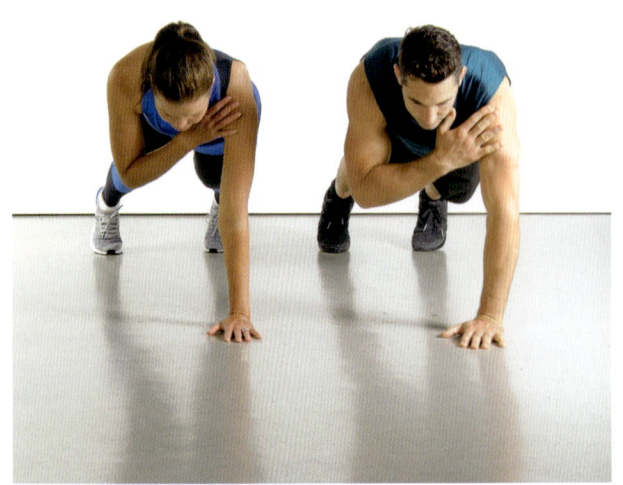

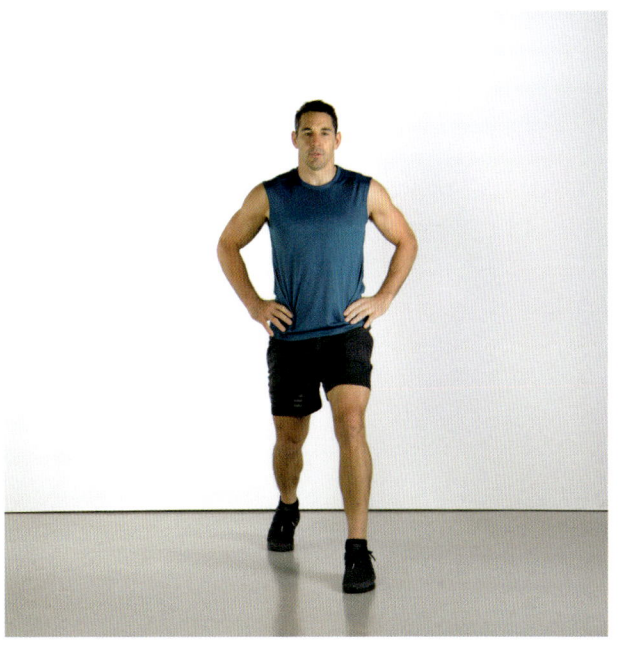

7 Plyometric split lunges

7.1 Start with your feet shoulder-width apart and your hands on your hips. Split your legs before dropping your back knee down in line with the heel of your leading foot – both legs should be at a 90-degree angle – then push up and repeat on the other side.

7.2 Alternatively, stand with your feet shoulder-width apart and your hands on your hips. Step one leg back and lower your back leg to a 90-degree position. Step forward to the starting position, then repeat on the other side.

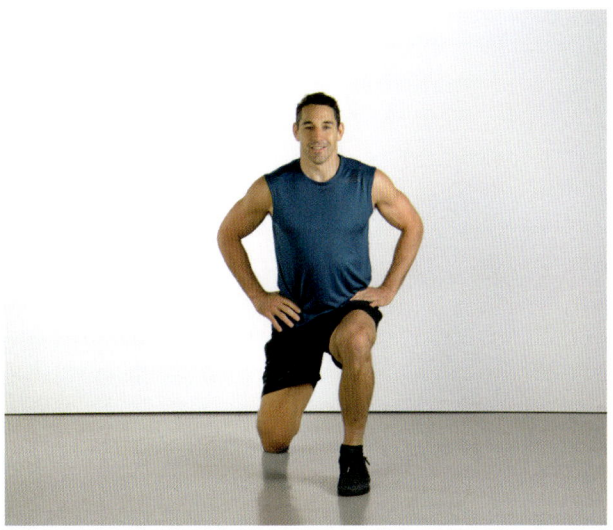

8 Sit-ups

Lie on your back, bend your legs and place your feet firmly on the ground to stabilise your lower body. Cross your arms over your chest and curl your upper body all the way up to touch your knees, then slowly lower yourself down to return to the starting point.

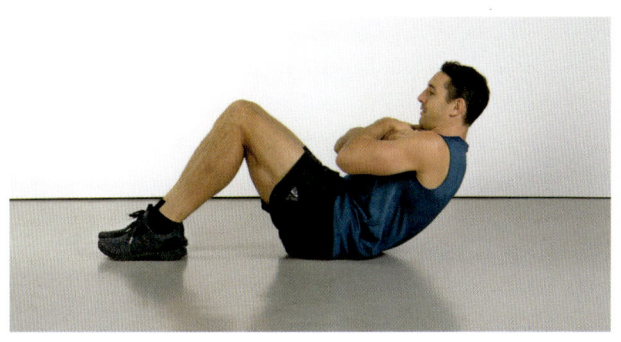

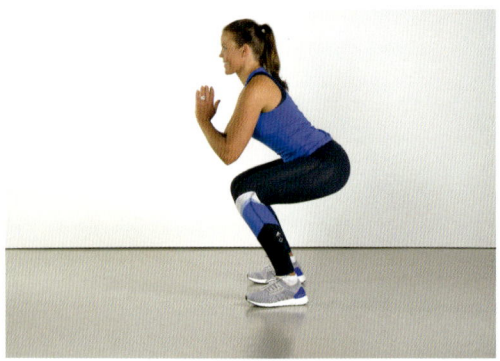

9 Sprawls

Stand with your feet shoulder-width apart, then squat until both your hands and both your feet are firmly on the ground. From this position transfer your weight into your shoulders and shoot your feet back so that your legs are out wide, then jump your feet back up and stand up into the starting position.

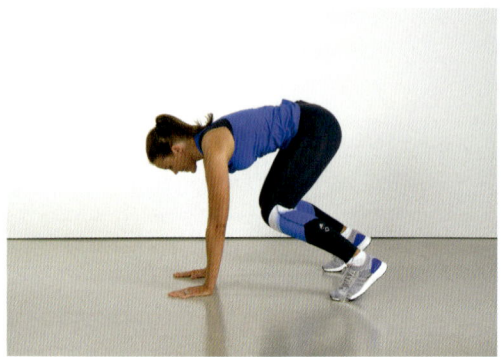
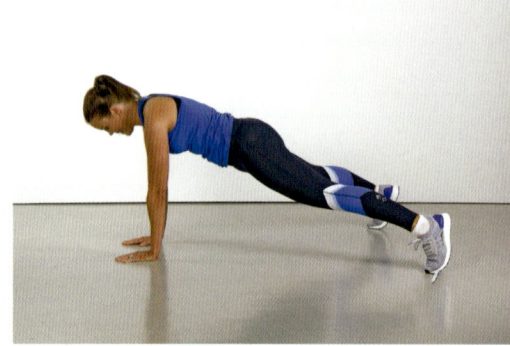

10 Star jumps

Begin in a relaxed stance with your arms close to your body. Jump your feet out wide past shoulder-width and raise both your arms above your head, then land back in the starting position.

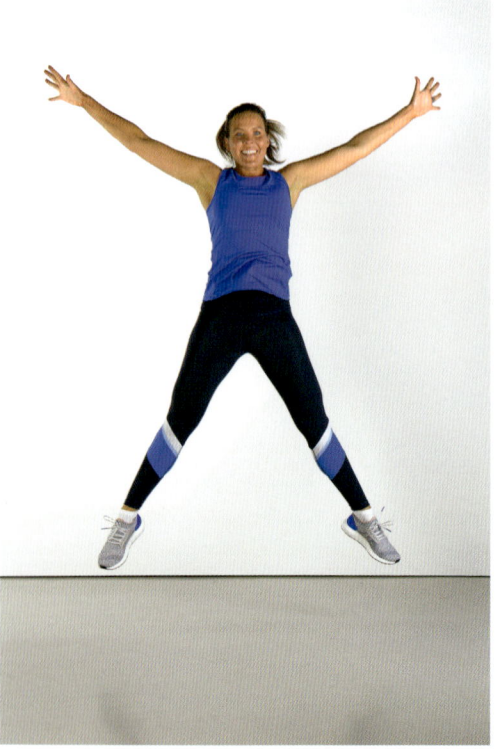

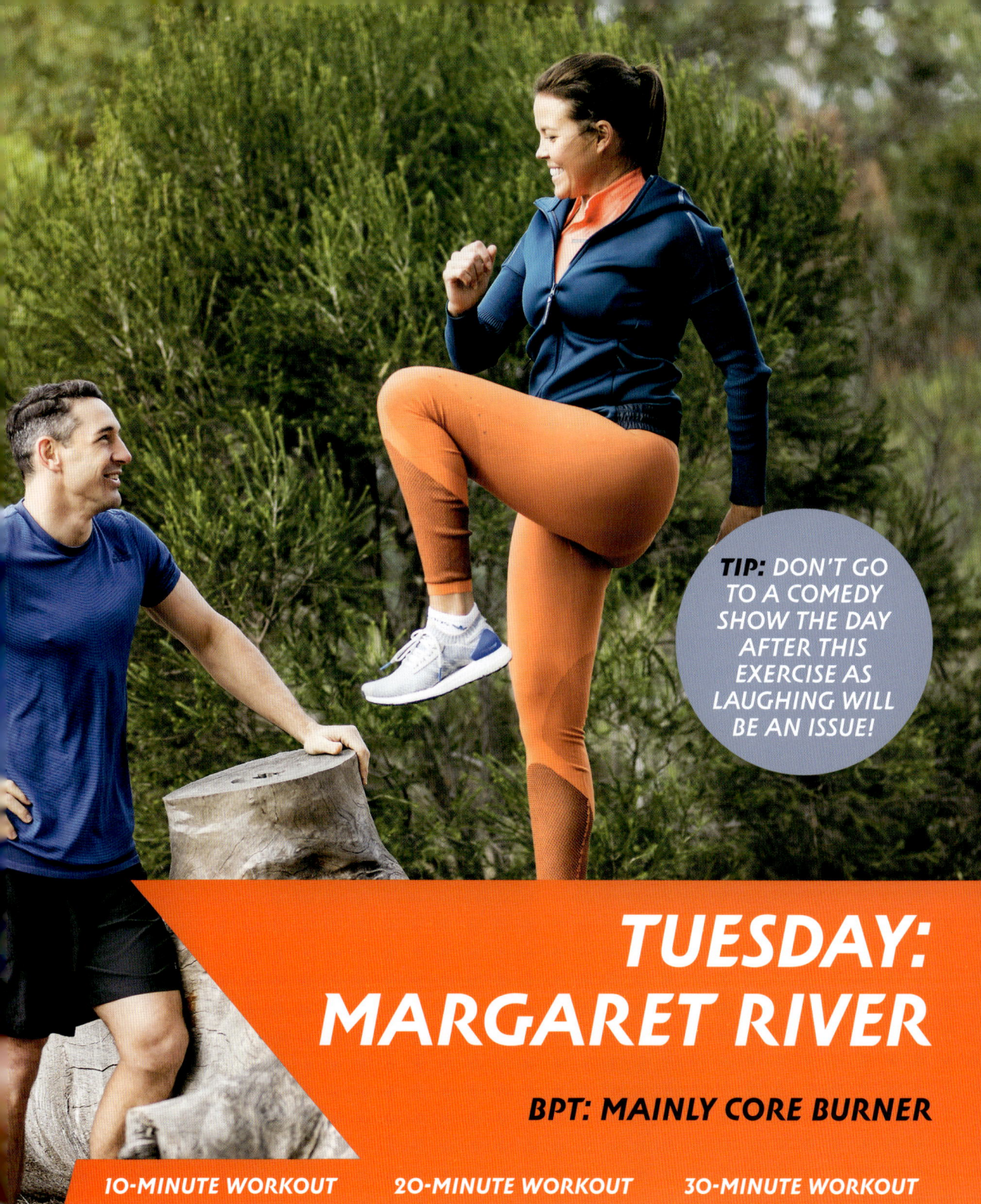

TIP: DON'T GO TO A COMEDY SHOW THE DAY AFTER THIS EXERCISE AS LAUGHING WILL BE AN ISSUE!

TUESDAY: MARGARET RIVER

BPT: MAINLY CORE BURNER

10-MINUTE WORKOUT

20 seconds movement /
10 seconds rest
2 sets of each exercise
(one lap)

20-MINUTE WORKOUT

20 seconds movement /
10 seconds rest
2 sets of each exercise
(two laps)

30-MINUTE WORKOUT

20 seconds movement /
10 seconds rest
2 sets of each exercise
(three laps)

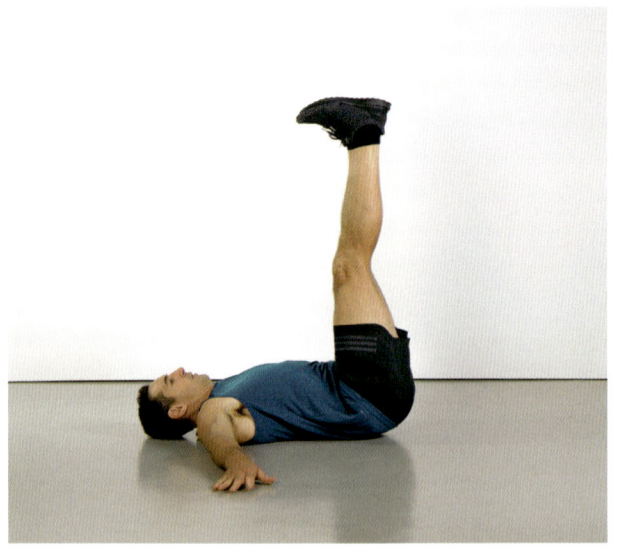

1 **Windscreen wipers**

Starting position is lying on the ground with your legs raised up straight and your arms by your sides. Rotate your hips and bring your legs down to one side without letting your shoulders lift off the ground. Squeezing your core, bring your legs back to the starting position. Repeat on the other side.

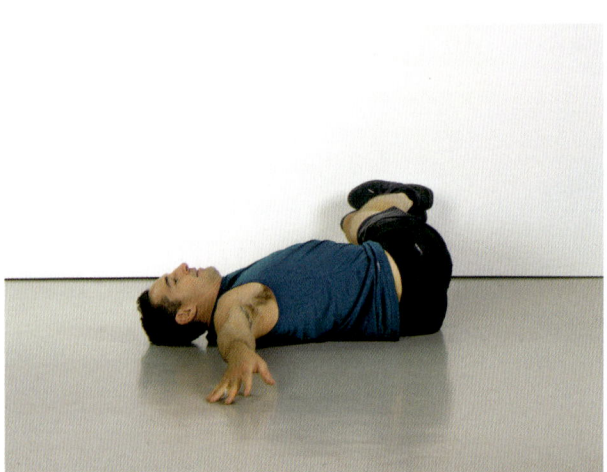

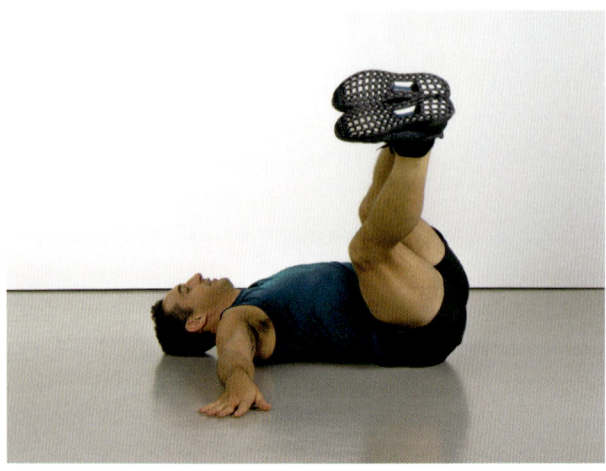

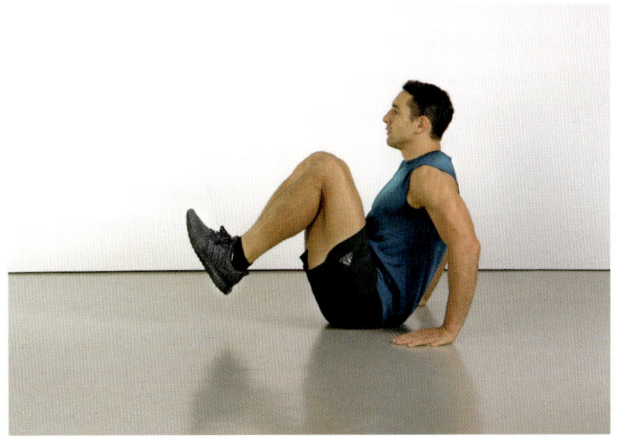

2 Full knee tucks

Starting position is sitting on the ground with your hands on the floor by your side and legs extended straight. Lean back and engage your core, then bring your knees to your chest, keeping your feet together. Extend your legs back out, keeping your heels off the ground.

Advanced: Take your hands off the ground and cross them over your chest.

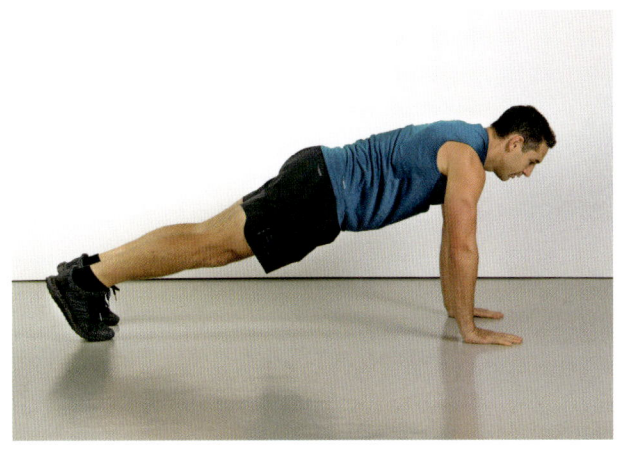

3 Mountain climbers

Start in a high plank position, with your shoulders over your wrists, your feet together and your core engaged. From here, bring one knee up towards your chest and then return it to the starting position. Repeat on the other side.

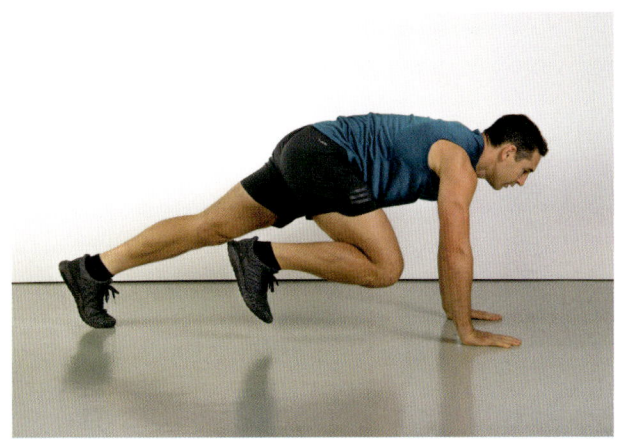

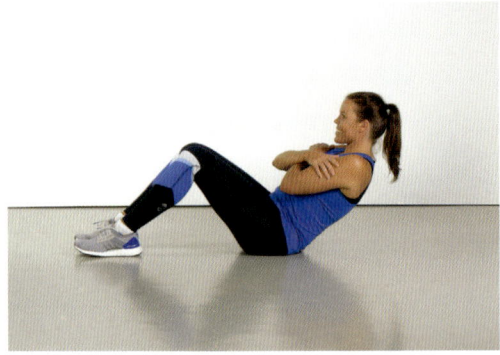

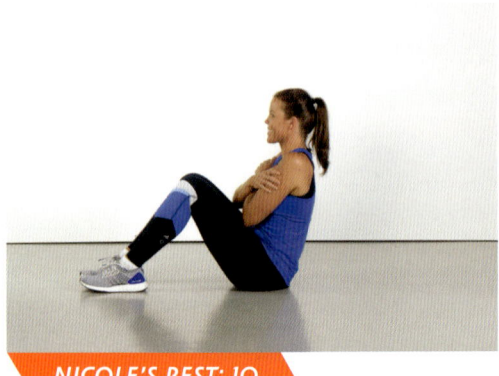

NICOLE'S BEST: 10

4   Sit-ups

Lie on your back, bend your legs and place your feet firmly on the ground to stabilise your lower body. Cross your arms over your chest, then curl your upper body all the way up to touch your knees. Slowly lower yourself down to return to the starting point.

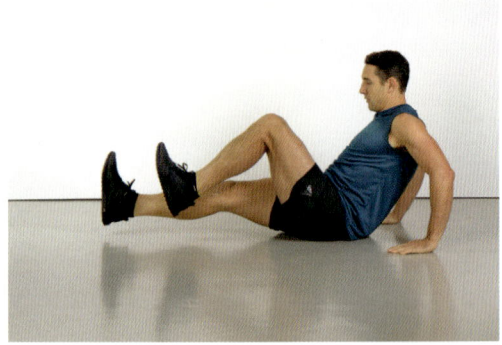

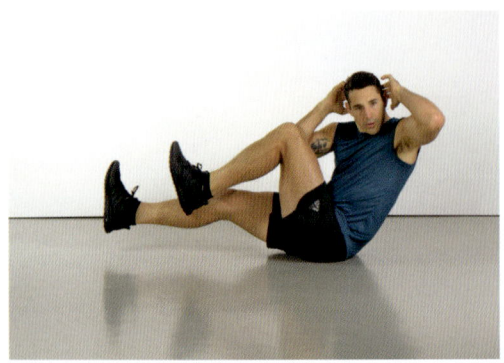

5   Bicycle crunches

Start by sitting on the ground with your hands on the floor by your side and your legs extended in front of you. From here, lean back, engaging your core so your feet are off the ground. Now bring one knee towards your chest, keeping the other leg straight. Return your knee to the earlier position and swap to bring your other knee towards your chest.

Advanced: Take your hands off the ground and bring the opposite elbow to your knee.

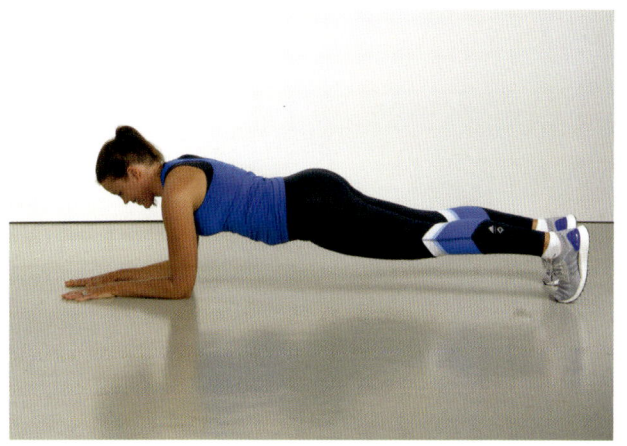

6   Plank

Place your forearms on the ground and lift your knees off the ground with your feet together and your toes touching the ground. From here, lean slightly forward to engage your core. Hold the position for the duration of time. (Note: Your back should not be sagging or bent.)

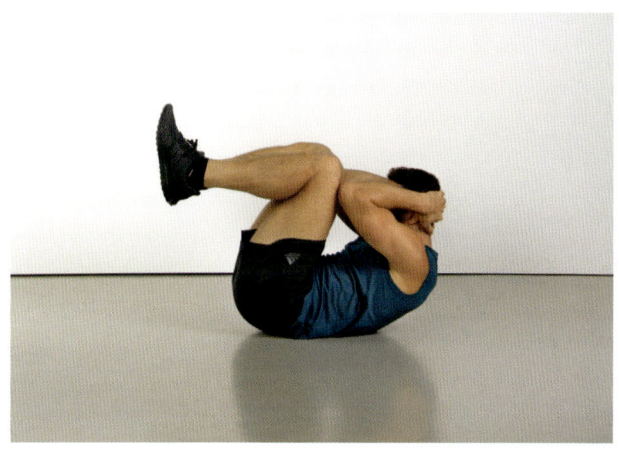

7   Crunches

Lie on your back with your legs off the ground and knees bent at a 90-degree angle to your body. With your hands crossed behind your head, bring your elbows in next to your ears. Bring your elbows up to your knees then return to the starting position.

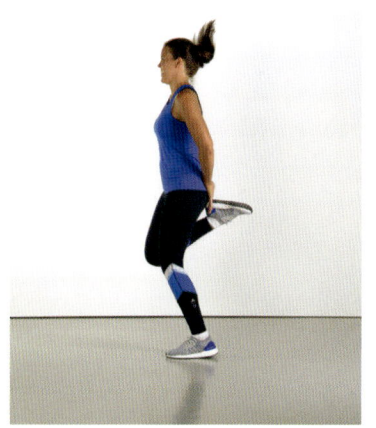

8   Butt kicks

Stand with your feet shoulder-width apart and your hands flat behind your back with your palms facing outwards. Bring one heel up to touch your butt, then do the same with the other heel. Try to keep your feet nice and soft and land back on the ball of your foot each time.

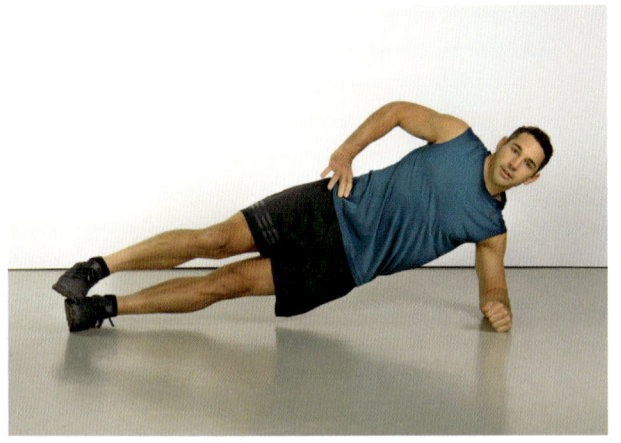

9   Side plank

Starting position is lying on your side with your feet together. With your lower forearm firmly on the ground, raise your hips up and place your other hand firmly on your waist. From here, press down into your shoulder and raise your hips, squeezing your core. Hold.

Advanced: Have your other hand raised straight up in the air instead of on your waist throughout the entire movement.

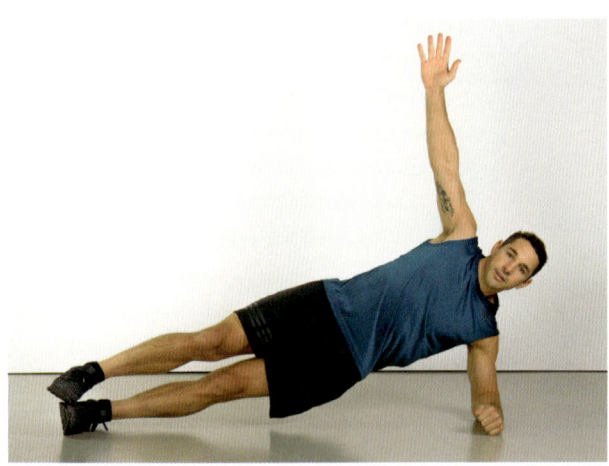

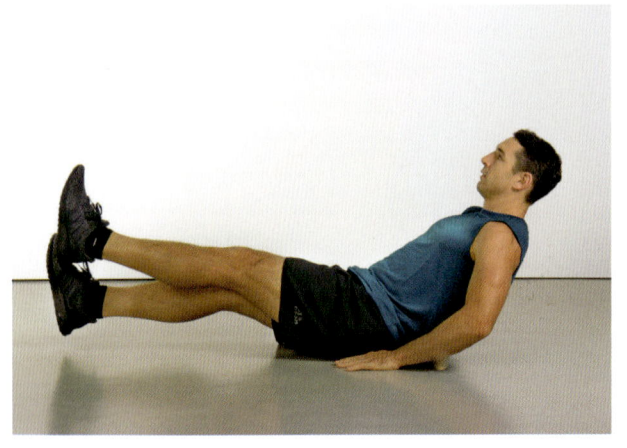

10   Flutter kicks

Starting position is lying on your back with your thumbs tucked under your lower lumbar (base of your back) on either side of your body. Raise your legs and kick them up and down in a small fluttering motion, engaging your core.

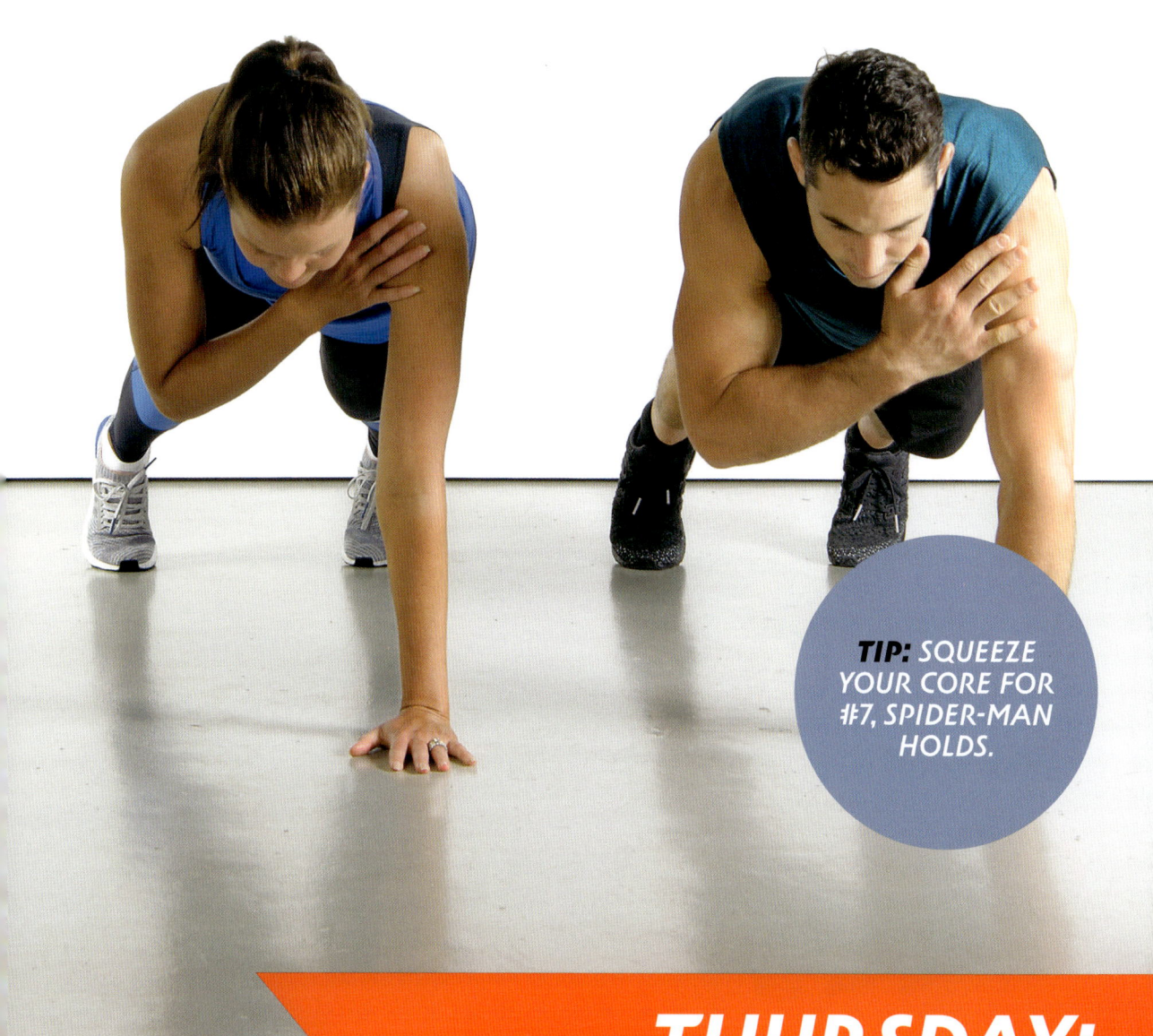

TIP: SQUEEZE YOUR CORE FOR #7, SPIDER-MAN HOLDS.

THURSDAY: BUNBURY

BPT: UPPER-BODY BLITZ

10-MINUTE WORKOUT

20 seconds movement /
10 seconds rest
2 sets of each exercise
(one lap)

20-MINUTE WORKOUT

20 seconds movement /
10 seconds rest
2 sets of each exercise
(two laps)

30-MINUTE WORKOUT

20 seconds movement /
10 seconds rest
2 sets of each exercise
(three laps)

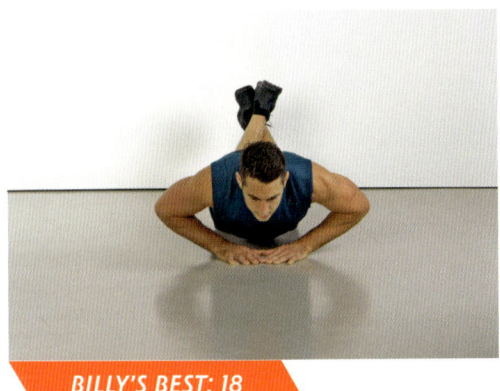

BILLY'S BEST: 18

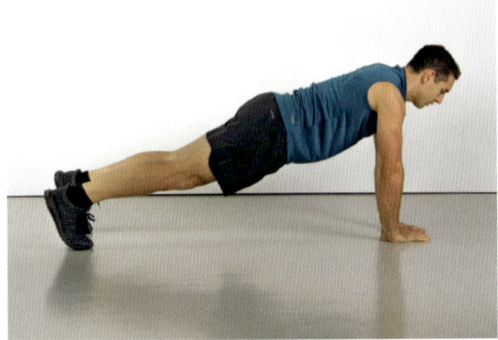

1 **Diamond push-ups**

Kneel on the ground with your ankles crossed, and set your hands so your thumbs and index fingers are touching. From here, lower your body towards the ground and then press back up to the starting position. You should feel this movement in your triceps.

Advanced: Do the exercise in high plank position with your knees off the ground.

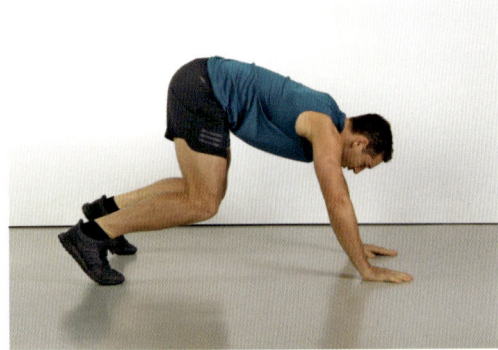

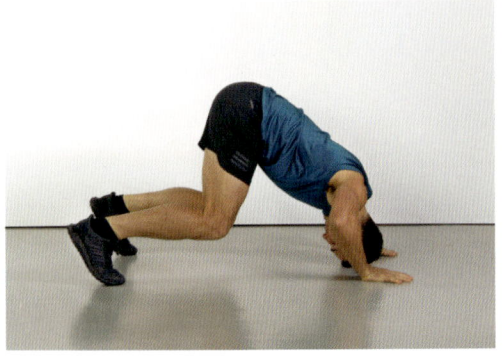

2 **A-frame push-ups**

Stand with your feet wide apart and slightly tracked out. With your hands shoulder-width apart, and bending at the hips, lean over to touch the ground with your legs straight or bent and your chin slightly tucked. From this starting position, lower yourself down till the top of your head is just off the ground and you're looking through your legs. Your head should be in line with your hands. From here, press back up to the starting position, transferring all the weight into your palms.

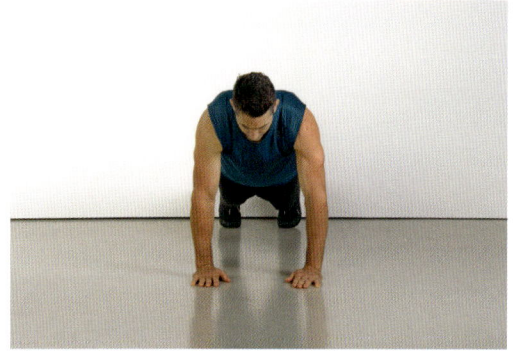

3   **Narrow width tempo push-ups**
    Get into high plank position with your hands a little bit in from shoulder width, and your feet elevated on your toes. Take 3 seconds to lower yourself down so that all your weight is transferred into your shoulders and triceps, then take 1 second to press back up to the starting position.

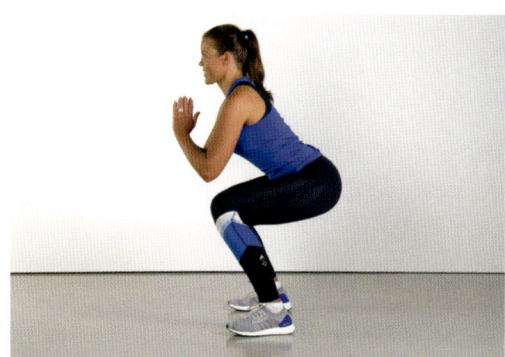

4   **Sprawls**
    Stand with your feet shoulder-width apart, then squat until both your hands and both your feet are firmly on the ground. From this position transfer your weight into your shoulders and shoot your feet back so that your legs are out wide, then jump your feet back up and stand up into the starting position.

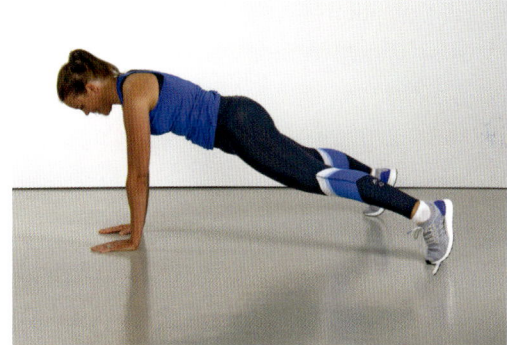

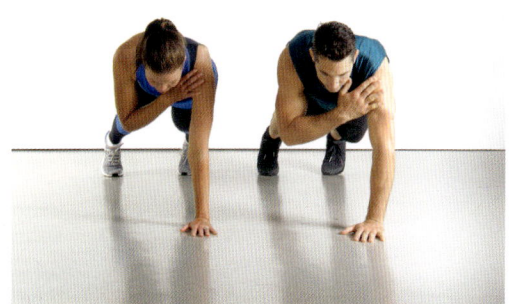

5   **Shoulder taps**
    Starting in plank position and engaging your core, transfer your weight into your right arm, and with your left hand touch your right shoulder. Return to the starting position and repeat on the left side.

BLOCK 1: WESTERN AUSTRALIA

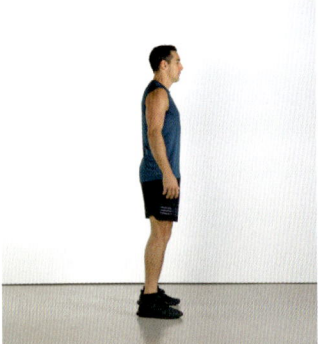

6 Burpees or sprawls

6.1 To begin a burpee, stand in a relaxed position with your feet shoulder-width apart. Squat and place your hands firmly on the ground with your feet back. Shoot your legs back so you are in a high plank position, then lower your body so your torso is just touching the ground. Release your hands and then, placing your hands back on the ground, raise your torso and jump your feet forward so both hands and both feet are on the ground. Stand back up, then jump up and raise your hands above your head.

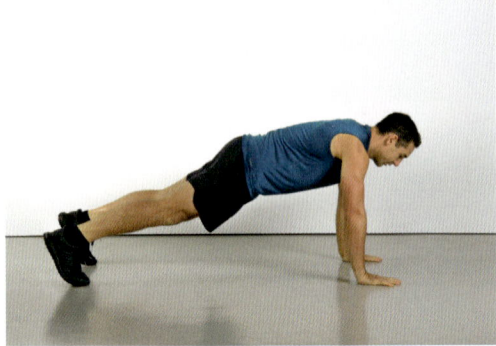

6.2 Alternatively, for a sprawl, stand with your feet shoulder-width apart, then squat until both your hands and both your feet are firmly on the ground. From this position transfer your weight into your shoulders and shoot your feet back so that your legs are out wide, then jump your feet back up and stand up into the starting position. (See page 20 for images.)

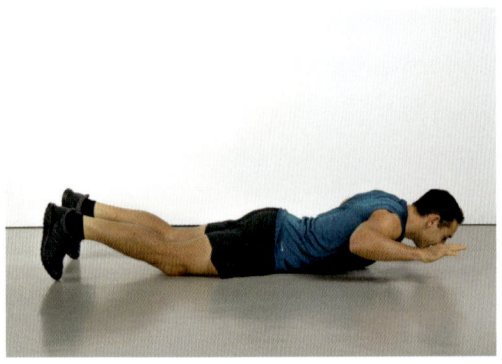

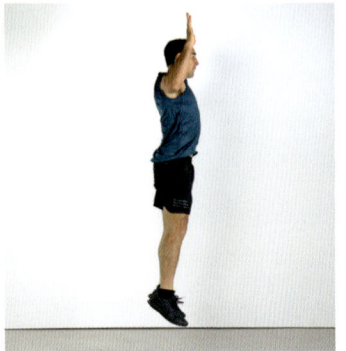

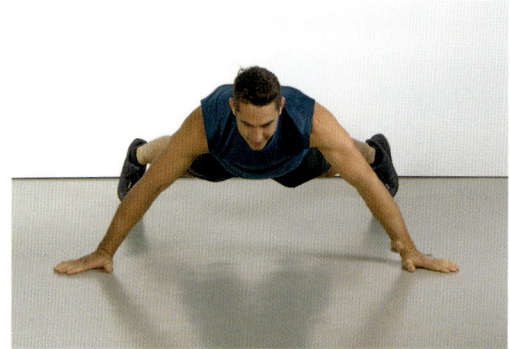

7 Spider-Man holds

Start in a high plank position but with your hands out nice and wide and your legs as wide as your hands. From here, raise your knees and lean forward slightly, engaging your core and squeezing your glutes. You should also feel this movement in your biceps and shoulders.

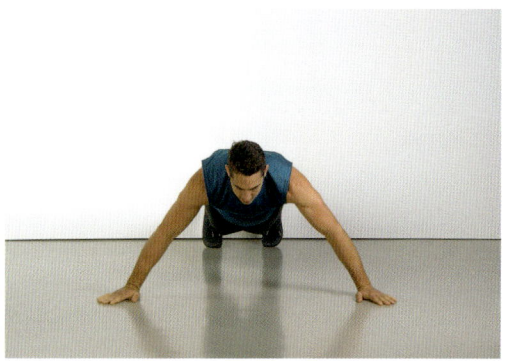

8 Wide push-ups

Get into a high plank position but with your hands slightly wider than shoulder-width, and lift yourself up so your shoulders are over your wrists and your feet are elevated on your toes. Now lower yourself to transfer all your weight into your shoulders and your back. Press back up to the starting position.

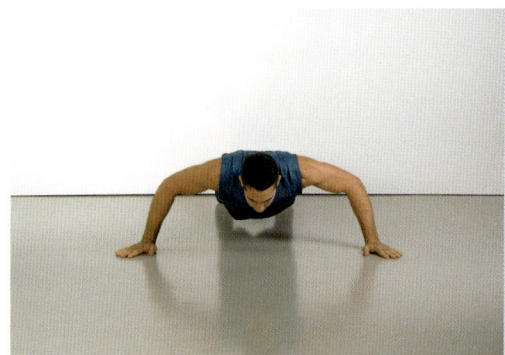

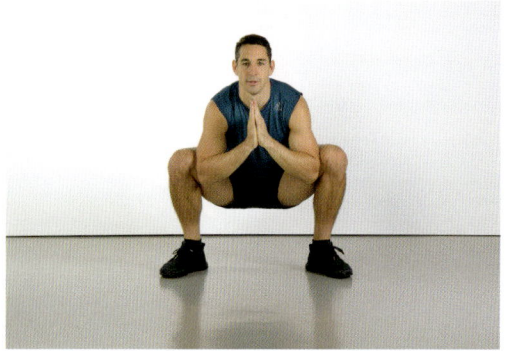

9 Frog squats

Stand with your feet shoulder-width apart and your feet slightly tracked out. Bend down to full squat position with your elbows tucked inside your legs. This is the starting position. From here, raise your hips and then lower them back to the starting position.

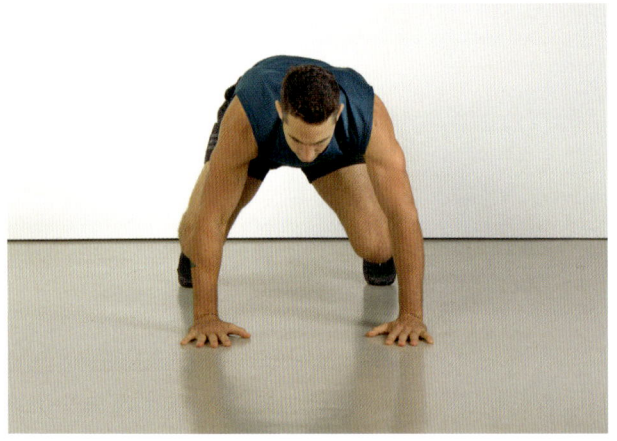

10 Lateral shoot-throughs

Start in high plank position with your hands firmly on the ground and your shoulders above your wrists. Bend your knees at a 90-degree angle and have your toes firmly on the ground and your knees off the ground. This is the starting position. Now turn your left foot so it is flat on the ground. Kick your right foot in front of your left foot and out to the side, so your right leg is now straight and your left foot is firmly on the ground. Now pull your right leg back to the starting position. Repeat on the other side.

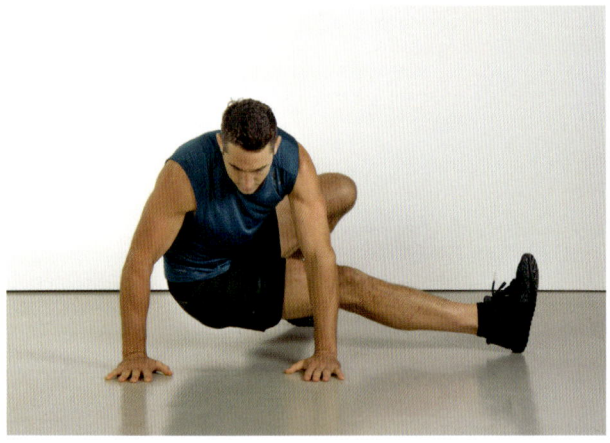

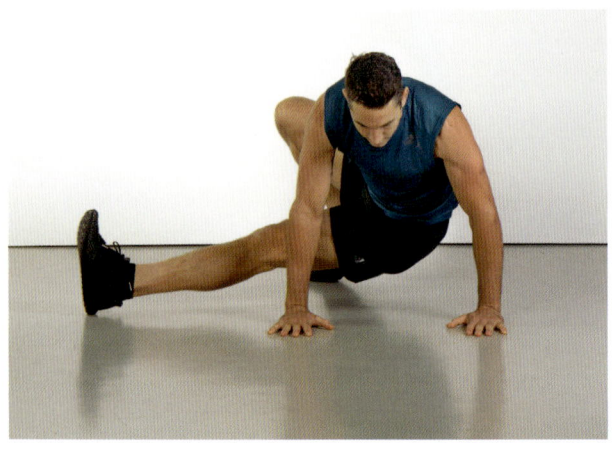

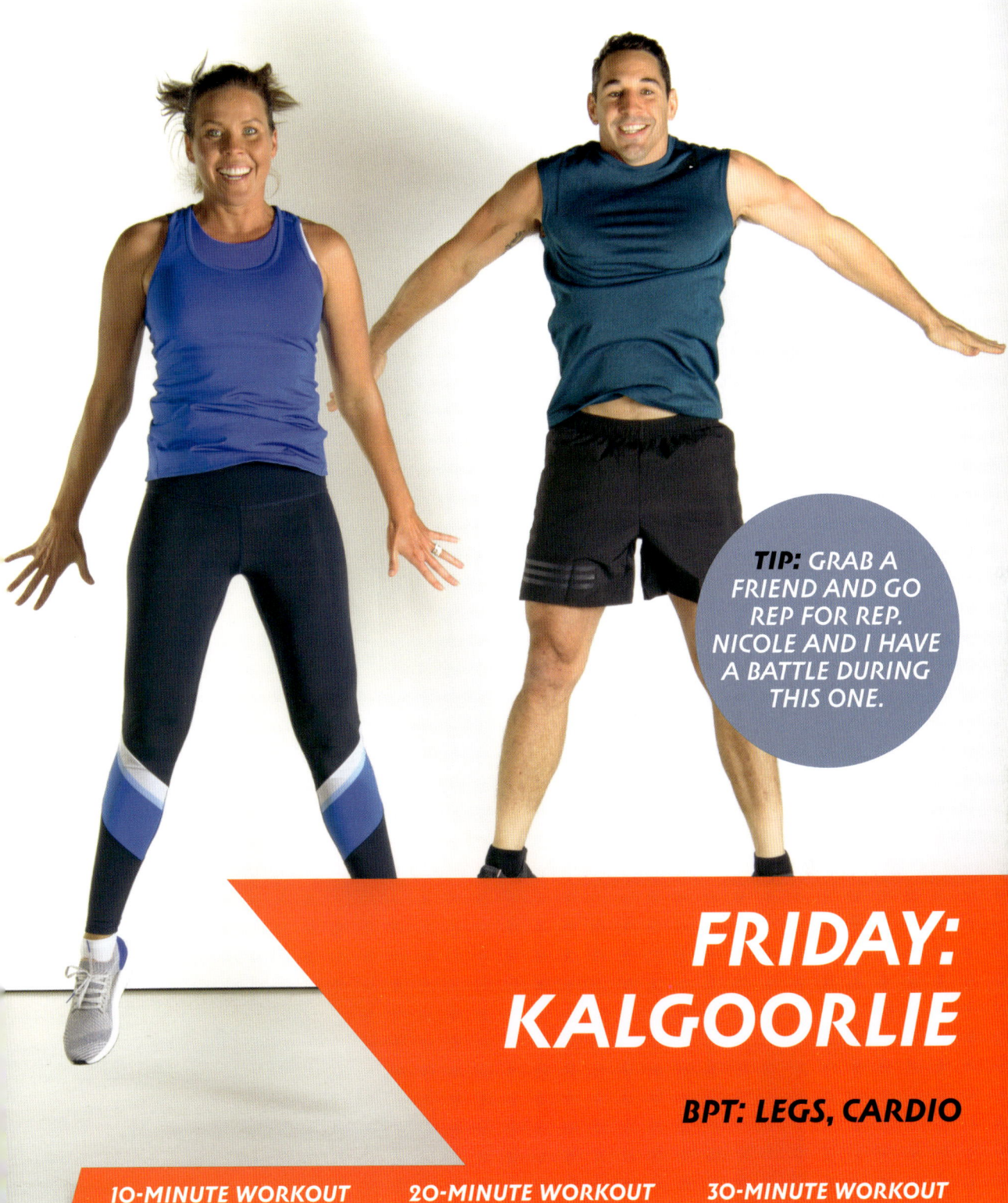

TIP: GRAB A FRIEND AND GO REP FOR REP. NICOLE AND I HAVE A BATTLE DURING THIS ONE.

FRIDAY: KALGOORLIE

BPT: LEGS, CARDIO

10-MINUTE WORKOUT	20-MINUTE WORKOUT	30-MINUTE WORKOUT
20 seconds movement / 10 seconds rest 2 sets of each exercise (one lap)	20 seconds movement / 10 seconds rest 2 sets of each exercise (two laps)	20 seconds movement / 10 seconds rest 2 sets of each exercise (three laps)

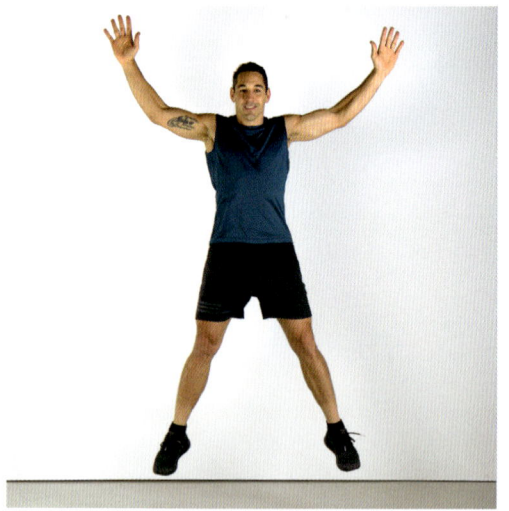

1 Star jumps

Begin in a relaxed stance with your arms close to your body. Jump your feet out wide past shoulder-width and raise both your arms above your head, then land back in the starting position.

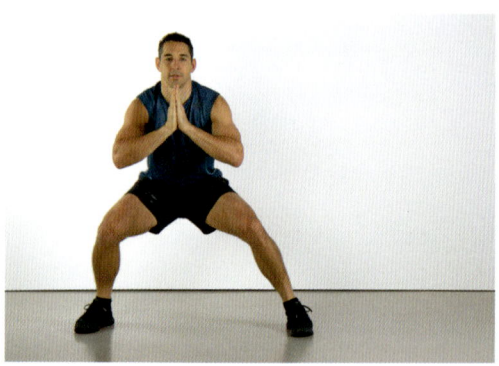

2 Crab walks

Stand with your feet shoulder-width apart and bend at the hips to come down into a squatting position. With your hands in front of your chest and staying low, step two to your left and then two to your right. Try to stay low throughout the time allocated.

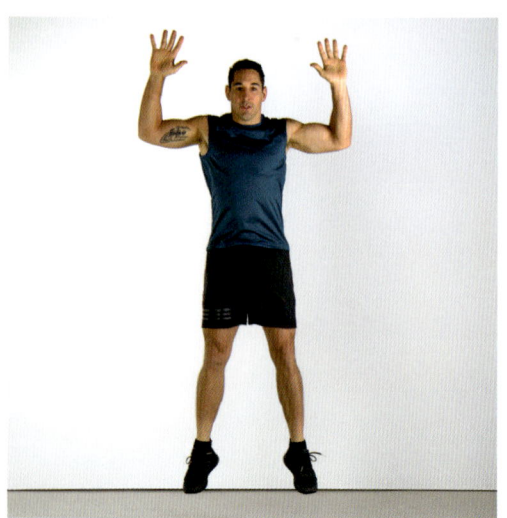

3 Burpees

Stand in a relaxed position with your feet shoulder-width apart. Squat and place your hands firmly on the ground with your feet back. Shoot your legs back so you are in a high plank position, then lower your body so your torso is just touching the ground. Release your hands and then, placing your hands back on the ground, raise your torso and jump your feet back so both hands and both feet are on the ground. Stand back up, then jump up and raise your hands above your head.

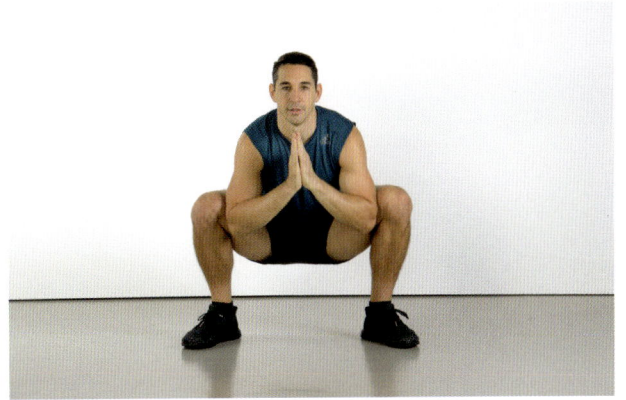

4 Frog squats

Stand with your feet shoulder-width apart and your feet slightly tracked out. Bend down to full squat position with your elbows tucked inside your legs. This is the starting position. From here, raise your hips and then lower them back to the starting position.

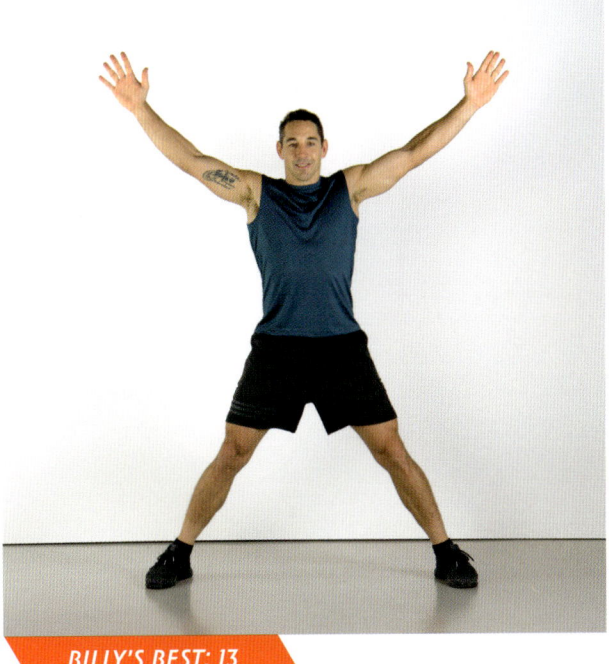

5 Star tucks

Stand with your feet shoulder-width apart. Jump your feet out wide with your arms straight above your head. Now jump your feet back together and squat into a ball as low as you can go before exploding back up to the starting position.

BILLY'S BEST: 13

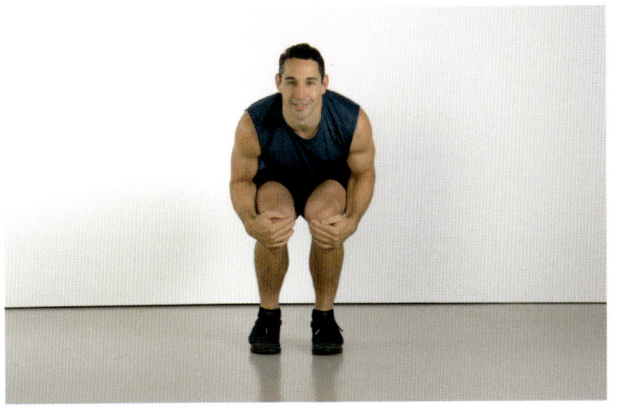

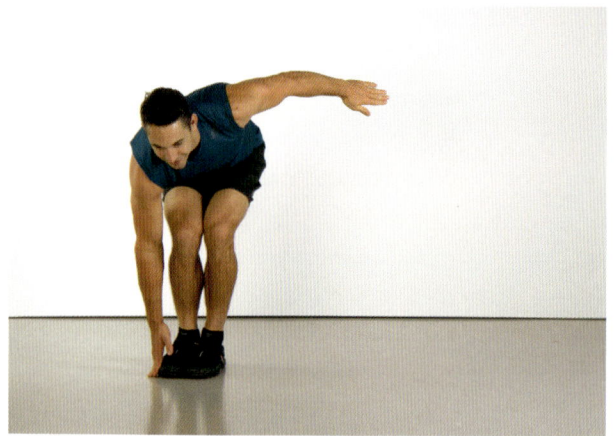

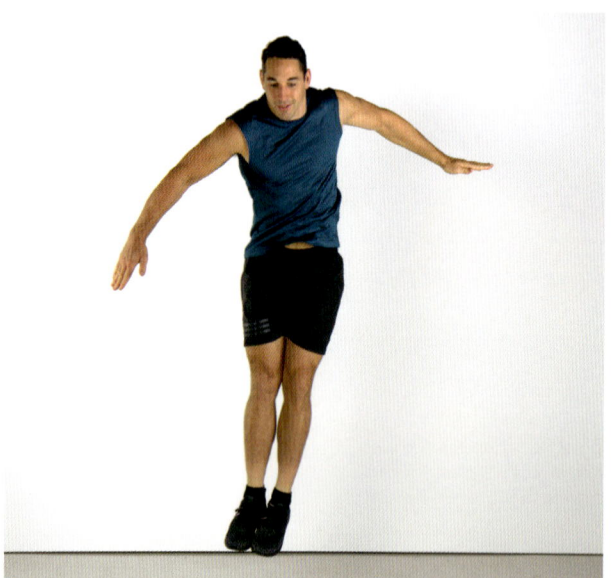

6 Slalom taps, 1 x burpee

For the slalom taps, start with your feet together, then jump to the left to land on both feet, touching your left hand down next to your left foot. Then jump to the right with both feet, touching your right hand to your right foot.

For the burpee, stand in a relaxed position with your feet shoulder-width apart. Squat and place your hands firmly on the ground with your feet back. Shoot your legs back so you are in a high plank position, then lower your body so your torso is just touching the ground. Release your hands and then, placing your hands back on the ground, raise your torso and jump your feet back so both hands and both feet are on the ground. Stand back up, then jump up and raise your hands above your head.

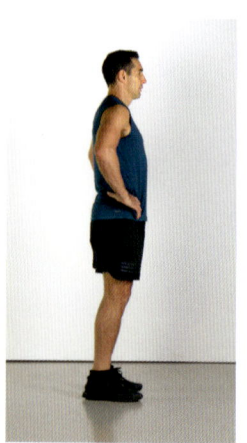 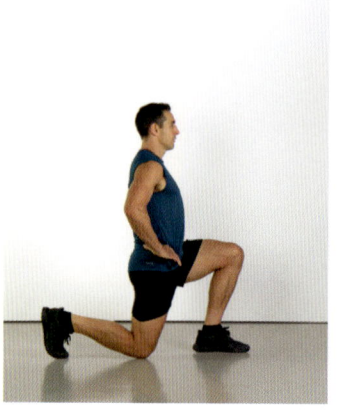

7 Reverse lunges

Stand with your feet shoulder-width apart and your hands on your hips. Step one leg back and then lower it until it is 90 degrees to the ground. Step forward to the starting position. Repeat on the other side to complete the movement.

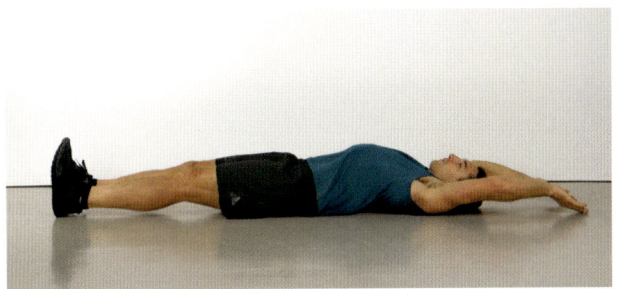

8 Jackknife

Lie on the ground with your legs out straight and your arms above your head. From here, raise your arms and legs until your hands and toes meet. This movement can be done with your knees bent.

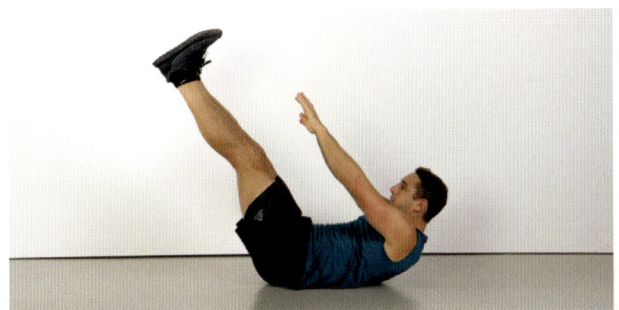

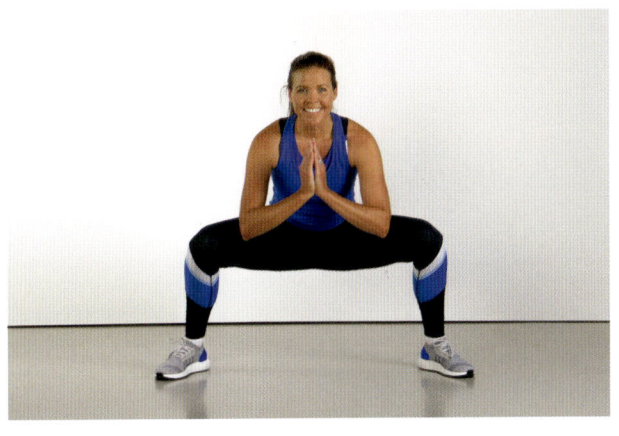

9 Mountain climbers

Start in a high plank position, with your shoulders over your wrists, your feet together and your core engaged. From here, bring one knee up towards your chest and then return it to the starting position. Repeat on the other side.

10 Sumo squats

Stand with your feet wide apart and slightly tracked out, and your hands on your hips. Bend at the hips, lower your butt towards the ground, bending your knees and keeping your shoulders back and your chest tight. Lower yourself down as far as is comfortable. Return to starting position.

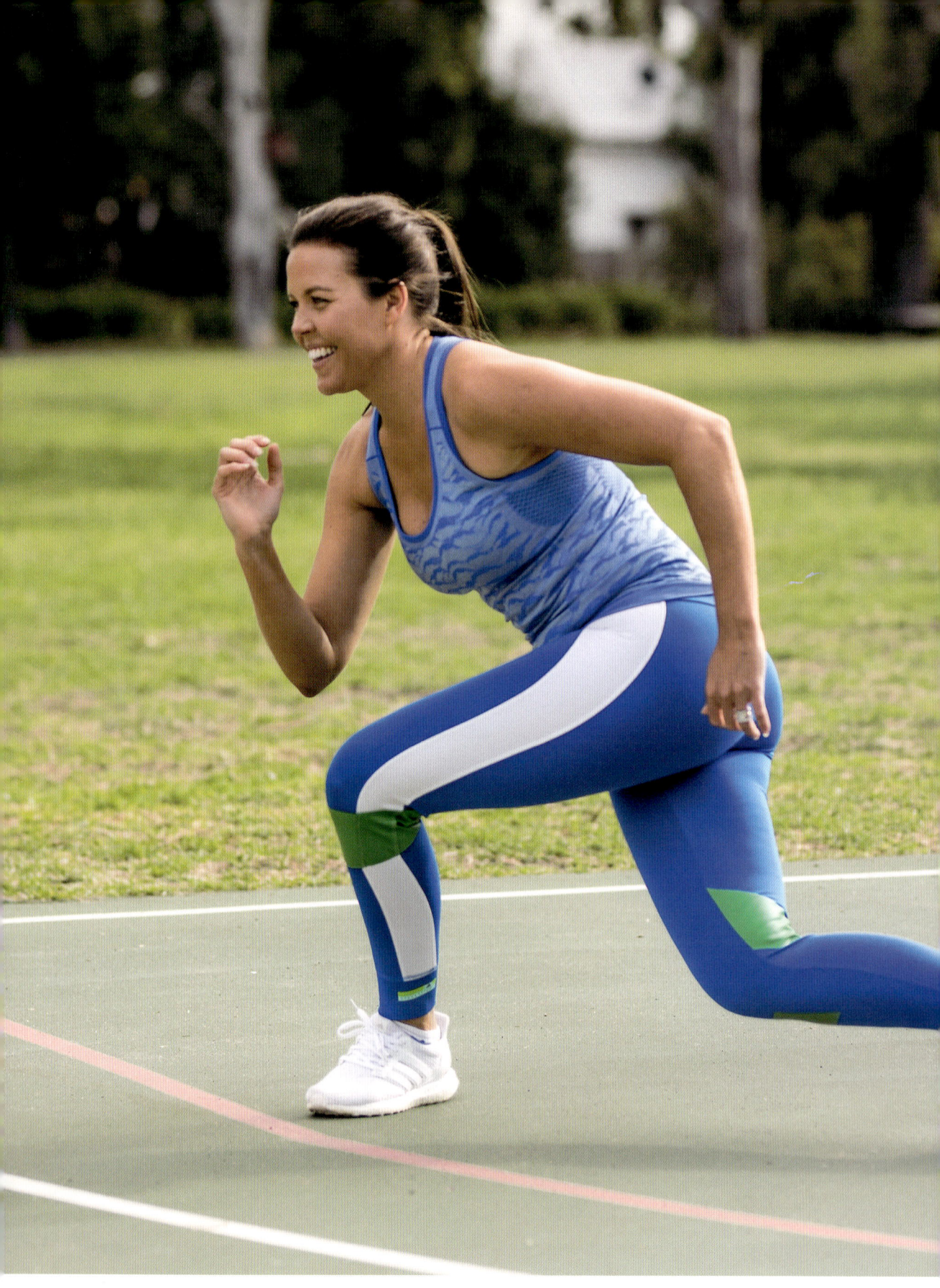

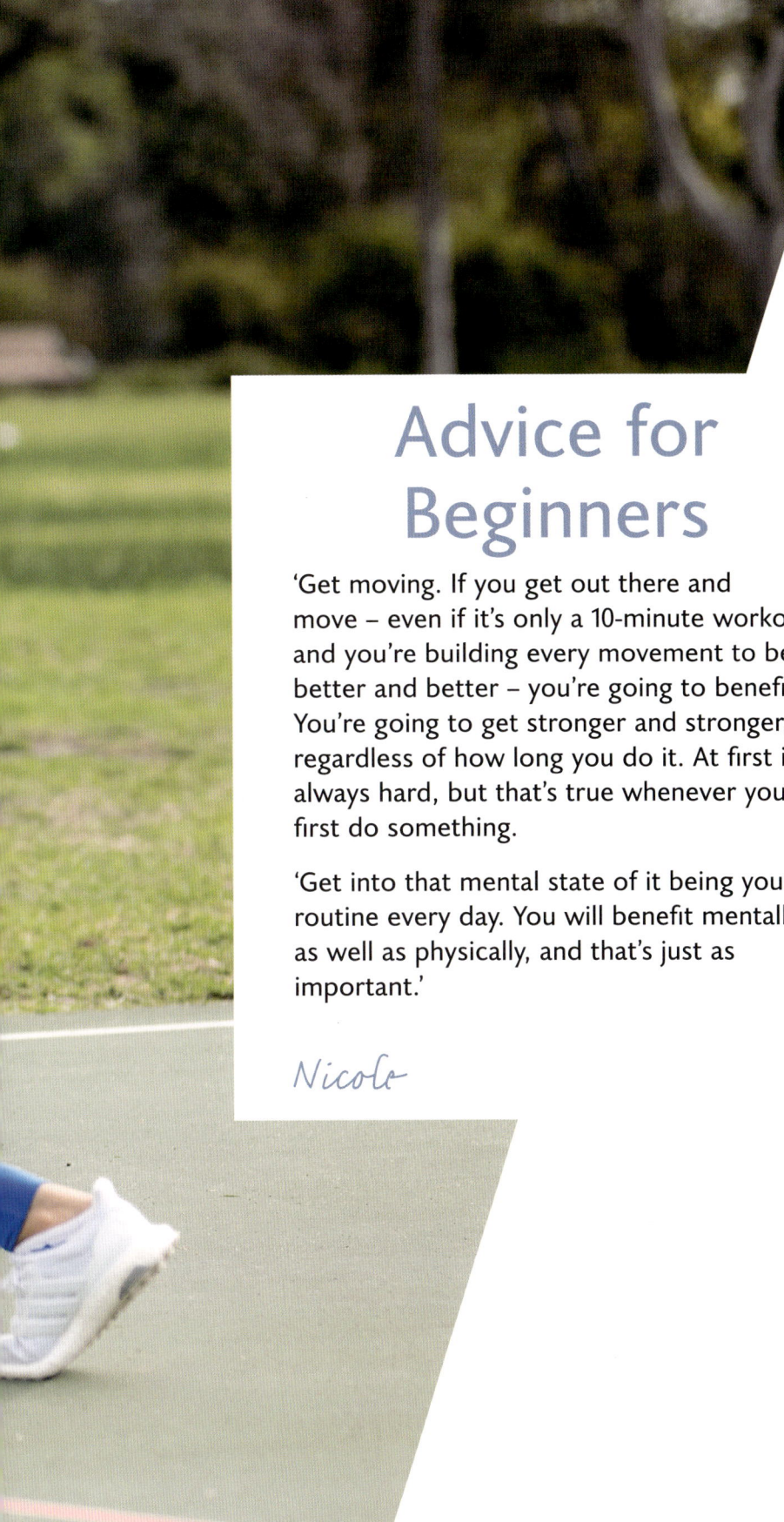

Advice for Beginners

'Get moving. If you get out there and move – even if it's only a 10-minute workout, and you're building every movement to be better and better – you're going to benefit. You're going to get stronger and stronger, regardless of how long you do it. At first it's always hard, but that's true whenever you first do something.

'Get into that mental state of it being your routine every day. You will benefit mentally as well as physically, and that's just as important.'

Nicole

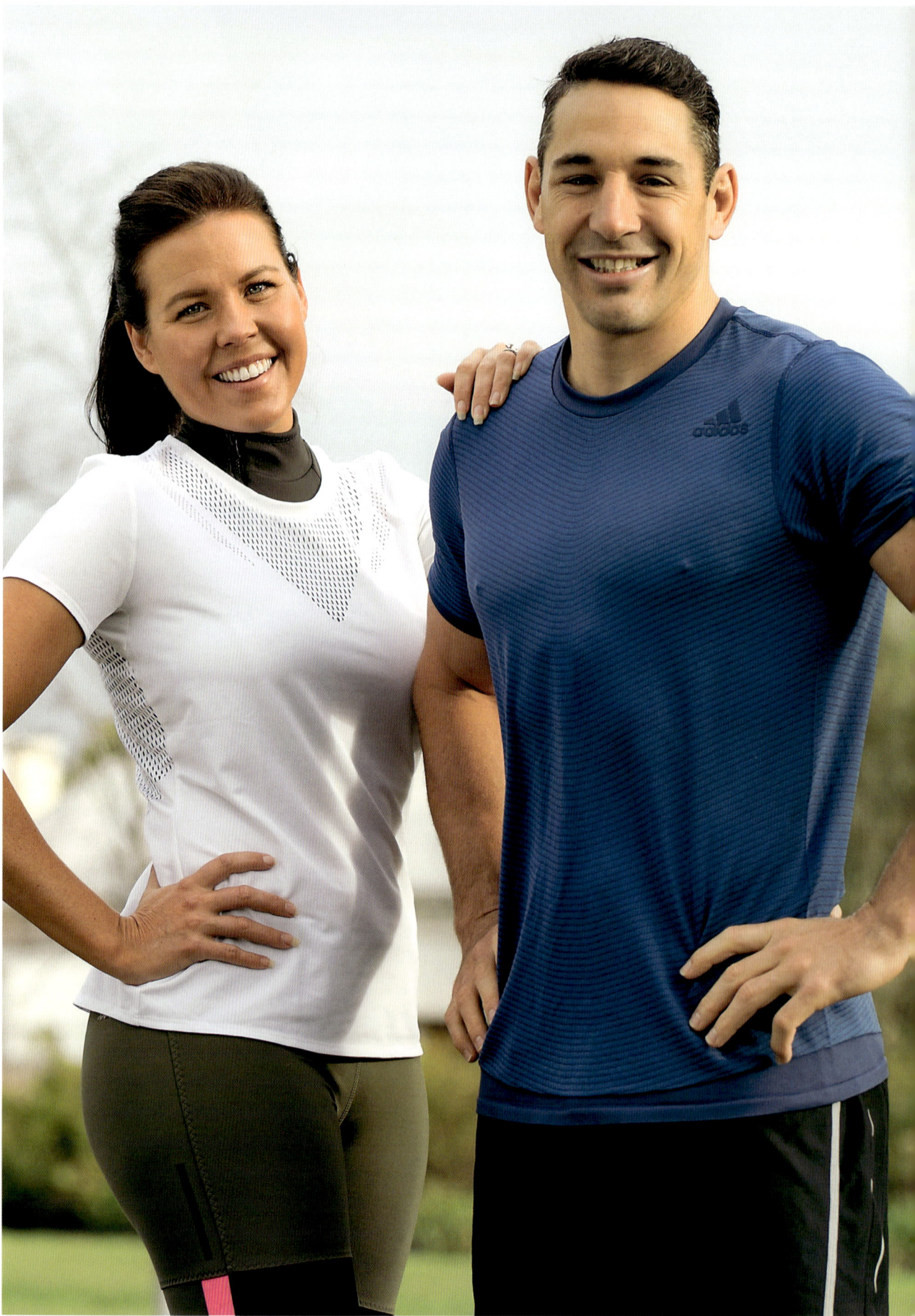

BLOCK 2: NEW SOUTH WALES

'Sydney's always a fantastic city to hit the beaches, get outdoors or see some great natural sites. I love going for a city run or a quick dip at Bondi. For something a little bit different, try running on the soft sand at one of the many beaches.'

Billy

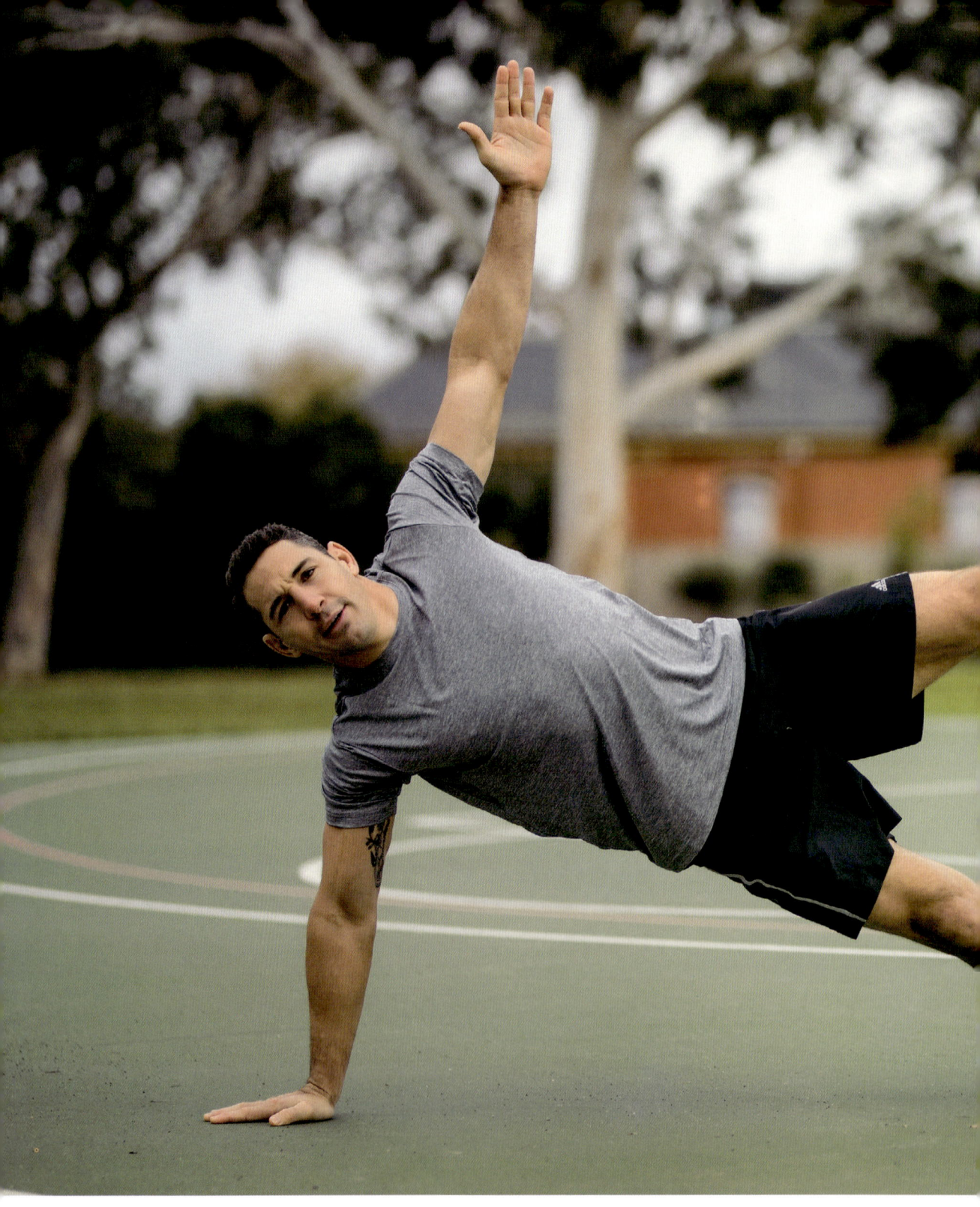

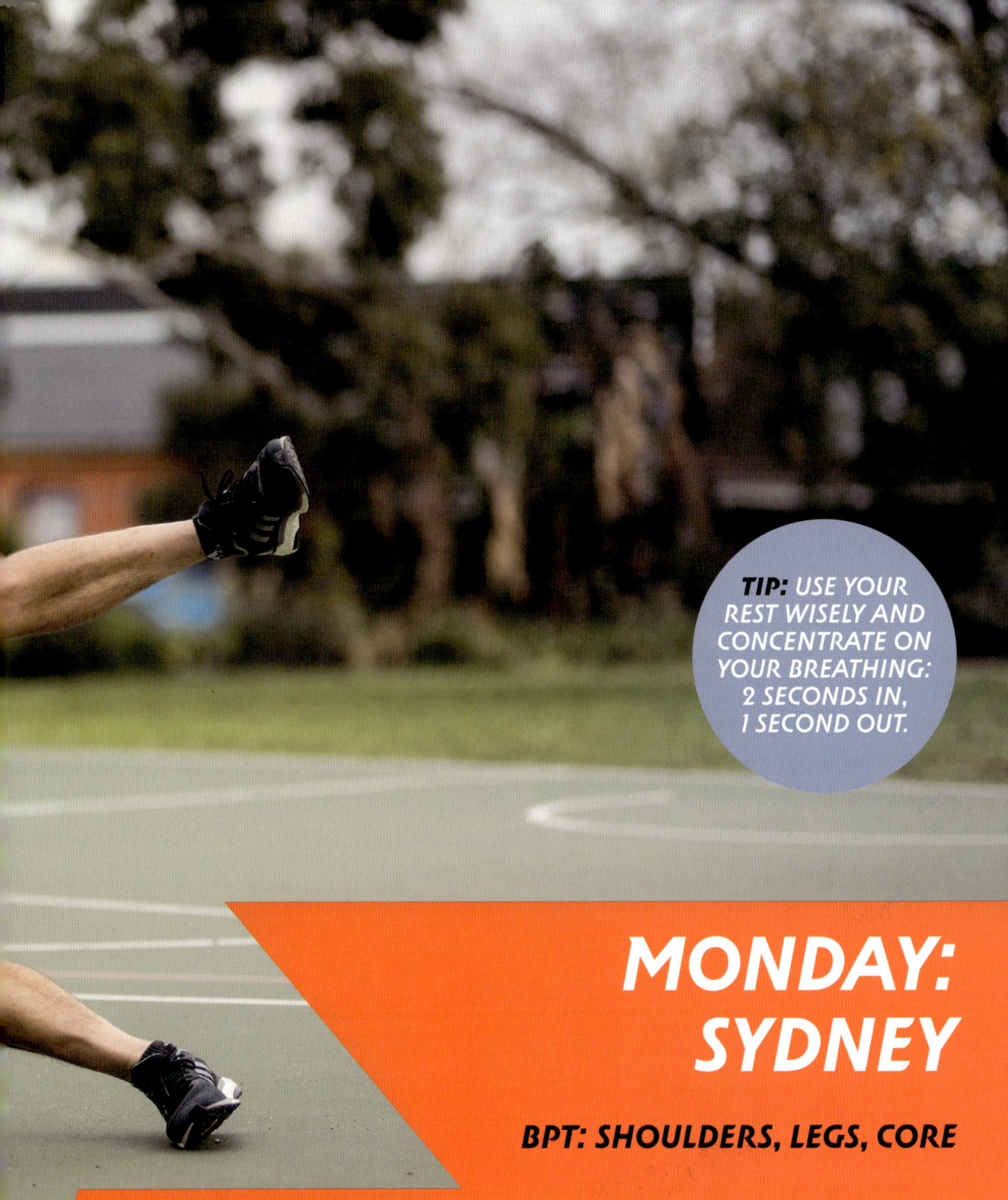

TIP: USE YOUR REST WISELY AND CONCENTRATE ON YOUR BREATHING: 2 SECONDS IN, 1 SECOND OUT.

MONDAY: SYDNEY

BPT: SHOULDERS, LEGS, CORE

10-MINUTE WORKOUT	20-MINUTE WORKOUT	30-MINUTE WORKOUT
20 seconds movement / 10 seconds rest 2 sets of each exercise (one lap)	20 seconds movement / 10 seconds rest 2 sets of each exercise (two laps)	20 seconds movement / 10 seconds rest 2 sets of each exercise (three laps)

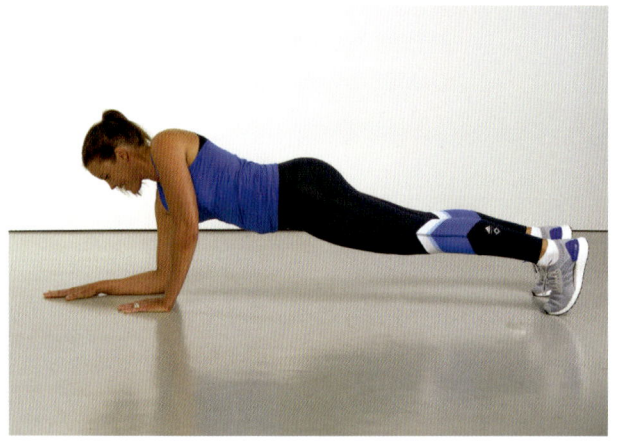

1. **Moving plank**

    Lie with your forearms on the ground, your knees off the ground and your feet together. From here, with your toes touching the ground, lean slightly forward to engage your core, lifting yourself up into the high plank position. Keep alternating between the high and low plank positions. (Note: Your back should not be sagging or bent.)

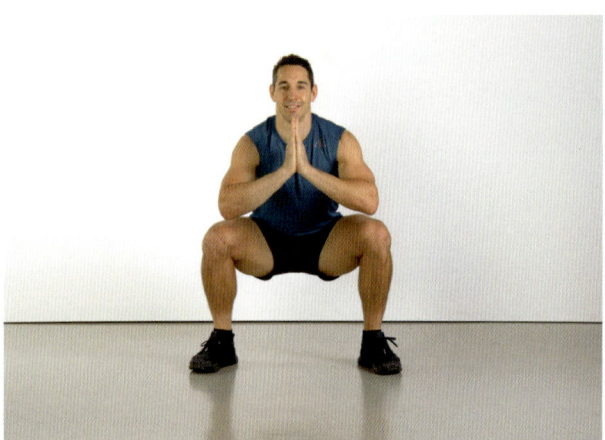

2. **2 x pulses, 1 x jump squat**

    For the pulses, stand with your feet just past shoulder-width apart and your feet slightly pointed outwards so your knees track with your feet. Bend at the hips, stick your butt out. Bend your knees until they are at a 90-degree angle. From here, pulse up and down twice before exploding upwards through your feet so that you are completely off the ground before returning to the pulse position.

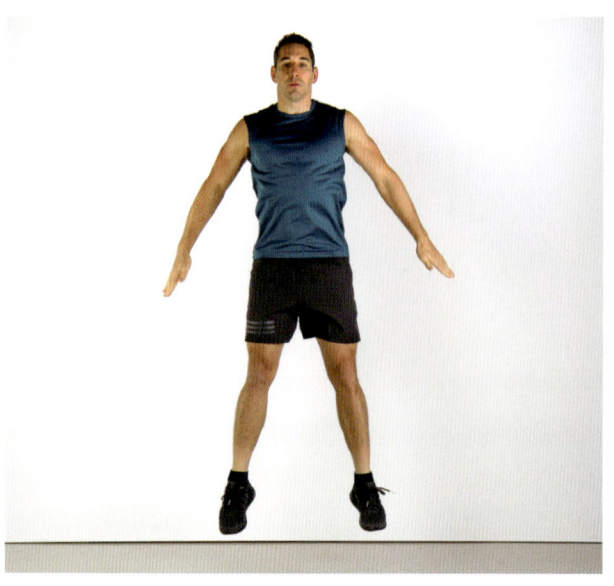

For the jump squat, stand with your feet just past shoulder-width apart and your feet slightly pointed outwards so your knees track with your feet. Bend at the hips, stick your butt out and bend your knees until they are at a 90-degree angle. Jump up either right or left 90 degrees (or 180 degrees for advanced). Repeat for one full circle going clockwise, and then go anticlockwise for one full circle.

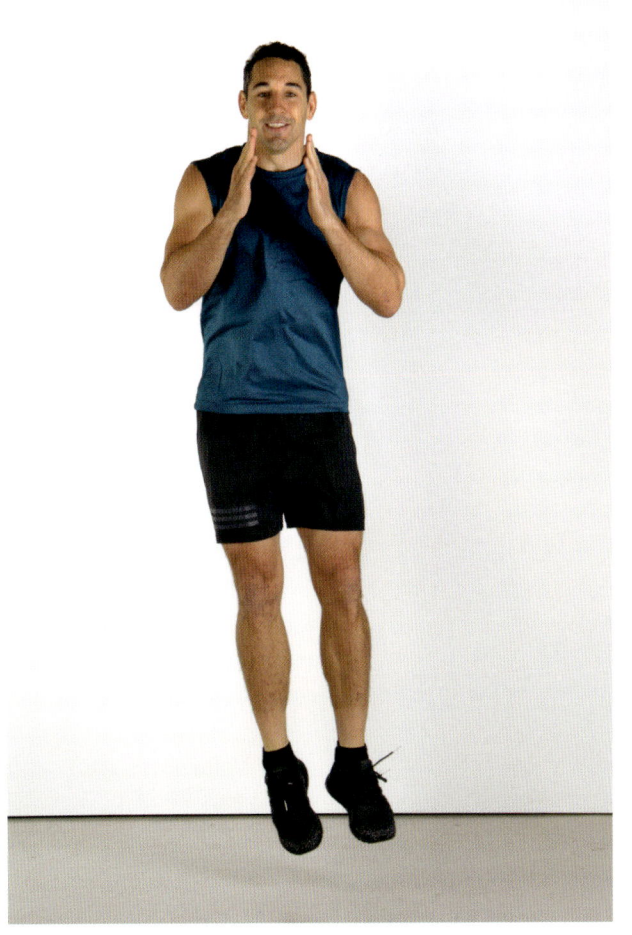

3 4 x lateral hops, 1 x burpee

For the lateral hops, stand with your feet together. From here, jump to the left to land on both feet, then jump to the right to land on both feet. Each side is one rep.

For the burpee, stand in a relaxed position with your feet shoulder-width apart. Squat and place your hands firmly on the ground with your feet back. Shoot your legs back so you are in a high plank position, then lower your body so your torso is just touching the ground. Release your hands and then, placing your hands back on the ground, raise your torso and jump your feet back so both hands and both feet are on the ground. Stand back up, then jump up and raise your hands above your head.

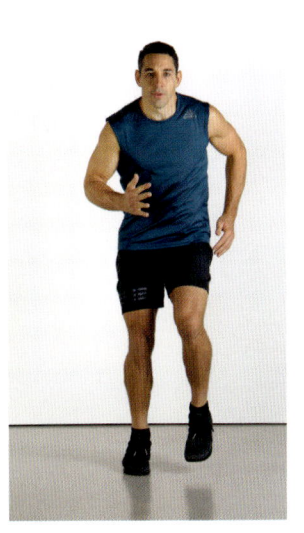 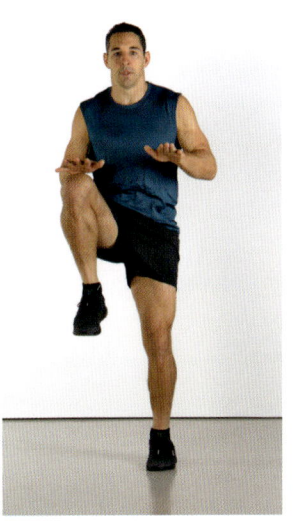

4 10 x fast feet, 10 x high knees

For the fast feet, stand with your feet shoulder-width apart, then transfer your weight from side to side in a small movement.

For the high knees, stand with your feet shoulder-width apart. One leg at a time, raise your left knee up as high as you can before alternating to the other leg.

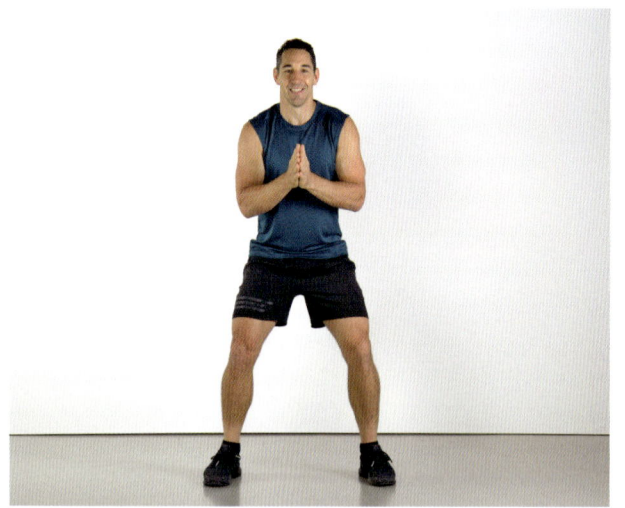

5 **Seal jacks**

Starting in a relaxed position with your hands touching together in the middle of your chest, jump out so your feet are in a wide stance and your arms split. Bring your feet and hands back together.

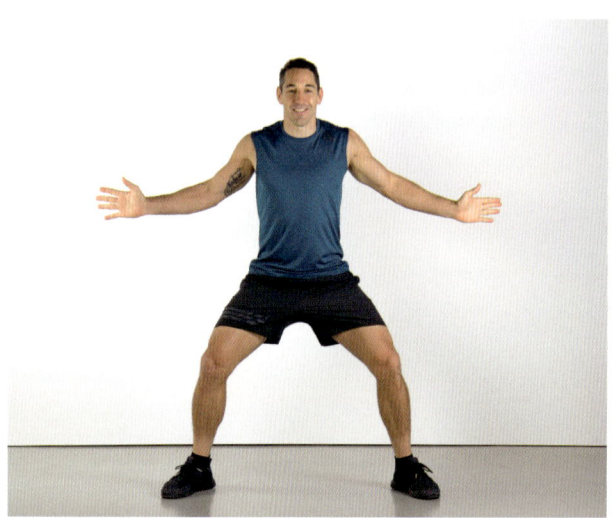

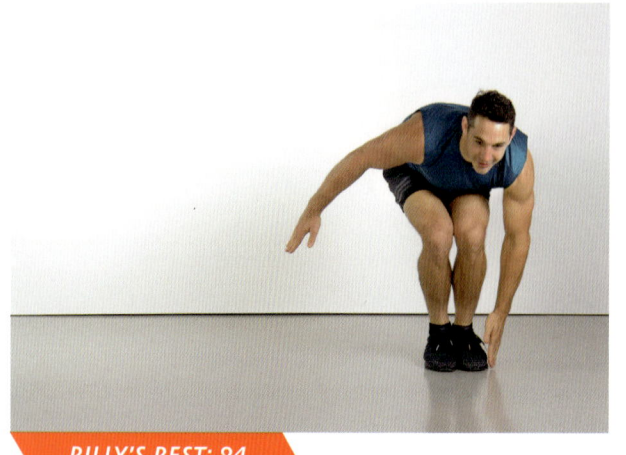

6 **Slalom taps**

Start with your feet together, then jump to the left to land on both feet, touching your left hand down next to your left foot. Then jump to the right with both feet, touching your right hand to your right foot.

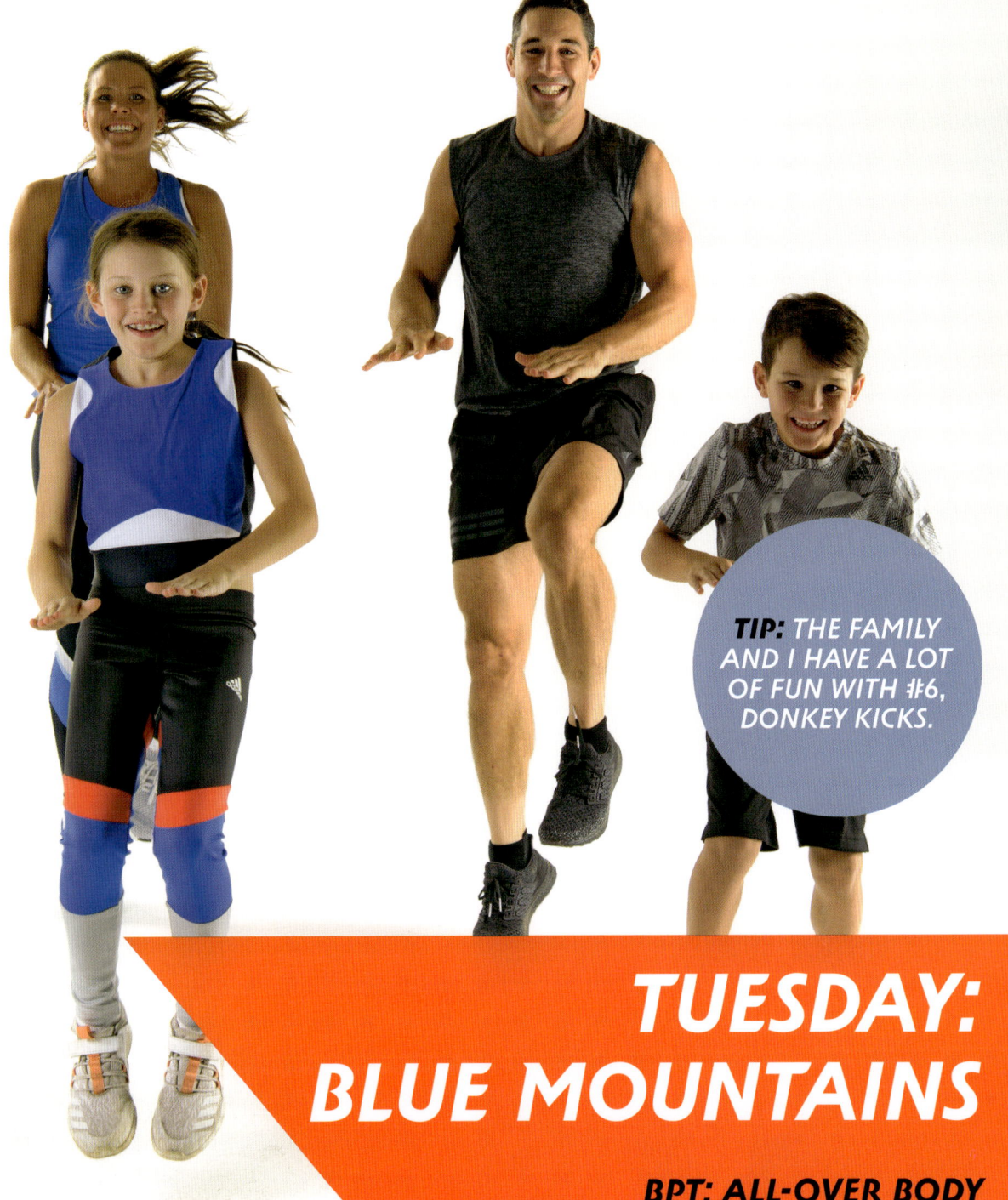

TIP: THE FAMILY AND I HAVE A LOT OF FUN WITH #6, DONKEY KICKS.

TUESDAY: BLUE MOUNTAINS

BPT: ALL-OVER BODY

10-MINUTE WORKOUT

20 seconds movement /
10 seconds rest
2 sets of each exercise
(one lap)

20-MINUTE WORKOUT

20 seconds movement /
10 seconds rest
2 sets of each exercise
(two laps)

30-MINUTE WORKOUT

20 seconds movement /
10 seconds rest
2 sets of each exercise
(three laps)

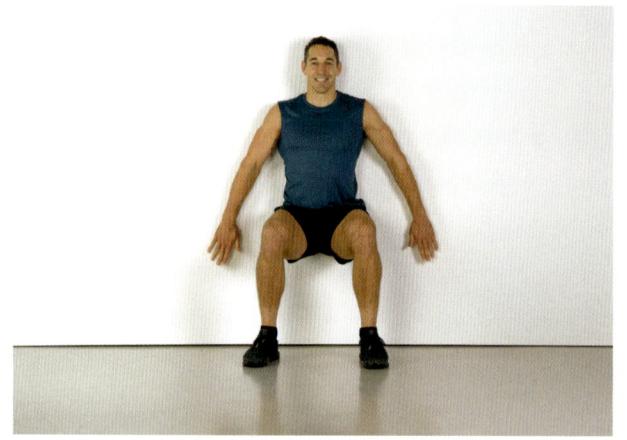

1 **Wall sit**

Put your back against a wall, feet shoulder-width apart and two steps away from the wall. With your hands firmly against the wall, lower your butt down the wall until your knees are at a 90-degree angle. Hold the position.

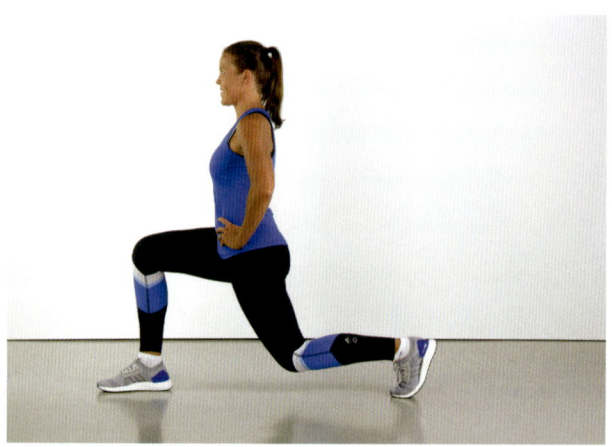

2 **Forward lunges**

Stand with your feet shoulder-width apart and your hands on your hips. Step one leg forward and lower your back leg to a 90-degree position so your knee is in line with the heel of your leading foot. Step back to the starting position and then repeat on the other side to complete the movement.

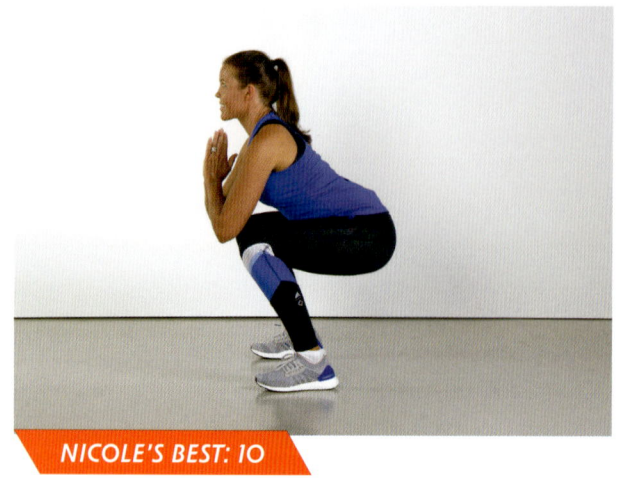

3 **Squats**

Stand with your feet just past shoulder-width apart and your feet slightly pointed outwards so your knees track with your feet. Bend at the hips, stick your butt out and bend your knees until they are at a 90-degree angle. Return to starting position.

NICOLE'S BEST: 10

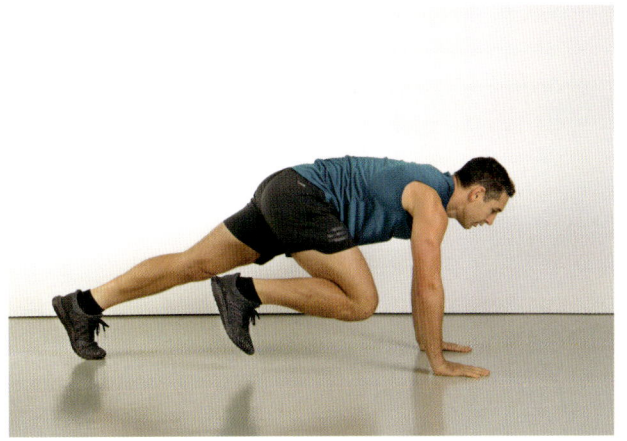

4 Mountain climbers

Start in a high plank position, with your shoulders over your wrists, your feet together and your core engaged. From here, bring one knee up towards your chest and then return it to the starting position. Repeat on the other side.

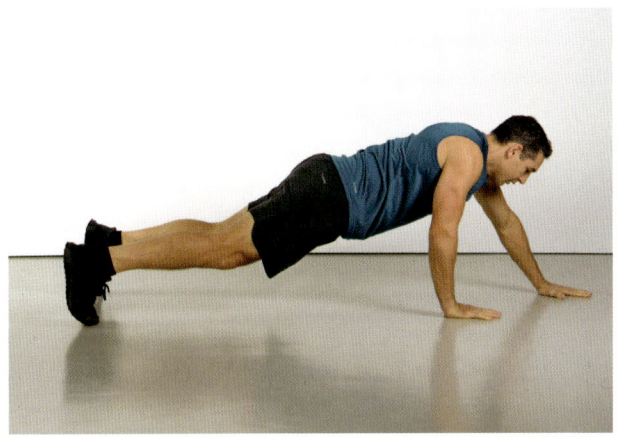

5 Inchworms

Stand with your feet just wide enough apart that when you bend forward to touch the ground your legs remain straight. From the bent position, walk your hands out until you are in a high plank position. Engage your core and squeeze your glutes. Now walk your hands back, keeping your legs straight, before engaging your core to stand up into the starting position.

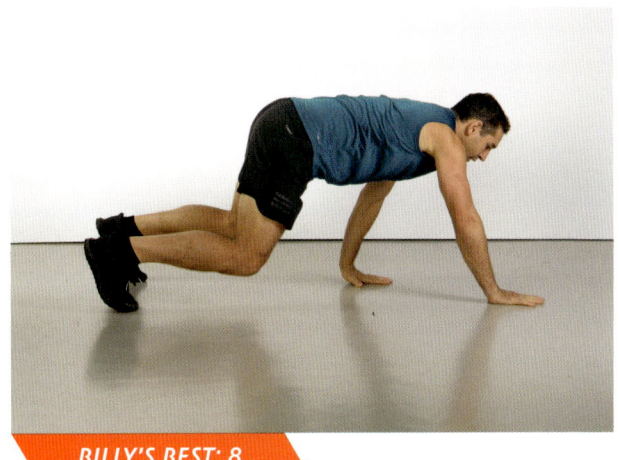

BILLY'S BEST: 8

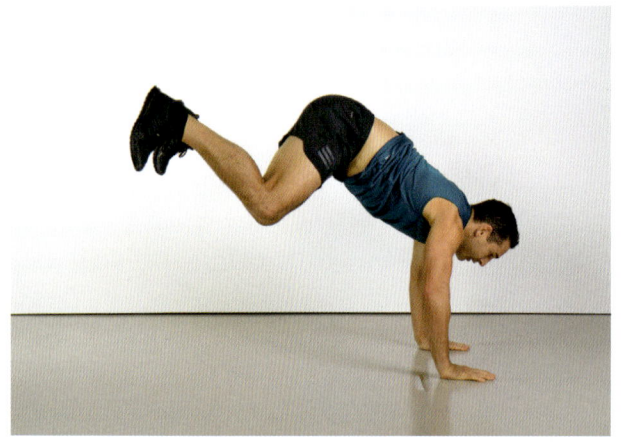

6   Donkey kicks
Bend over and place your hands on the ground with your shoulders over your wrists. From here, bend your knees at a 90-degree angle and lean forward. Take your feet off the ground and then kick out your legs to a comfortable distance before returning to the starting position.

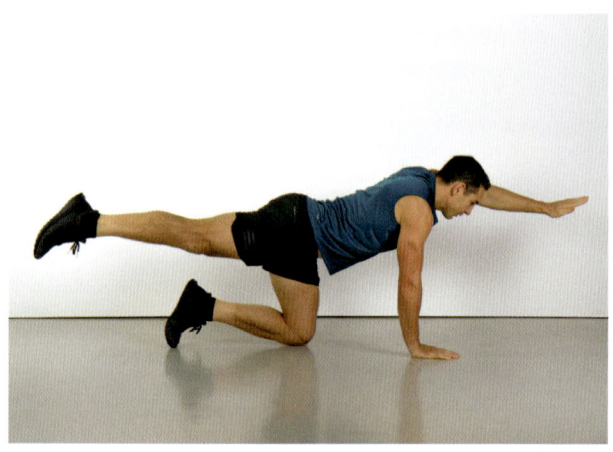

7   Contralateral limb raises
Place your hands, knees and toes firmly on the ground. From here, raise one arm and the opposite leg. Kick the leg out straight, squeezing your core, and then return to the starting position. Repeat on the other side.

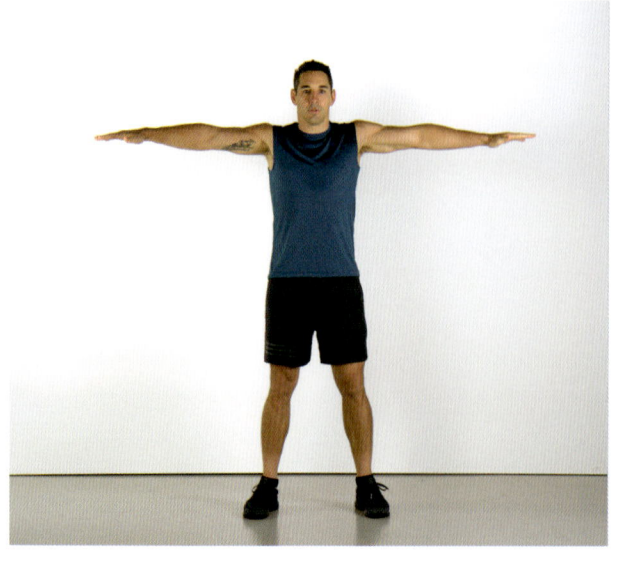

8   Arm circles
Stand with your feet shoulder-width apart and raise your arms so they are straight and in line with your shoulders. From here, rotate your arms in a circular motion forwards and backwards.

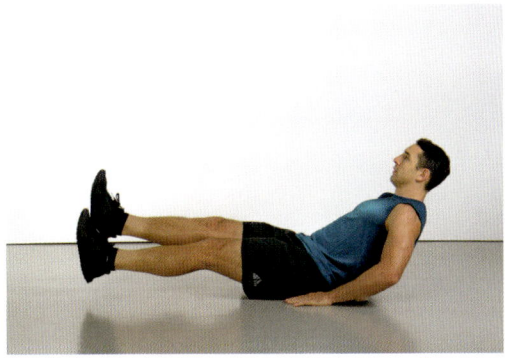

9   **Flutter kicks**

Starting position is lying on your back with your thumbs tucked under your lower lumbar (base of your back) on either side of your body. Raise your legs and kick them up and down in a small fluttering motion, engaging your core.

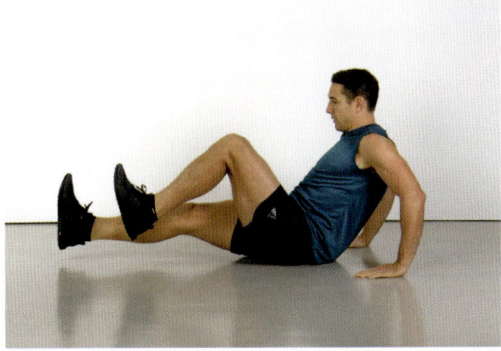

10 **Bicycle crunches**

Start by sitting on the ground with your hands on the floor by your side and your legs extended in front of you. From here, lean back, engaging your core so your feet are off the ground. Now bring one knee towards your chest, keeping the other leg straight. Return your knee to the earlier position and swap to bring your other knee towards your chest.

Advanced: Take your hands off the ground and bring the opposite elbow to your knee.

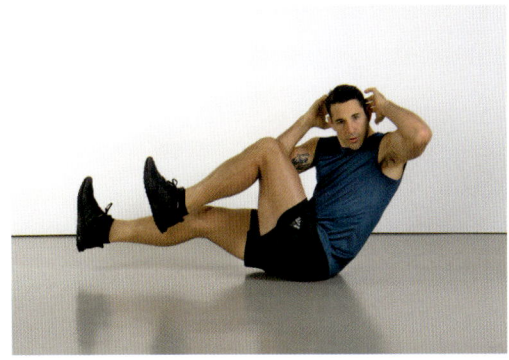

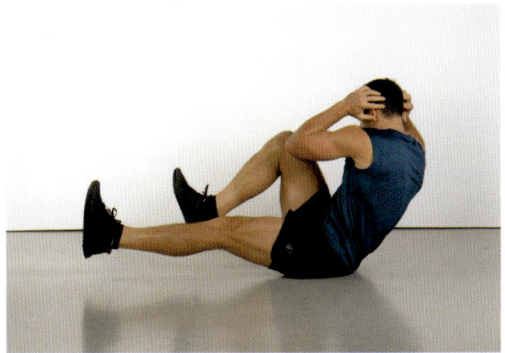

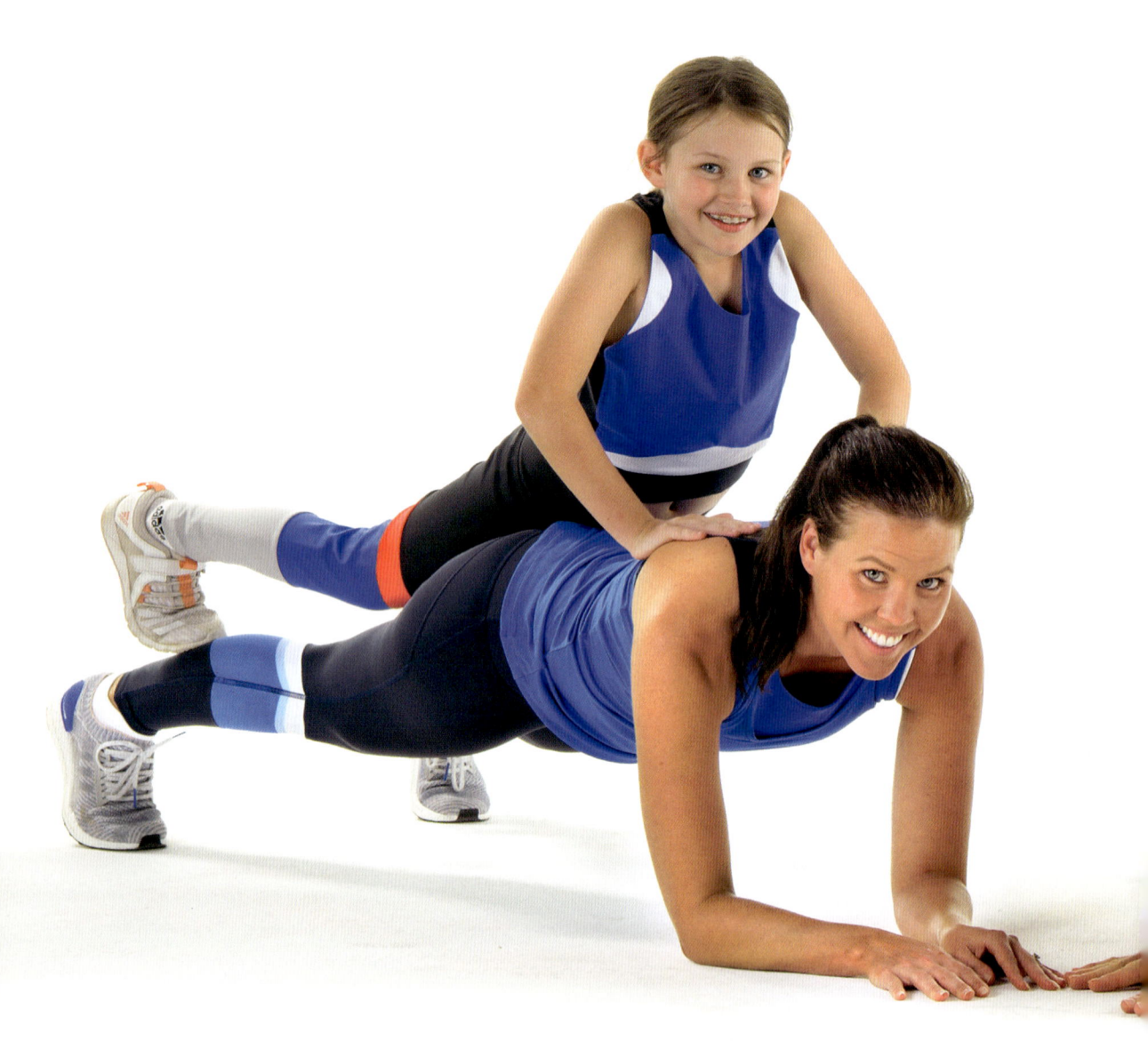

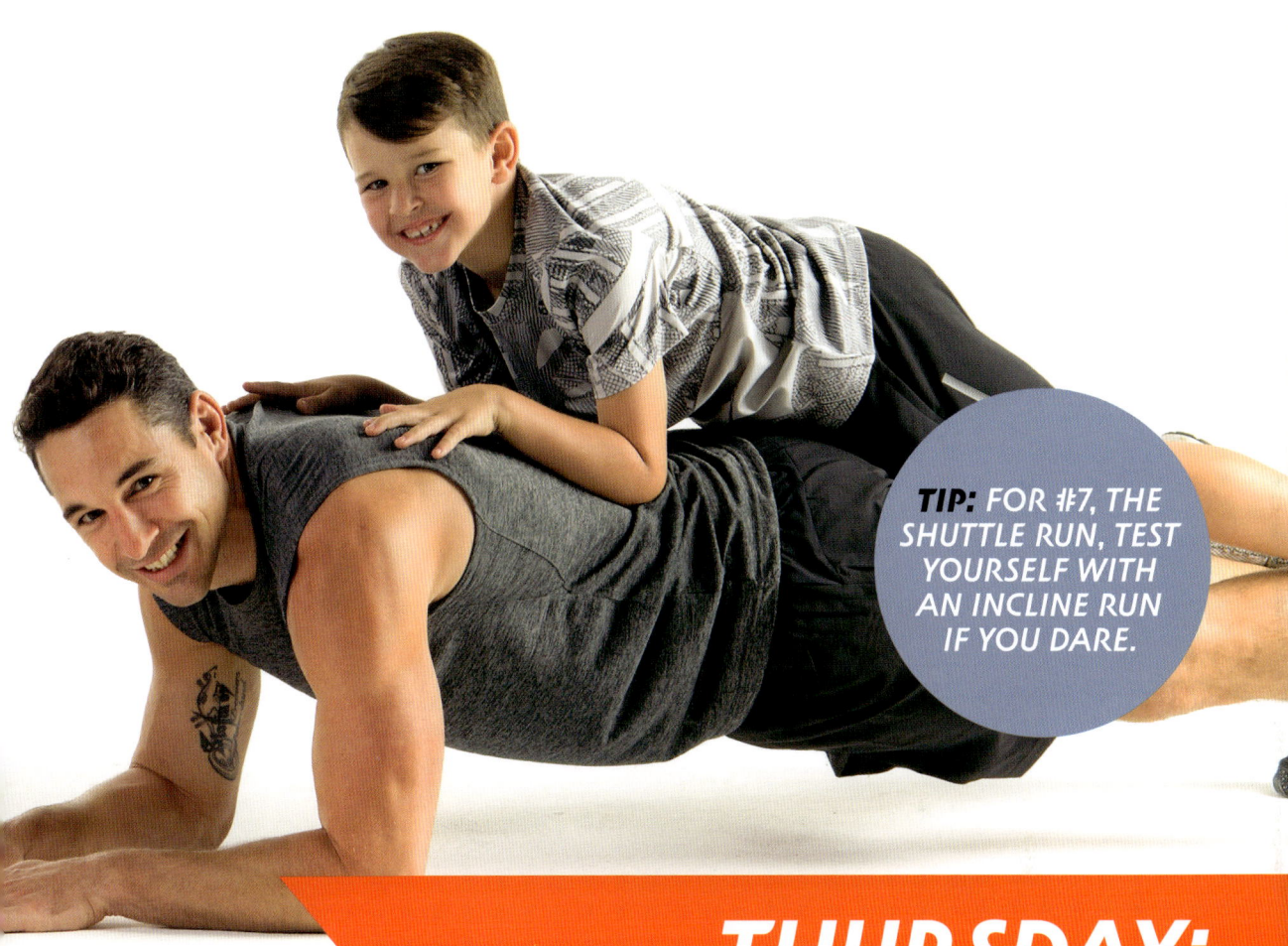

TIP: FOR #7, THE SHUTTLE RUN, TEST YOURSELF WITH AN INCLINE RUN IF YOU DARE.

THURSDAY: COFFS HARBOUR

BPT: BACK, CORE, CARDIO

10-MINUTE WORKOUT

20 seconds movement /
10 seconds rest
2 sets of each exercise
(one lap)

20-MINUTE WORKOUT

20 seconds movement /
10 seconds rest
2 sets of each exercise
(two laps)

30-MINUTE WORKOUT

20 seconds movement /
10 seconds rest
2 sets of each exercise
(three laps)

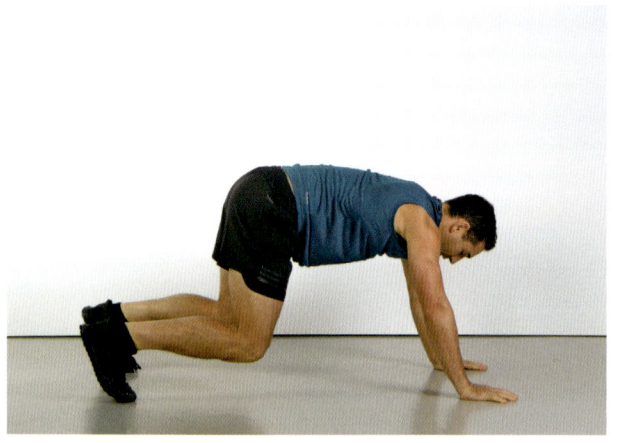

1 **Bear crawl**

Start in the push-up position with your knees bent at a 90-degree angle and positioned directly under your hips. Engage your core and do not raise or round your back. This is the starting position. Walk your right hand and your left foot forward, and then your left hand and your right foot forward. Continue until you reach 5 metres. Now, keeping your hips down and your core engaged, reverse the movement by walking your left arm and your right foot back, and then your right arm and your left leg back. Continue until you have returned to your starting position.

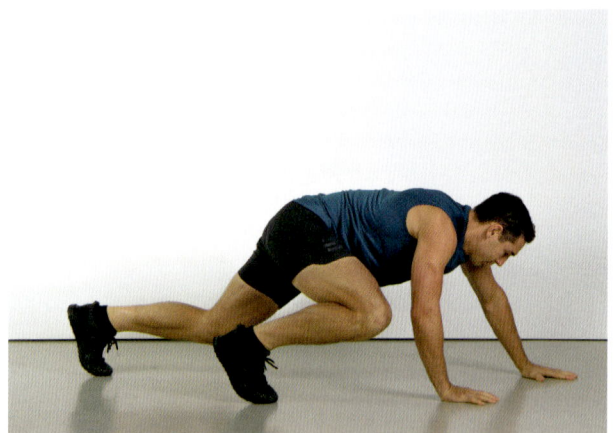

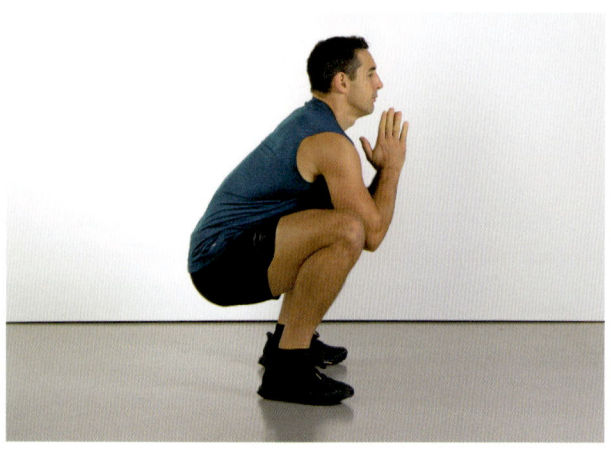

2 **Frog squats**

Stand with your feet shoulder-width apart and your feet slightly tracked out. Bend down to full squat position with your elbows tucked inside your legs. This is the starting position. From here, raise your hips and then lower them back to the starting position.

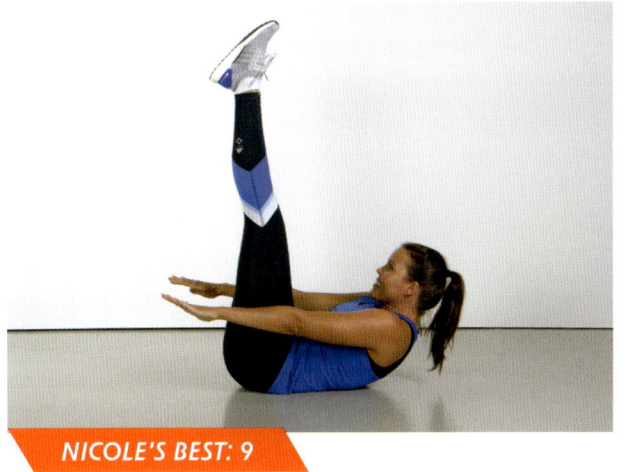

NICOLE'S BEST: 9

3 **Toe touches**

Lie on your back with your legs up in the air and your toes flexed. Run your hands up your shins as far as you can go towards your toes, then release back to the starting position.

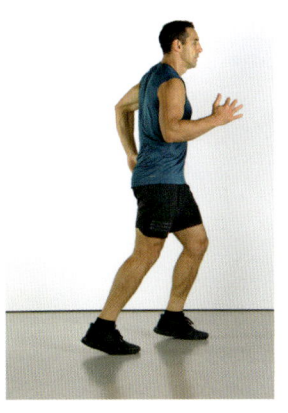 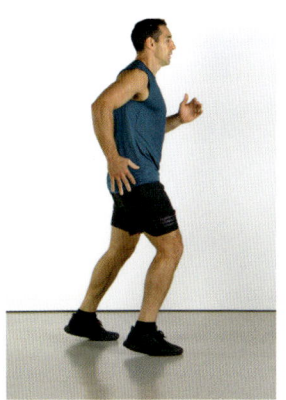

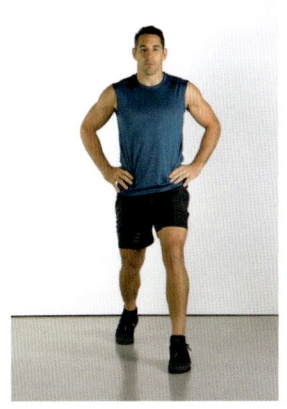 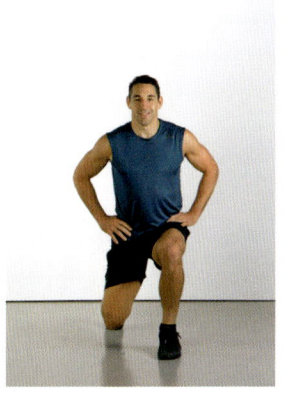

4 **4 x shuffles,
2 x plyometric split lunges**

For the shuffles, stand with your feet shoulder-width apart and your hands on your hips. Split your feet so your back toe is in line with your front heel. Alternate four times.

4.1 For the plyometric split lunges, start with your feet shoulder-width apart and your hands on your hips. Split your legs before dropping your back knee down in line with the heel of your leading foot – both legs should be at a 90-degree angle – then push up and repeat on the other side.

4.2 Alternatively, stand with your feet shoulder-width apart and your hands on your hips. Step one leg back and then lower it until it is 90 degrees to the ground. Step forward to the starting position. Repeat on the other side to complete the movement.

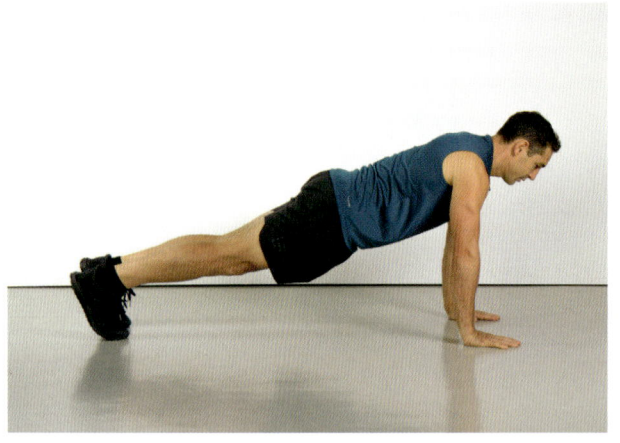

5 Push-ups

5.1 Get into high plank position with your hands shoulder-width apart, your shoulders over your wrists and your feet elevated on your toes. This is the starting position. Now lower yourself down to transfer all your weight into your shoulders and back. Press back up to the starting position.

5.2 Alternatively, place one ankle over the other while your knees are on the floor in the starting position. Now lift yourself up so your shoulders are over your wrists. Lower yourself down to the ground and then press back up to the starting position.

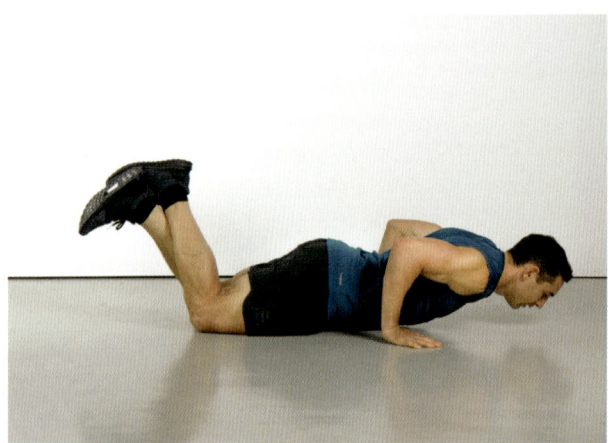

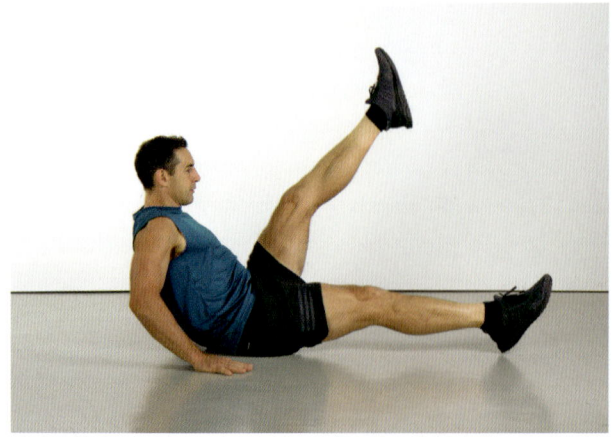

6 Scissor kicks

Sit on the ground with your legs extended in front and lean back with your hands in a comfortable position by your side. Raise one leg as high as you can, keeping it straight, then return it to the ground. Repeat with the other leg.

7   **Shuttle run**
    Picking a distance that suits your environment, run up and back for the duration of time.

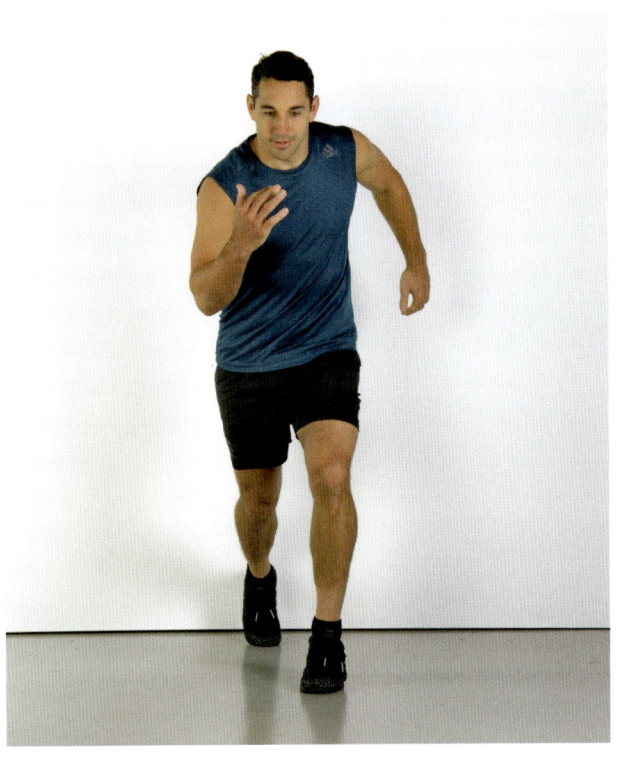

8   **Sprawls**
    Stand with your feet shoulder-width apart, then squat until both your hands and both your feet are firmly on the ground. From this position transfer your weight into your shoulders and shoot your feet back so that your legs are out wide, then jump your feet back up and stand up into the starting position.

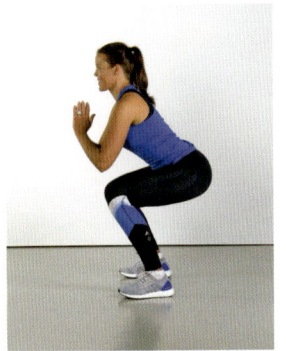 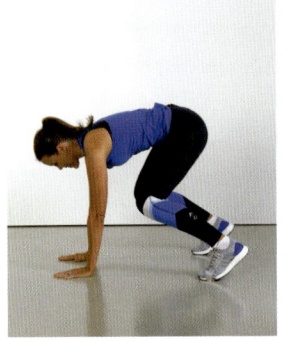

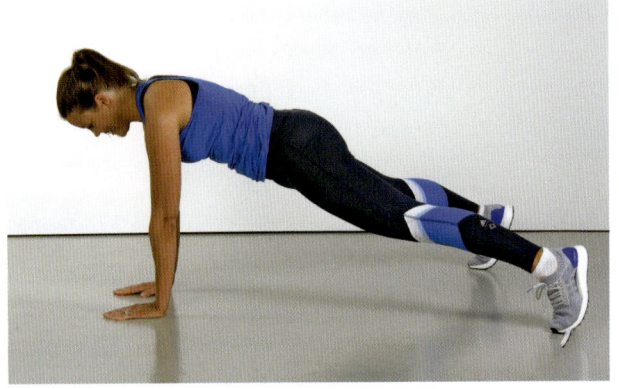

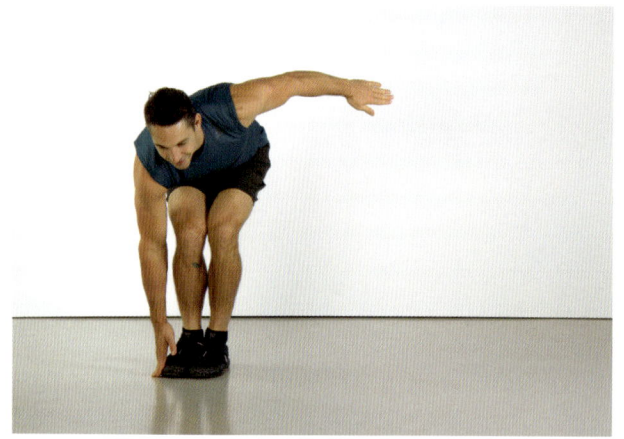

9 Slalom taps

Start with your feet together, then jump to the left to land on both feet, touching your left hand down next to your left foot. Then jump to the right with both feet, touching your right hand to your right foot.

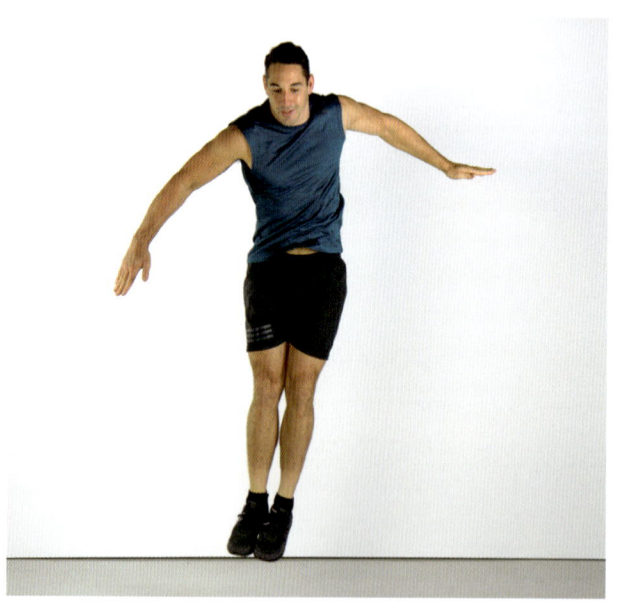

10 Elbow to knee

Lie on your back with your arms stretched out above your head. Bring your right knee up towards your chest and your right elbow towards your knee. Go as far as you can before returning to the starting position. Repeat with your left knee and elbow.

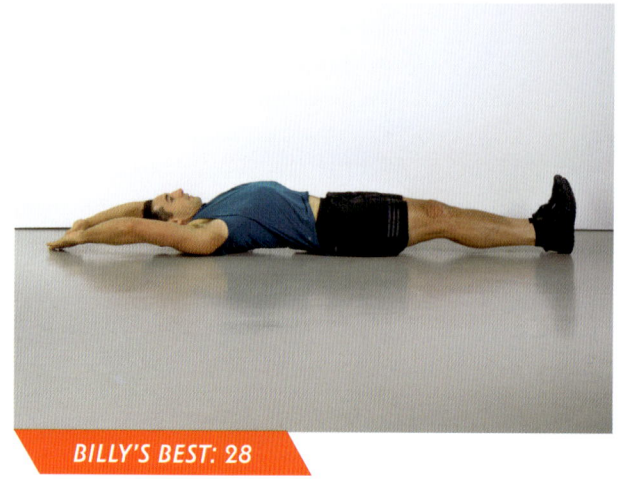

BILLY'S BEST: 28

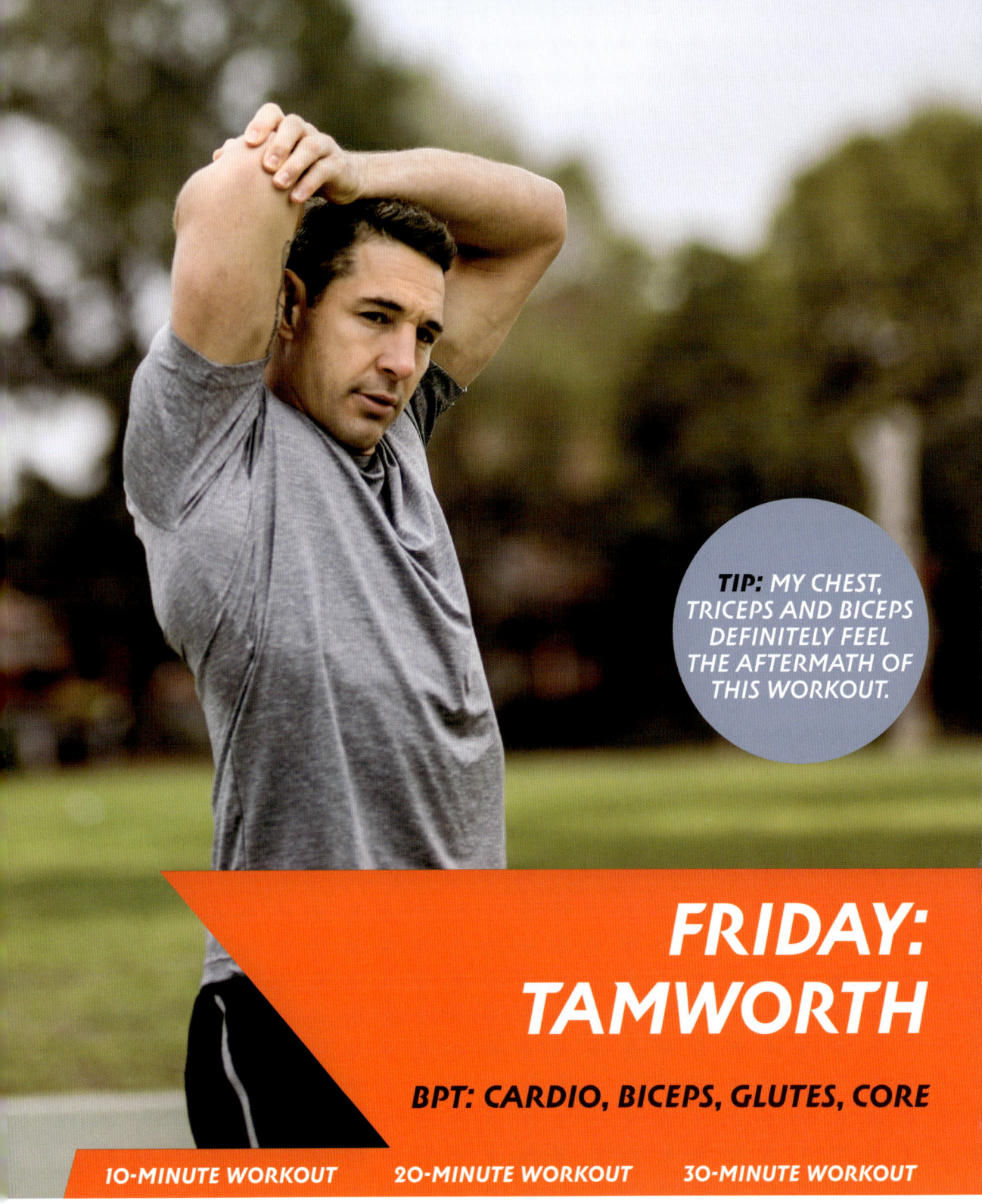

TIP: MY CHEST, TRICEPS AND BICEPS DEFINITELY FEEL THE AFTERMATH OF THIS WORKOUT.

FRIDAY: TAMWORTH

BPT: CARDIO, BICEPS, GLUTES, CORE

10-MINUTE WORKOUT	20-MINUTE WORKOUT	30-MINUTE WORKOUT
20 seconds movement / 10 seconds rest 2 sets of each exercise (one lap)	20 seconds movement / 10 seconds rest 2 sets of each exercise (two laps)	20 seconds movement / 10 seconds rest 2 sets of each exercise (three laps)

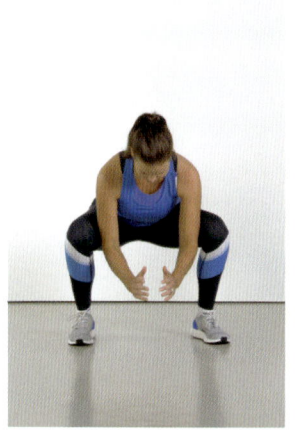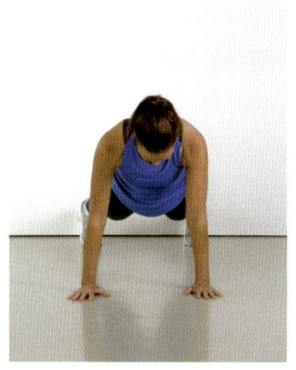

1 Jump sprawls

Stand with your feet just past shoulder-width apart, then jump forward and land softly on both feet before going into a sprawl. Squat until both your hands and both your feet are firmly on the ground. From this position, transfer your weight into your shoulders and shoot your feet back so that your legs are out wide, then jump your feet back up and return to the starting position.

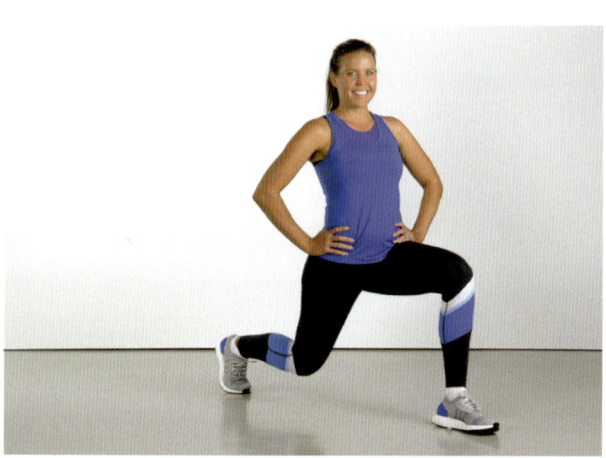

2 Side lunges

Stand with your feet shoulder-width apart and your hands on your hips or by your side. Take a half-step to one side and then bend at the knee and lunge, sticking your butt out and keeping your chest up and your core tight. Lunge back to the starting position. Repeat on the other side.

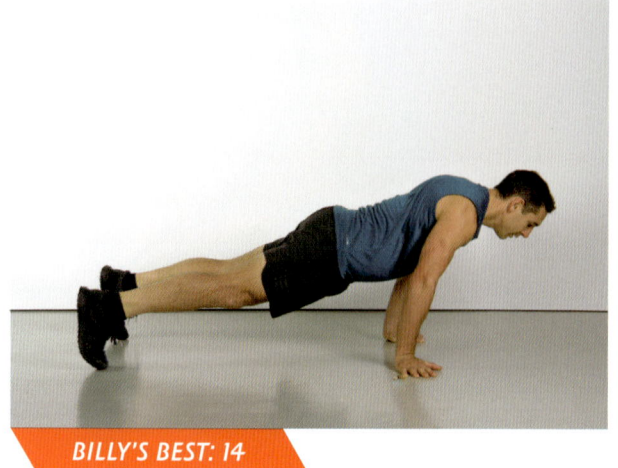

3 Planche push-ups

Start in an assisted or full push-up position with your hands slightly tracked out. Lean forward so that your arms are straight and you are comfortable. From here, lower yourself until your chest is just off the ground, and then press back up. You should feel this movement in your shoulders and biceps.

BILLY'S BEST: 14

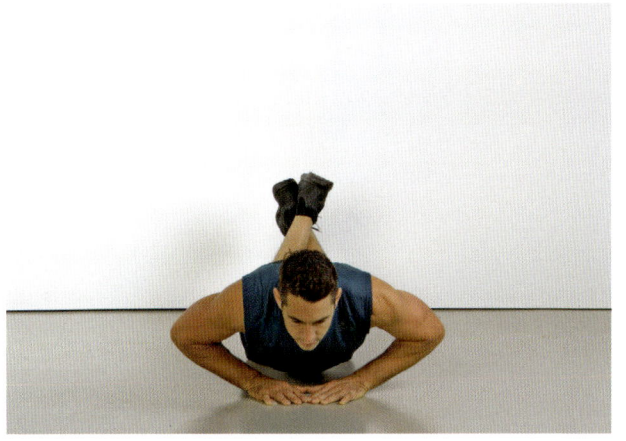

4 **Diamond push-ups**

Kneel on the ground with your ankles crossed and set your hands so your thumbs and index fingers are touching in line with your chin. From here, lower your body towards the ground and then press back up to the starting position. You should feel this movement in your triceps.

Advanced: Do the exercise in high plank position with your knees off the ground.

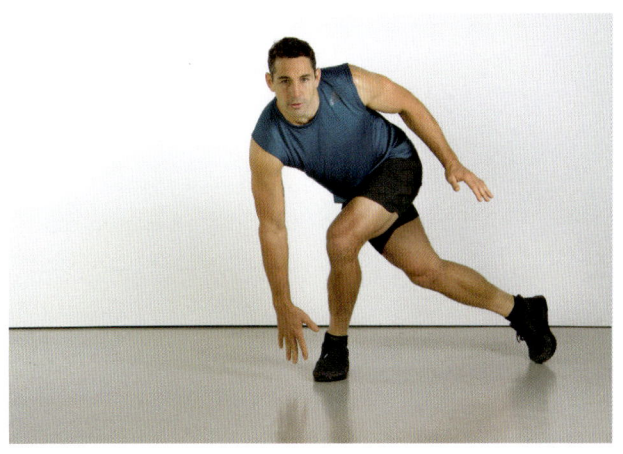

5 **Ice skaters**

Start with your feet shoulder-width apart. Step half a foot to your left, swing your right leg behind your left leg, and with your right hand touch your left toe. From here, step to your right, swing your left leg behind your right leg, and with your left hand touch your right toe.

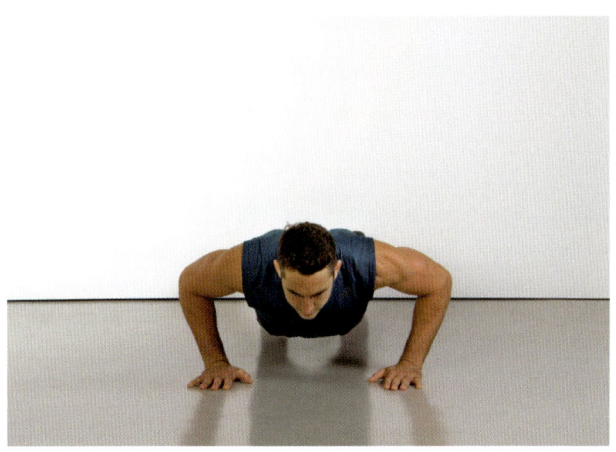

6 **2 x push-ups into 10 x crunches**

6.1 Get into high plank position with your hands shoulder-width apart, your shoulders over your wrists and your feet elevated on your toes. This is the starting position. Now lower yourself down to transfer all your weight into your shoulders and back. Press back up to the starting position.

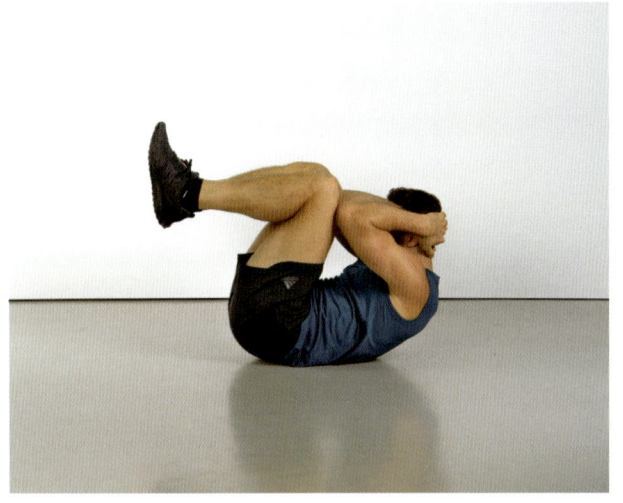

6.2 Alternatively, place one ankle over the other while your knees are on the floor in the starting position. Lift yourself up so your shoulders are over your wrists. Lower yourself down to the ground and then press back up to the starting position.

For the crunches, lie on your back with your legs off the ground at a 90-degree angle to your body. With your hands crossed behind your head, bring your elbows in next to your ears. Bring your elbows up to your knees, then return to the starting position.

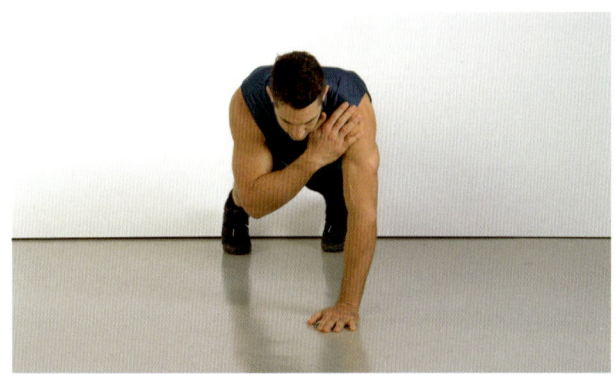

7 Shoulder taps

Starting in plank position and engaging your core, transfer your weight into your right arm, and with your left hand touch your right shoulder. Return to the starting position and repeat on the left side.

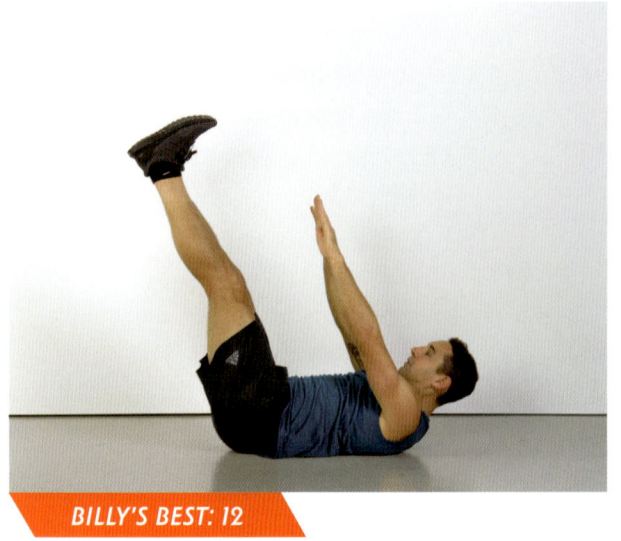

8 Jackknife

Lie on the ground with your legs out straight and your arms above your head. From here, raise your arms and legs until your hands and toes meet. This movement can be done with your knees bent.

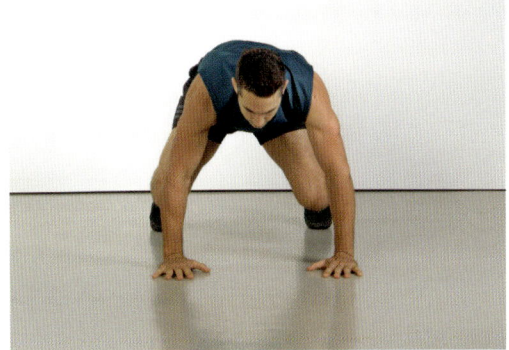

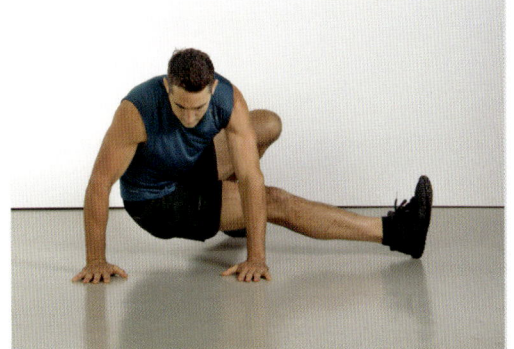

9   **Lateral shoot-throughs**

Start in high plank position with your hands firmly on the ground and your shoulders above your wrists. Bend your knees at a 90-degree angle and have your toes firmly on the ground and your knees off the ground. This is the starting position. Now turn your left foot so it is flat on the ground. Kick your right foot in front of your left foot and out to the side, so your right leg is now straight and your left foot is firmly on the ground. Now pull your right leg back to the starting position. Repeat on the other side.

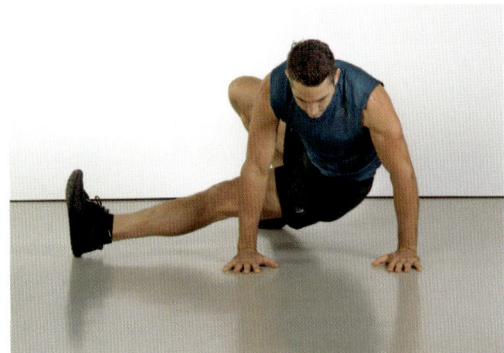

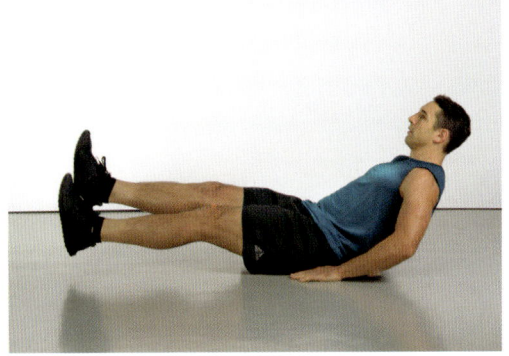

10 **Flutter kicks**

Starting position is lying on your back with your thumbs tucked under your lower lumbar (base of your back) on either side of your body. Raise your legs and kick them up and down in a small fluttering motion, engaging your core.

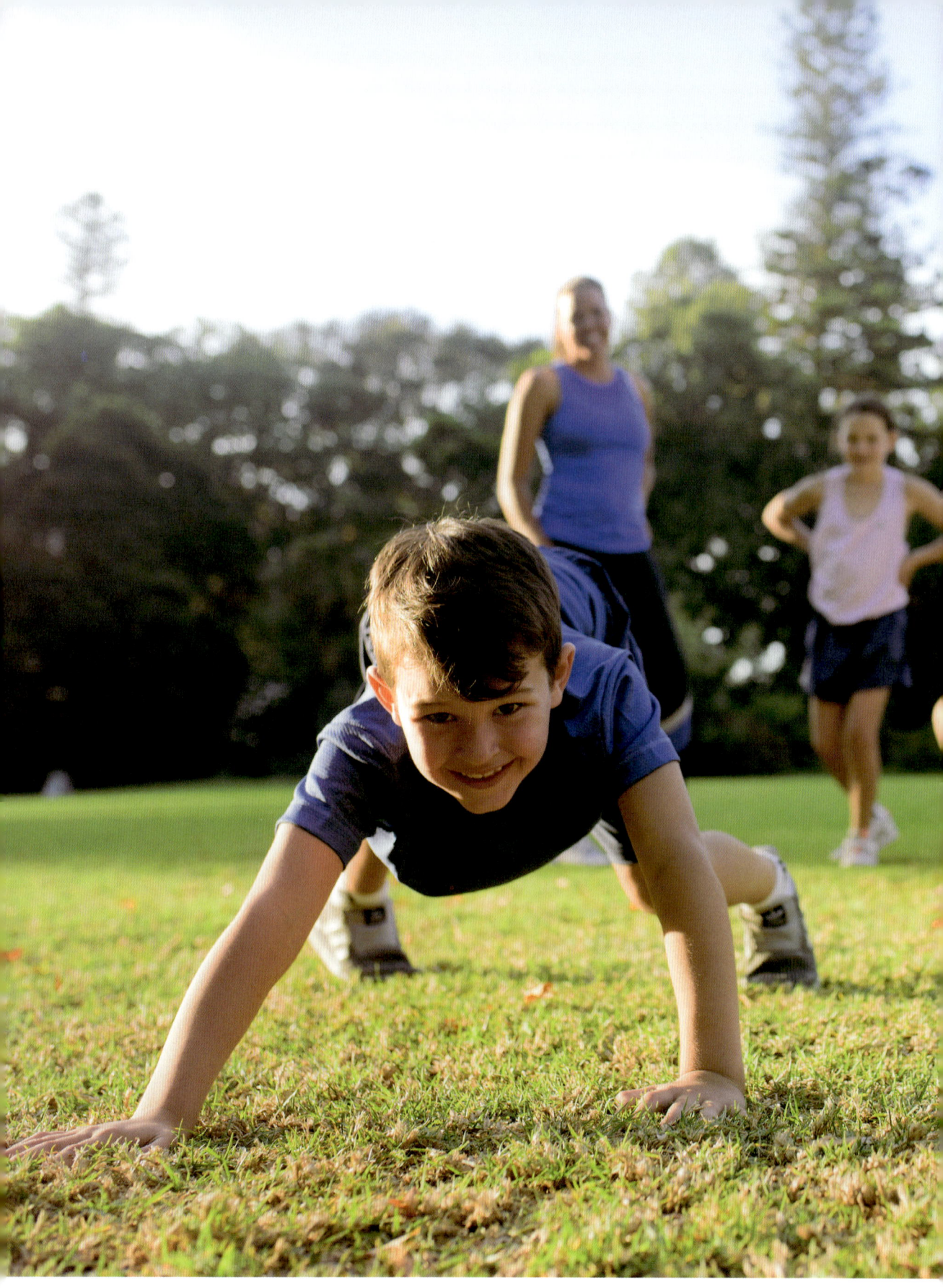

Getting the Kids Fired Up

'Kids are creatures of habit. They get used to something – whether it's a good thing or a bad thing, they get in that routine. This is all about teaching them a good routine, and creating good habits. If you can do that from an early age, whether it's eating, whether it's exercise, whether it's manners, it's likely to stick. It's all about bringing your kids up in a way that you'd like them to live the rest of their life.

'You make it fun – that's your reward system. Exercising can be going through the program with them and having fun with it, or it can be kicking a ball around at the park. A lot of people think of exercising as a chore, but it doesn't have to be. We exercise as a family all the time, and the kids enjoy it.'

Billy

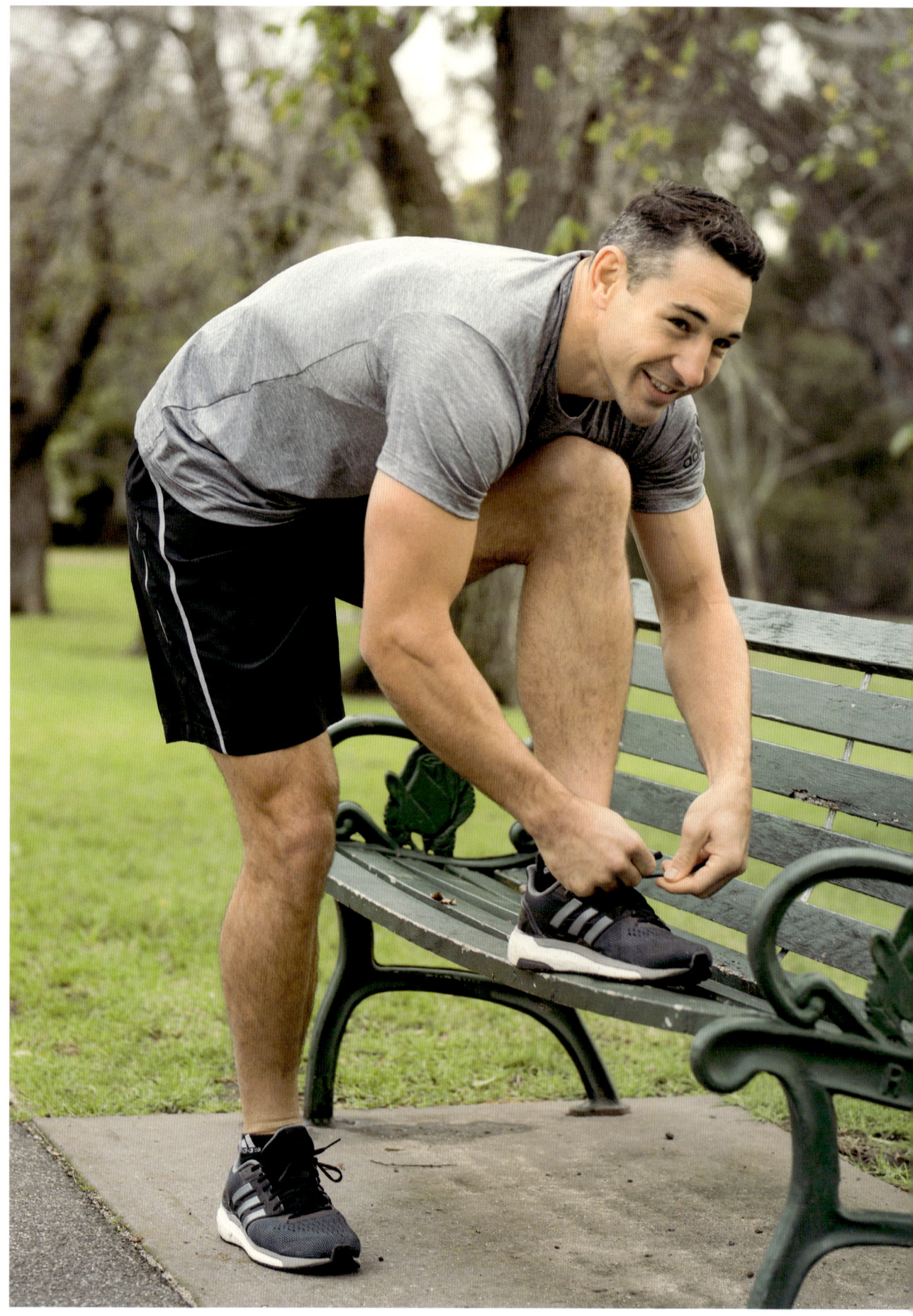

BLOCK 3: QUEENSLAND

'It all started in Innisfail, Queensland. I have heaps of great memories from my childhood, running around barefoot, playing outside and generally having fun. I love the relaxed environment and being able to get back to basics.'

Billy

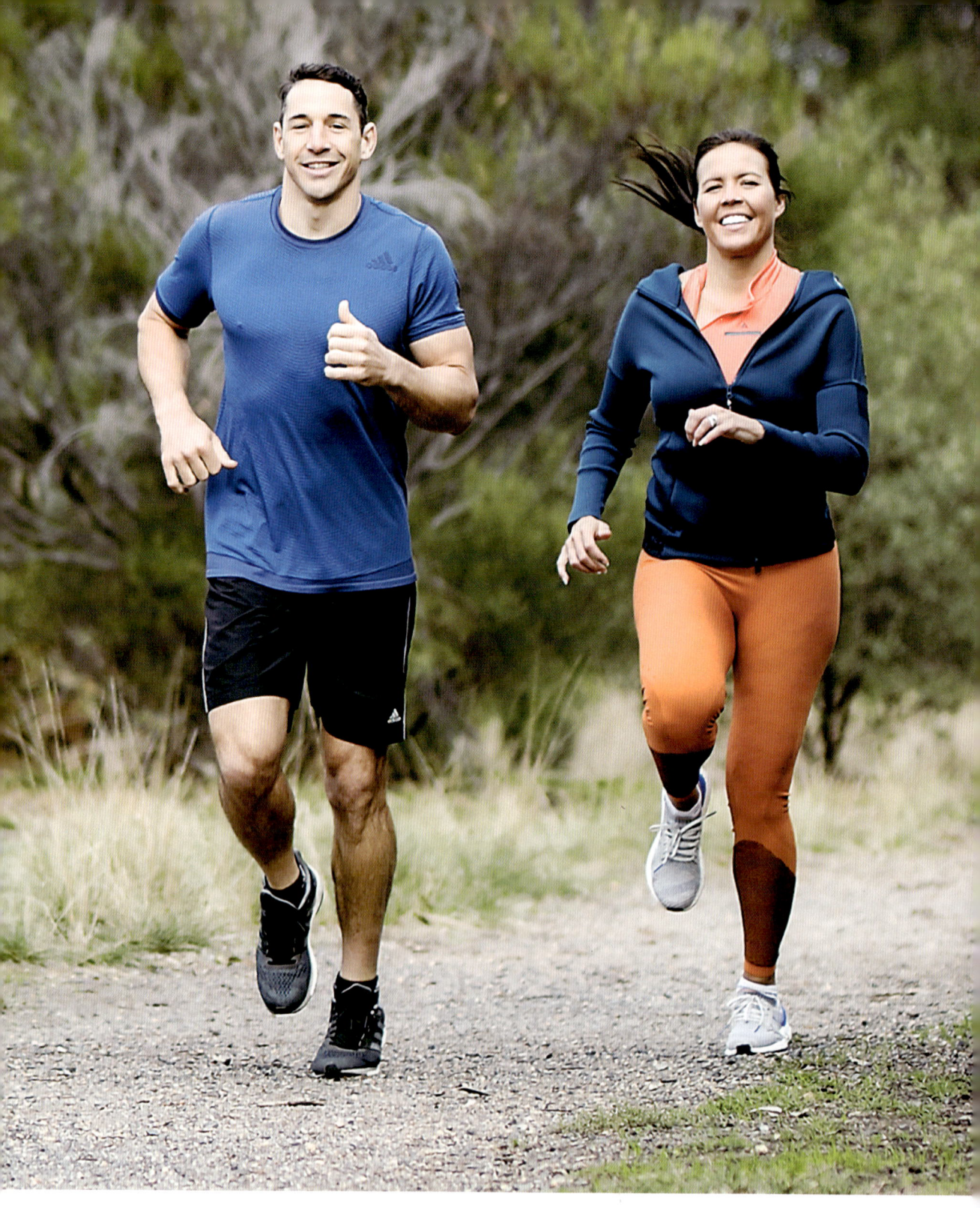

MOVE WITH BILLY SLATER

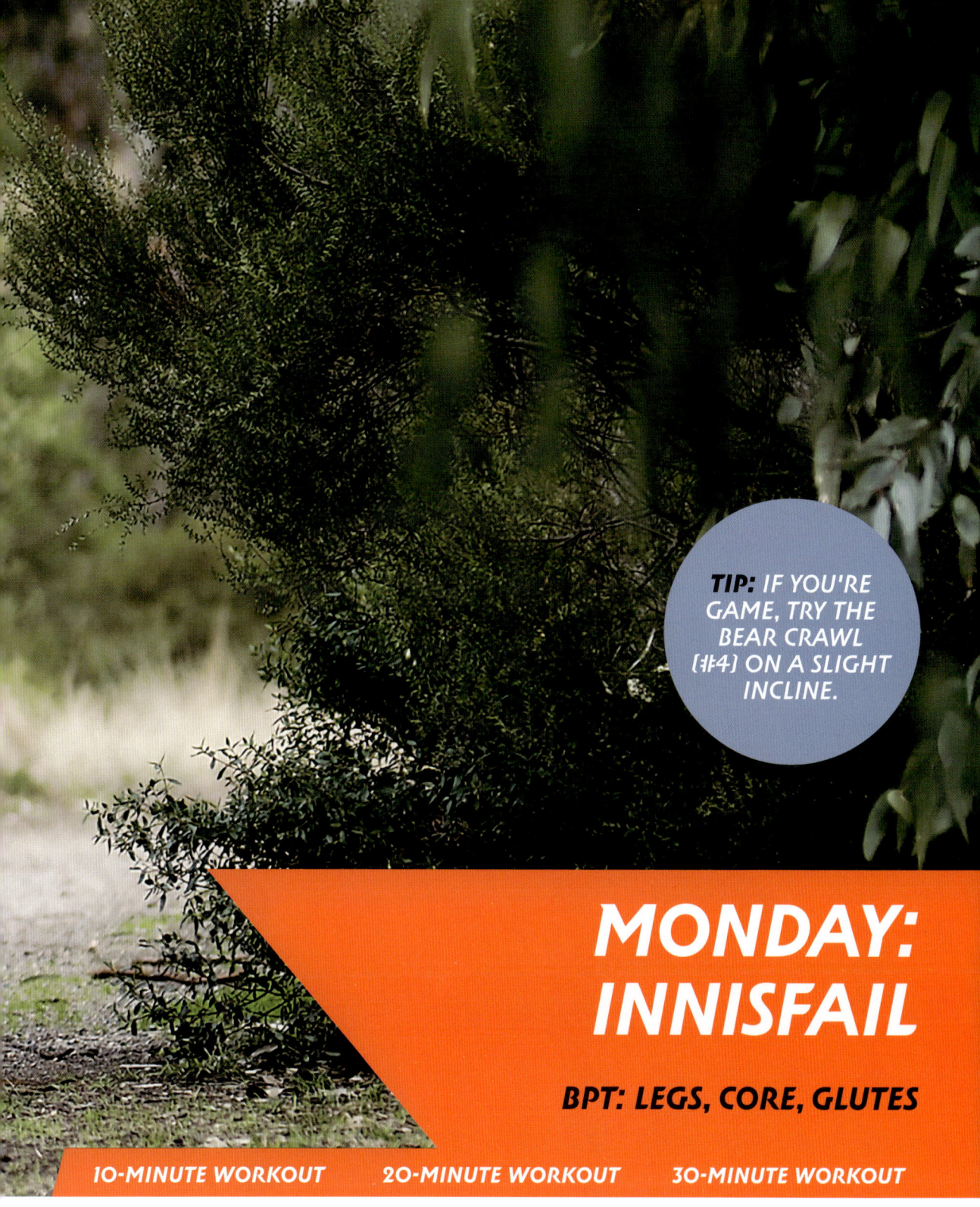

TIP: IF YOU'RE GAME, TRY THE BEAR CRAWL (#4) ON A SLIGHT INCLINE.

MONDAY: INNISFAIL

BPT: LEGS, CORE, GLUTES

10-MINUTE WORKOUT	20-MINUTE WORKOUT	30-MINUTE WORKOUT
20 seconds movement / 10 seconds rest 2 sets of each exercise (one lap)	20 seconds movement / 10 seconds rest 2 sets of each exercise (two laps)	20 seconds movement / 10 seconds rest 2 sets of each exercise (three laps)

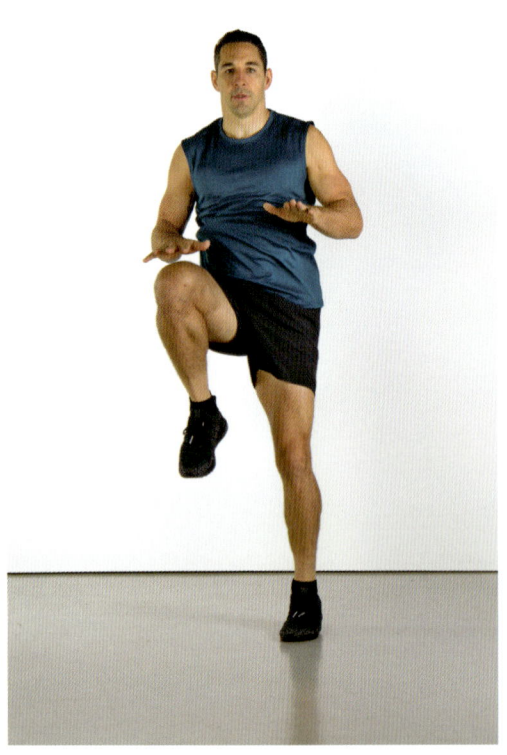

1. **10 x high knees, 1 x burpee**

   For the high knees, stand with your feet shoulder-width apart. One leg at a time, raise your left knee up as high as you can before alternating to the other leg.

   For the burpee, stand in a relaxed position with your feet shoulder-width apart. Squat and place your hands firmly on the ground with your feet back. Shoot your legs back so you are in a high plank position, then lower your body so your torso is just touching the ground. Release your hands and then, placing your hands back on the ground, raise your torso and jump your feet back so both hands and both feet are on the ground. Stand back up, then jump up and raise your hands above your head.

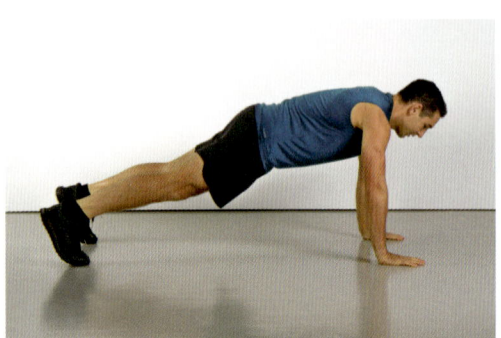

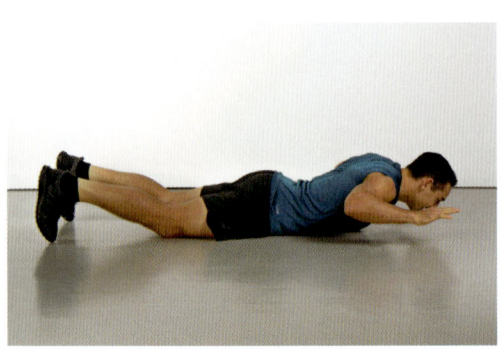

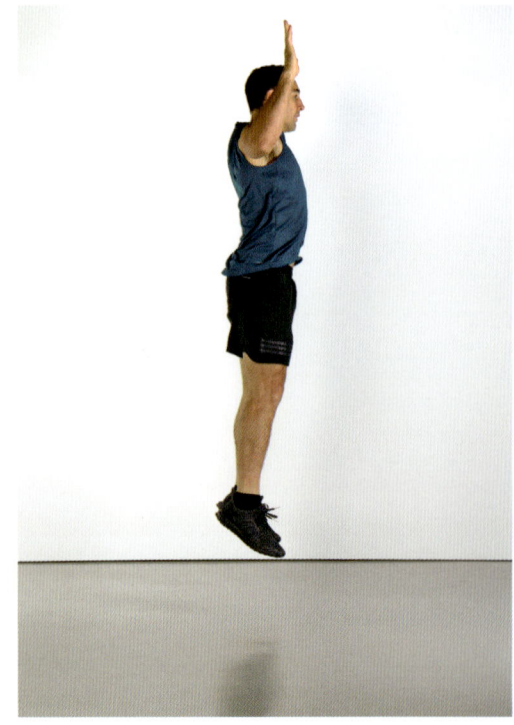

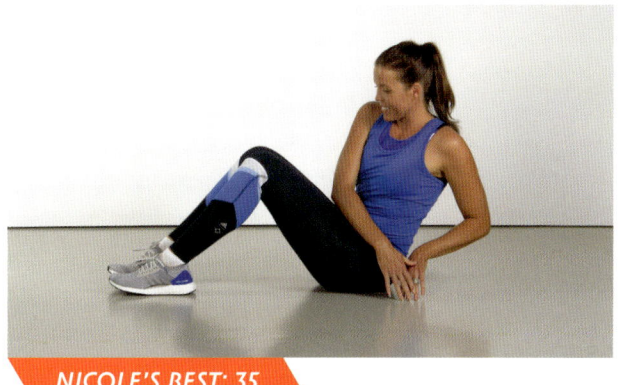

NICOLE'S BEST: 35

2. **Russian twists**

   Sit on the ground with your knees bent and your feet flat on the ground. Clasping your hands in front of your chest, twist your torso to one side and touch the ground with your fingertips, engaging your core. Then shift your weight and twist your torso to touch the ground on the other side.

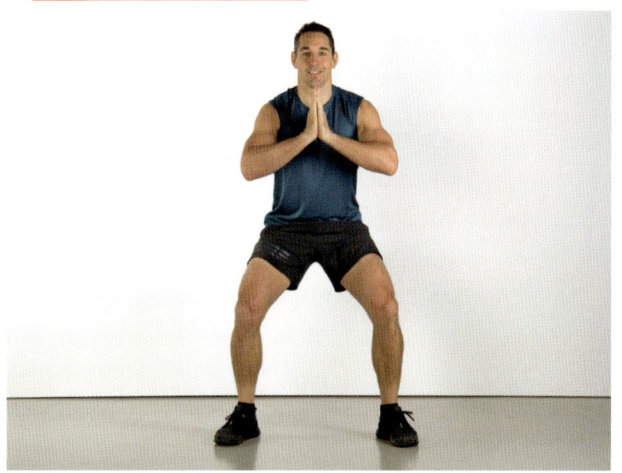

3. **Pulse squats**

   Stand with your feet just past shoulder-width apart and slightly tracked out. Squat with your hips back and your legs at a 90-degree angle, then pulse up and down.

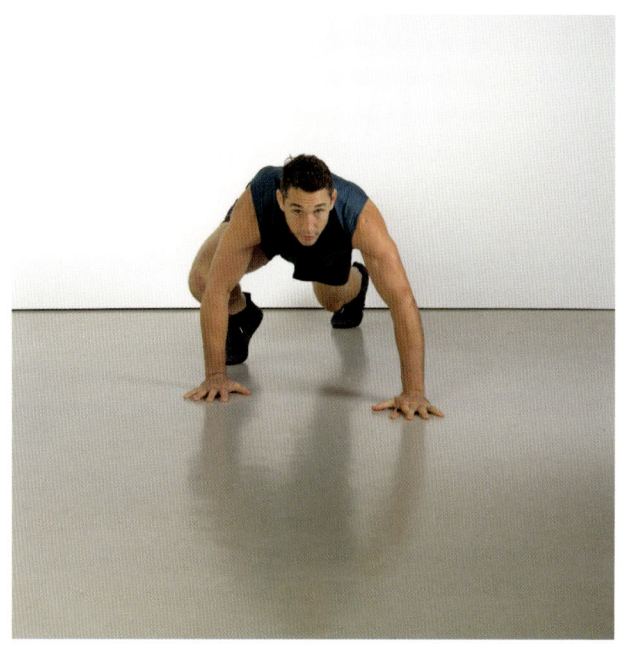

4. **Bear crawl**

   Start in the push-up position with your knees bent at a 90-degree angle and positioned directly under your hips. Engage your core and do not raise or round your back. This is your starting position. Walk your right hand and your left foot forward, and then your left hand and your right foot forward. Continue until you reach 5 metres. Now, keeping your hips down and your core engaged, reverse the movement by walking your left arm and your right foot back, and then your right arm and your left leg back. Continue until you have returned to your starting position.

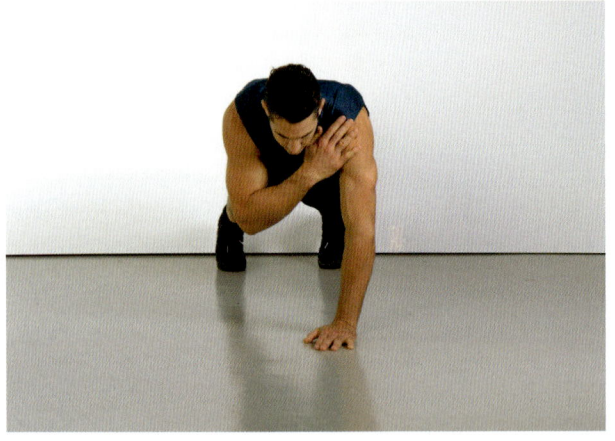

5   **4 x shoulder taps, 1 x push-up**
    For the shoulder taps, start in plank position. Engaging your core, transfer your weight into your right arm, and with your left hand touch your right shoulder. Return to the starting position and repeat on the left side.

5.1 Remain in the starting position. Now lower yourself down to transfer all your weight into your shoulders and back. Press back up to the starting position.

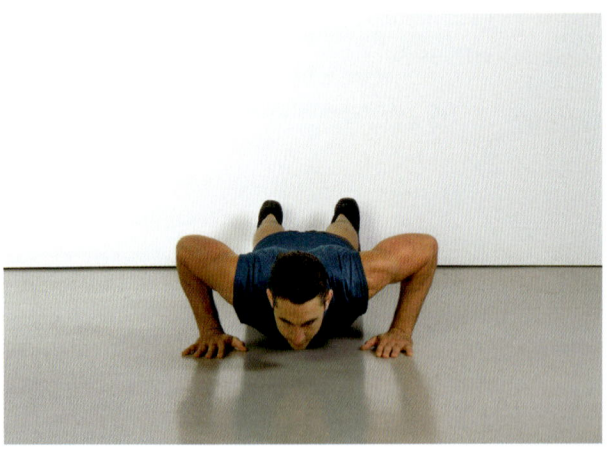

5.2 Alternatively, place one ankle over the other while your knees are on the floor in the starting position. Now lift yourself up so your shoulders are over your wrists. Lower yourself down to the ground and then press back up to the starting position.

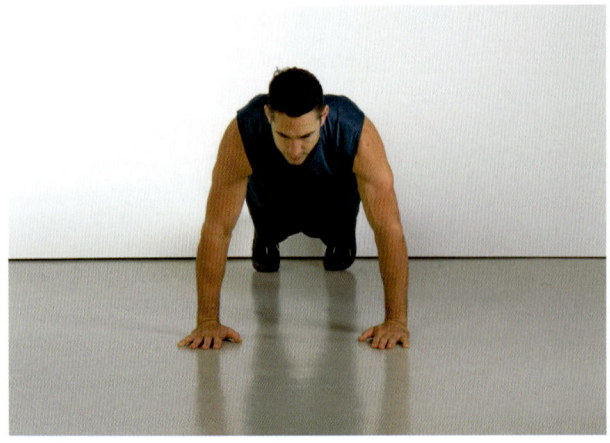

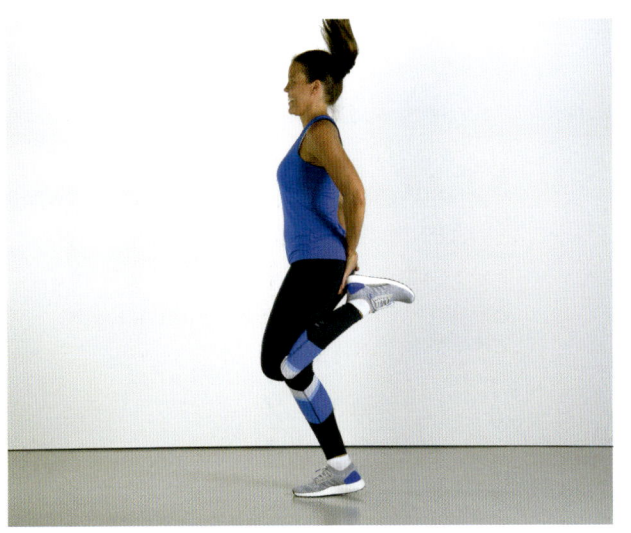

6 Butt kicks

Stand with your feet shoulder-width apart and your hands flat behind your back with your palms facing outwards. Bring one heel up to touch your butt, then do the same with the other heel. Try to keep your feet nice and soft and land back on the ball of your foot each time.

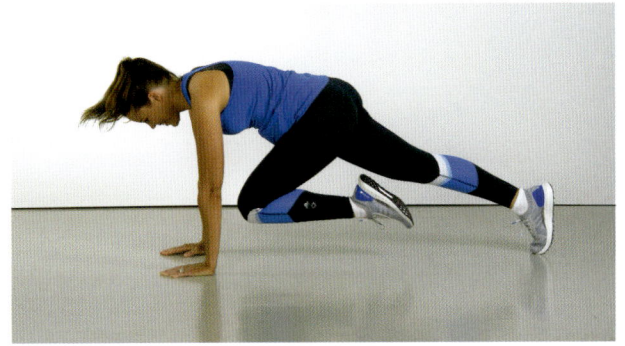

7 Mountain climbers

Start in a high plank position, with your shoulders over your wrists, your feet together and your core engaged. From here, bring one knee up towards your chest and then return it to the starting position. Repeat on the other side.

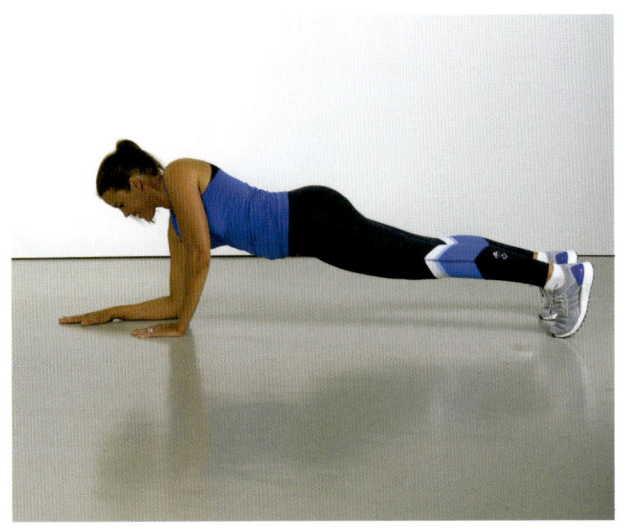

8 Moving plank

Lie with your forearms on the ground, your knees off the ground and your feet together. From here, with your toes touching the ground, lean slightly forward to engage your core, lifting yourself up into the high plank position. Keep alternating between the high and low plank positions. (Note: Your back should not be sagging or bent.)

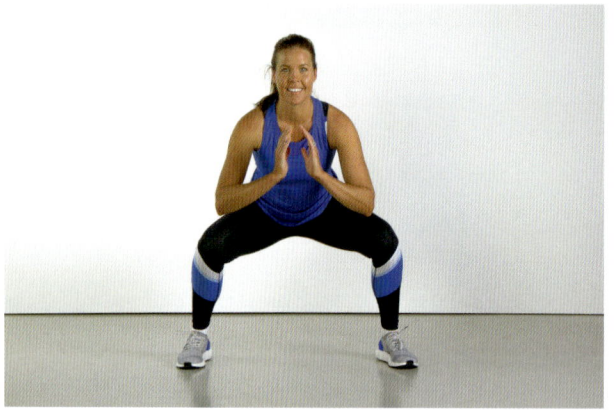

9 In/out jump squats

Squat so your knees are bent, hands up to chest and elbows to knees. Then explode up, bringing your feet together and your arms out to your sides before returning to the starting position.

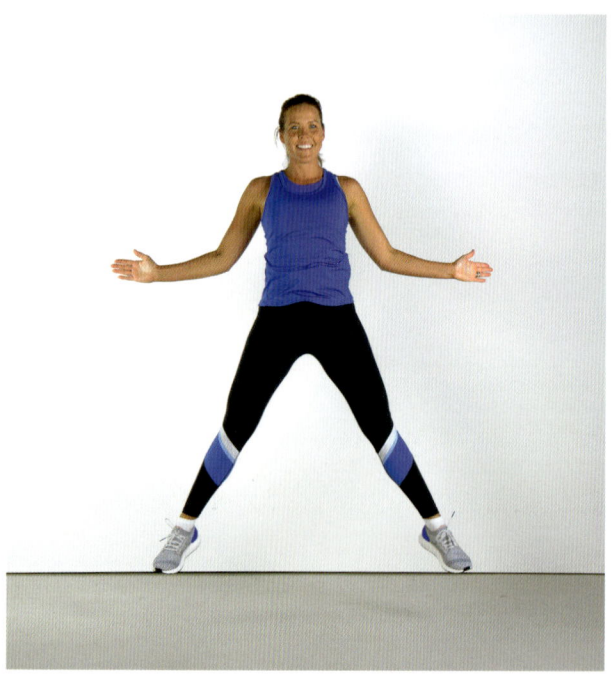

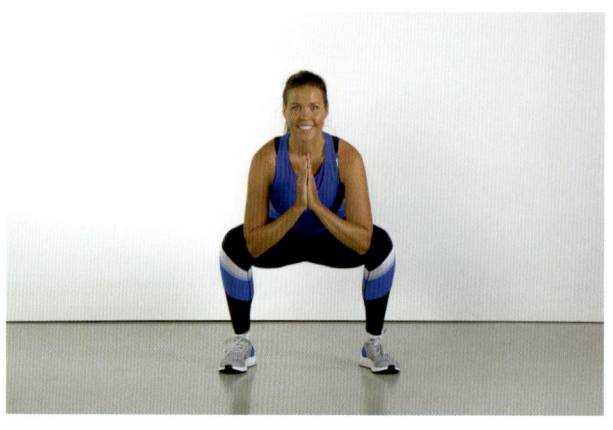

10 Frog squats

Stand with your feet shoulder-width apart and your feet slightly tracked out. Bend down to full squat position with your elbows tucked inside your legs. This is the starting position. From here, raise your hips and then lower them back to the starting position.

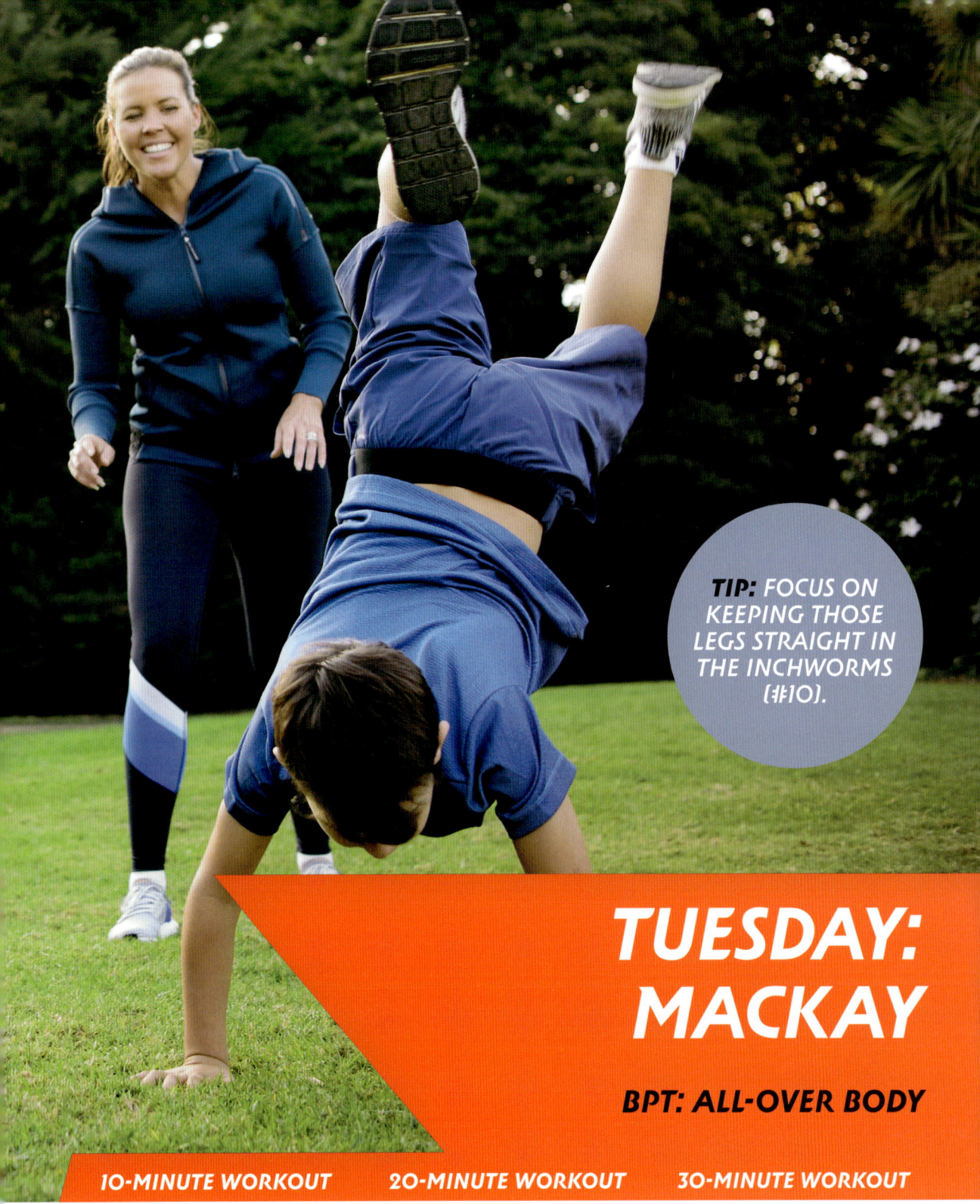

TIP: FOCUS ON KEEPING THOSE LEGS STRAIGHT IN THE INCHWORMS (#10).

TUESDAY: MACKAY

BPT: ALL-OVER BODY

10-MINUTE WORKOUT	20-MINUTE WORKOUT	30-MINUTE WORKOUT
20 seconds movement / 10 seconds rest 2 sets of each exercise (one lap)	20 seconds movement / 10 seconds rest 2 sets of each exercise (two laps)	20 seconds movement / 10 seconds rest 2 sets of each exercise (three laps)

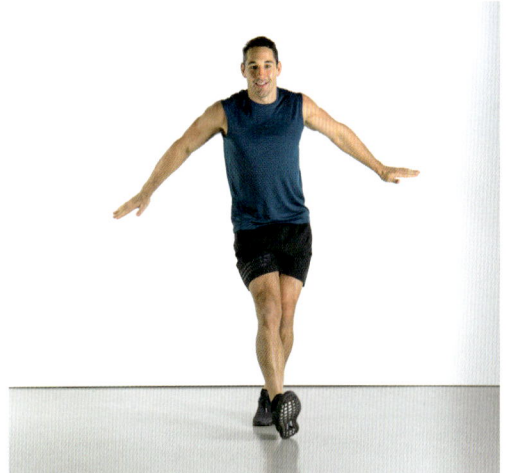

1 **Squat kick-outs**

Stand with your feet shoulder-width apart and slightly tracked out. Bend at the hips and bring your butt towards the ground so your knees are at a 90-degree angle. Explode back up to standing position, crossing one foot in front of the other and tapping the heel of your front foot in front of the toe of your back foot. Return to the starting position and repeat with your other foot in front.

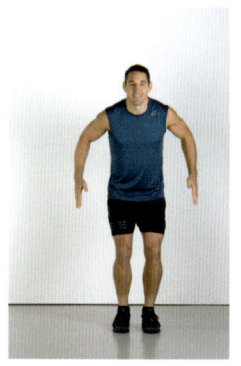 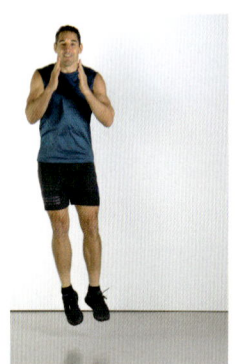

2 **4 x lateral hops, 1 x burpee**

For the lateral hops, stand with your feet together. From here, jump to the left to land on both feet, then jump to the right to land on both feet.

For the burpee, stand in a relaxed position with your feet shoulder-width apart. Squat and place your hands firmly on the ground with your feet back. Shoot your legs back so you are in a high plank position, then lower your body so your torso is just touching the ground. Release your hands and then, placing your hands back on the ground, raise your torso and jump your feet back so both hands and both feet are on the ground. Stand back up, then jump up and raise your hands above your head.

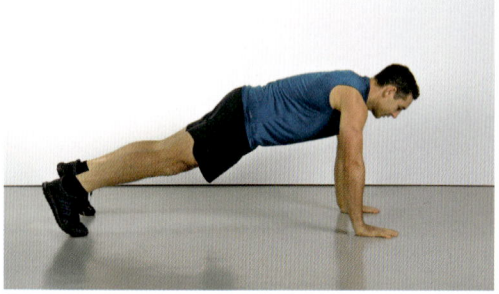

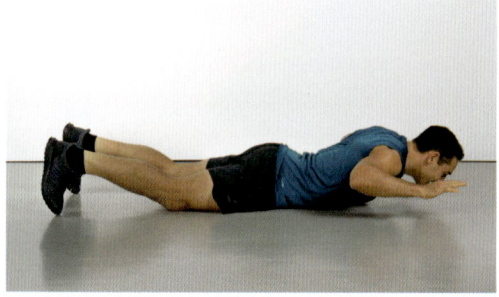

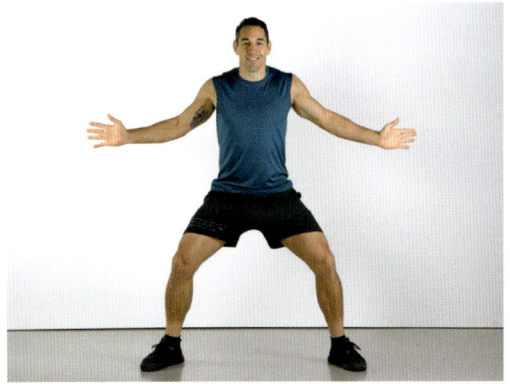

3 Seal jacks

Starting in a relaxed position with your hands touching together in the middle of your chest, jump out so your feet are in a wide stance and your arms split. Bring your feet and hands back together.

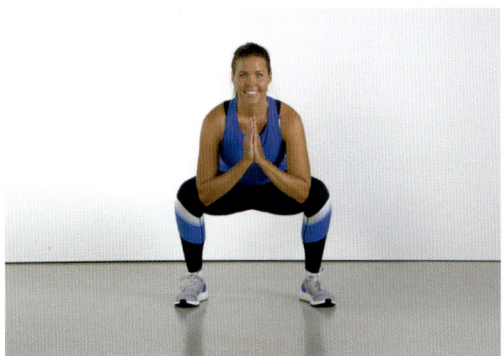

4 Frog squats

Stand with your feet shoulder-width apart and your feet slightly tracked out. Bend down to full squat position with your elbows tucked inside your legs. This is the starting position. From here, raise your hips and then lower them back to the starting position.

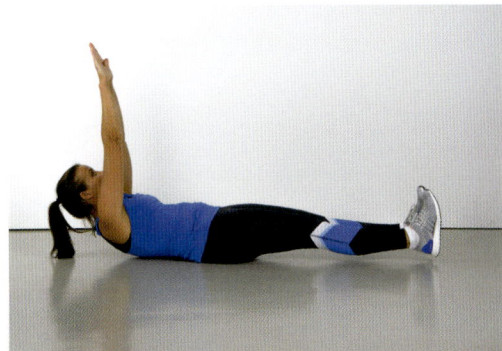

5 Straight-leg sit-ups

Lie flat on the ground with your arms by your sides. Lifting your head up and engaging your core, reach towards your toes, keeping your arms and legs straight. Return to the starting position.

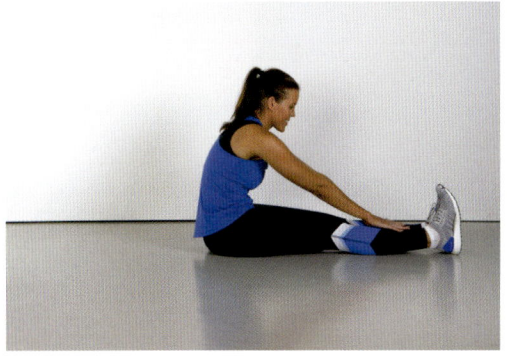

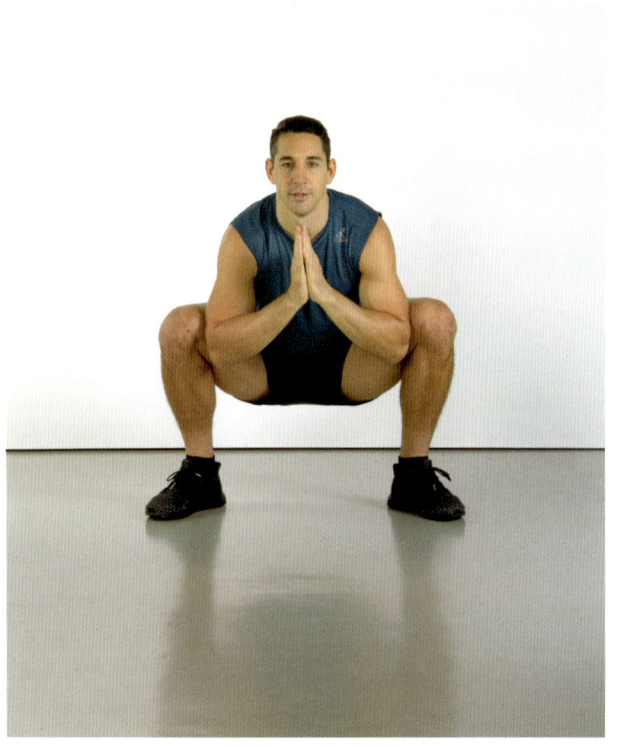

6. **1 x squat, 2 x reverse lunges**

   Stand with your feet shoulder-width apart and slightly pointed outwards so your knees track with your feet. Hinging at the hips, stick your butt out and bend your knees until they are at a 90-degree angle. Drive through with your feet and squeeze your glutes to finish the squat movement.

   For the reverse lunges, stand with your feet shoulder-width apart and your hands on your hips. Step one leg back and then lower it until it is 90 degrees to the ground. Step forward to the starting position. Repeat on the other side to complete the movement.

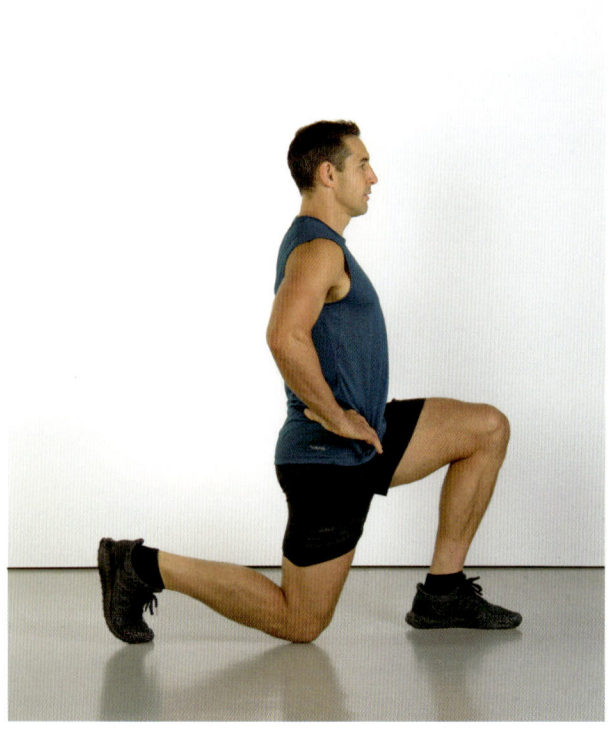

7 Burpees or sprawls

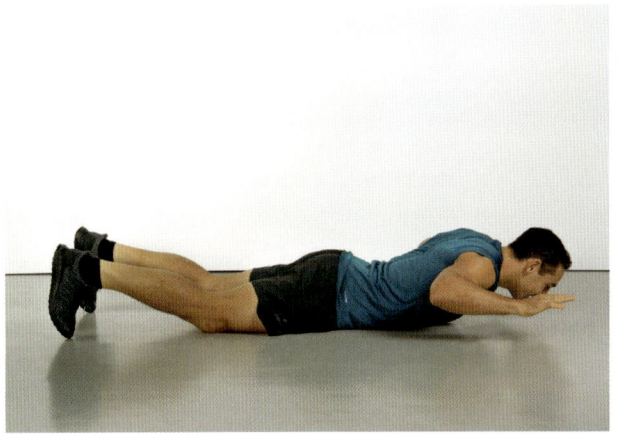

7.1 To begin a burpee, stand in a relaxed position with your feet shoulder-width apart. Squat and place your hands firmly on the ground with your feet back. Shoot your legs back so you are in a high plank position, then lower your body so your torso is just touching the ground. Release your hands and then, placing your hands back on the ground, raise your torso and jump your feet back so both hands and both feet are on the ground. Stand back up, then jump up and raise your hands above your head.

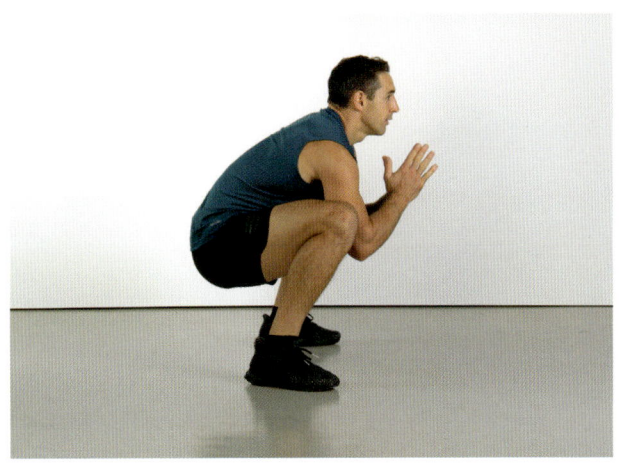

7.2 Alternatively, for a sprawl, stand with your feet shoulder-width apart, then squat until both your hands and both your feet are firmly on the ground. From this position transfer your weight into your shoulders and shoot your feet back so that your legs are out wide, then jump your feet back up and stand up into the starting position.

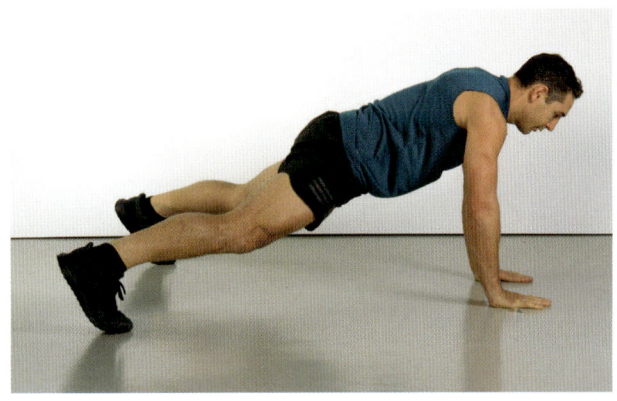

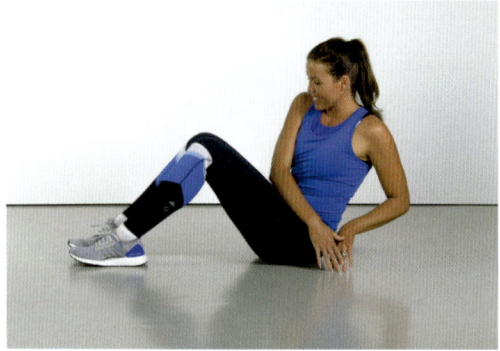

8 Russian twists

Sit on the ground with your knees bent and your feet flat on the ground. Clasping your hands in front of your chest, twist your torso to one side and touch the ground, engaging your core. Then shift your weight and twist your torso to touch the ground on the other side.

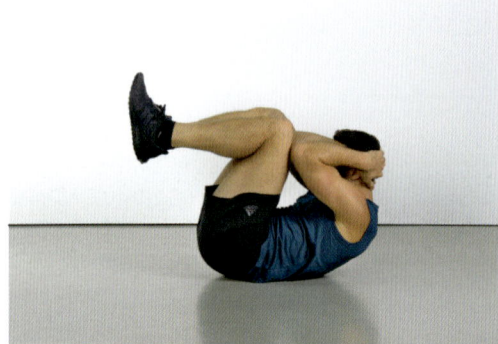

9 Crunches

Lie on your back with your legs off the ground, with knees bent at a 90-degree angle to your body. With your hands crossed behind your head, bring your elbows in next to your ears. Bring your elbows up to your knees and then return to the starting position.

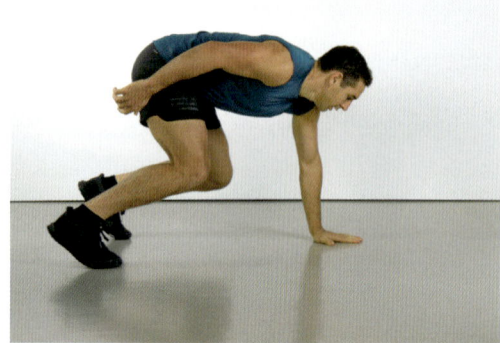

10 Inchworms

Stand with your feet just wide enough apart that when you bend forward to touch the ground your legs remain straight. From the bent position, walk your hands out until you are in a high plank position. Engage your core and squeeze your glutes. Now walk your hands back, keeping your legs straight, before engaging your core to stand up into the starting position.

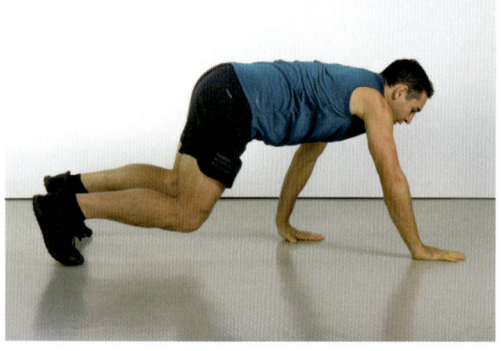

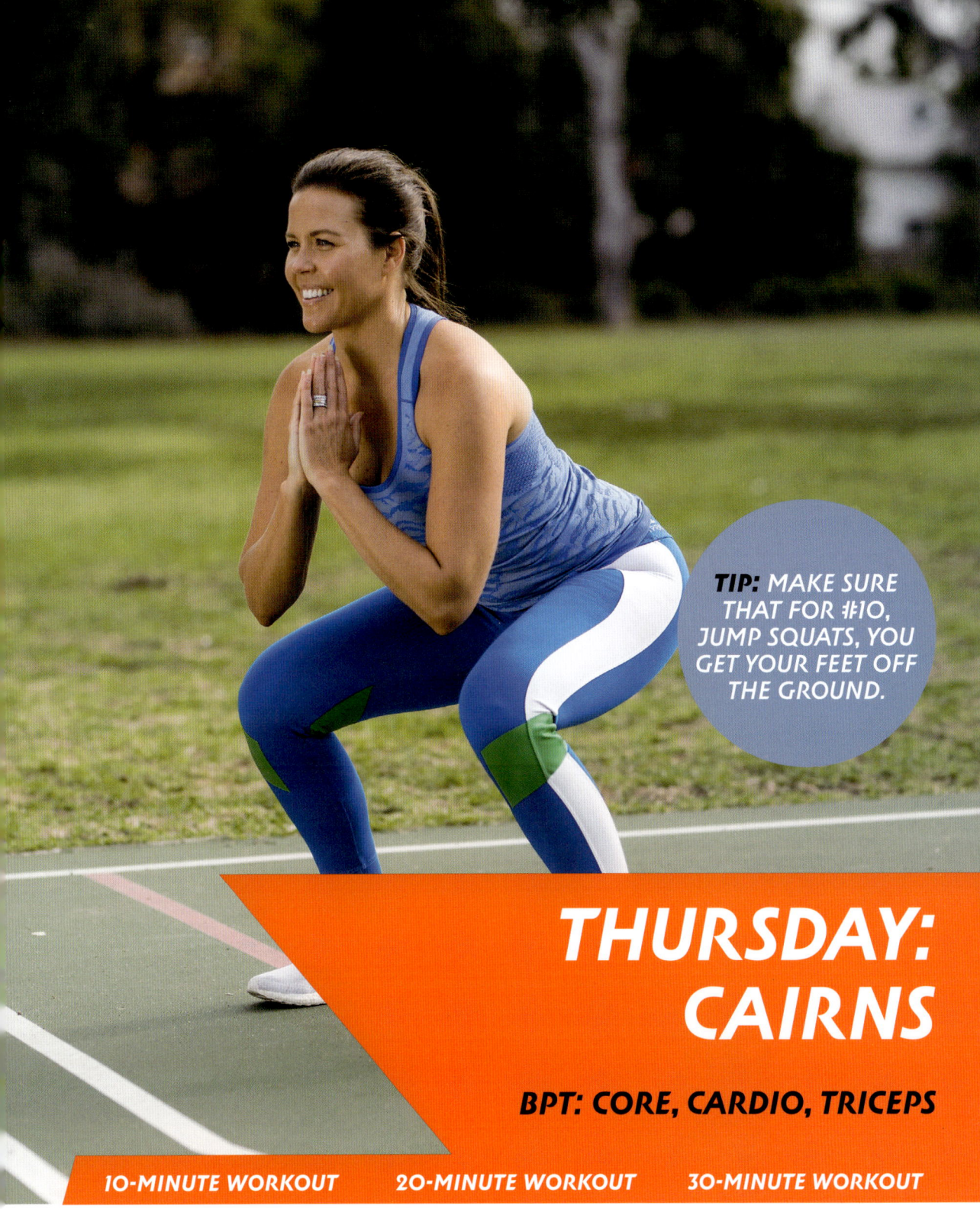

TIP: MAKE SURE THAT FOR #10, JUMP SQUATS, YOU GET YOUR FEET OFF THE GROUND.

THURSDAY: CAIRNS

BPT: CORE, CARDIO, TRICEPS

10-MINUTE WORKOUT	20-MINUTE WORKOUT	30-MINUTE WORKOUT
20 seconds movement / 10 seconds rest 2 sets of each exercise (one lap)	20 seconds movement / 10 seconds rest 2 sets of each exercise (two laps)	20 seconds movement / 10 seconds rest 2 sets of each exercise (three laps)

BLOCK 3: QUEENSLAND

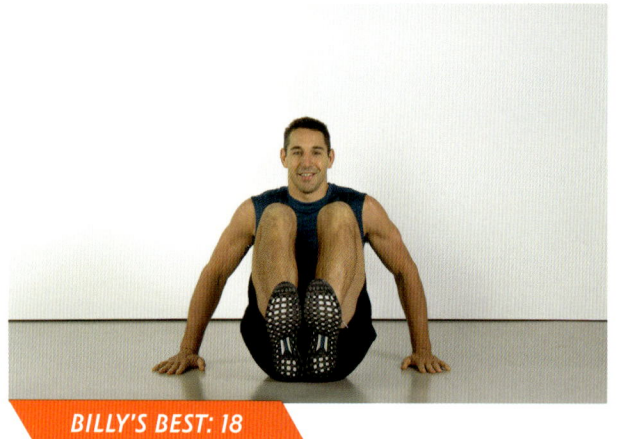

BILLY'S BEST: 18

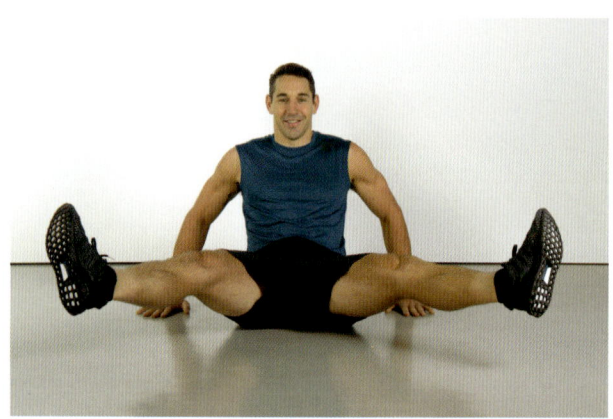

1 **Kick-in/outs**

Sit on the ground with your hands just behind your butt, your knees bent and your feet just above the ground. Kick your legs out until they are straight and split them before bringing them back together and to the starting position.

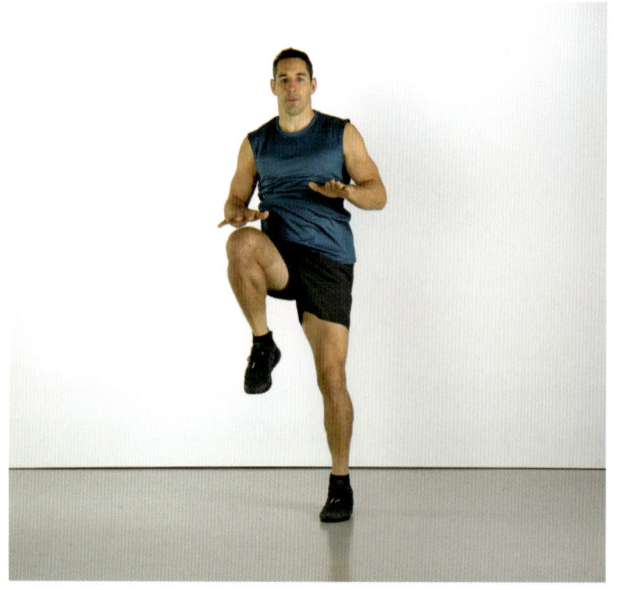

2 **High knees**

Stand with your feet shoulder-width apart. One leg at a time, raise your left knee up as high as you can before alternating to the other leg.

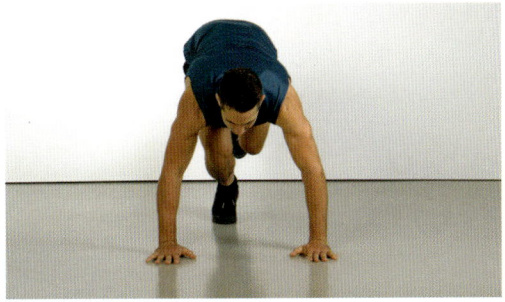

3 Single-leg burpees

Stand in a relaxed position with your feet shoulder-width apart. Squat and place your hands firmly on the ground with your feet back. Shoot your legs back so you are in a high plank position with one leg off the ground, then lower your body so your torso is just touching the ground. Release your hands and then, placing your hands back on the ground, raise your torso and jump your feet forward, keeping the one leg off the ground throughout the whole movement. Stand back up, then jump up and raise your hands above your head.

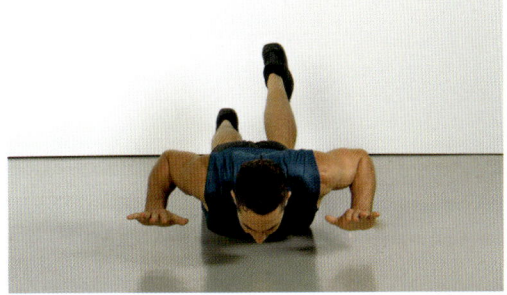

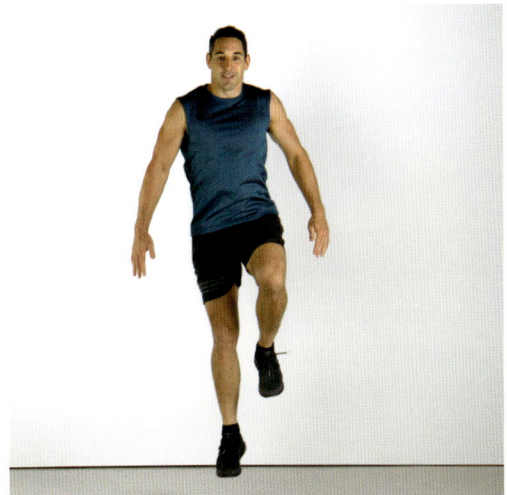

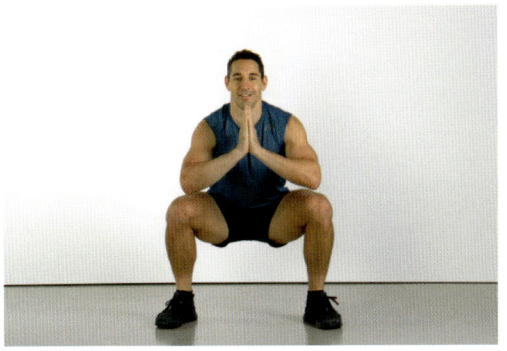

4 Pulse squats

Stand with your feet just past shoulder-width apart and slightly tracked out. Squat with your hips back and your legs at a 90-degree angle, then pulse up and down.

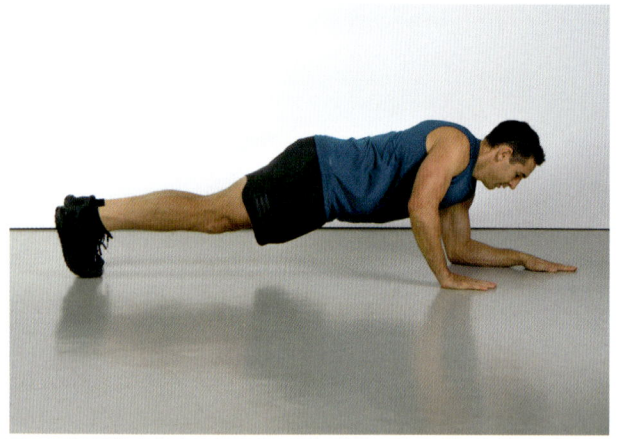

5 Moving plank

Lie with your forearms on the ground, your knees off the ground and your feet together. From here, with your toes touching the ground, lean slightly forward to engage your core, lifting yourself up into the high plank position. Keep alternating between the high and low plank positions. (Note: Your back should not be sagging or bent.)

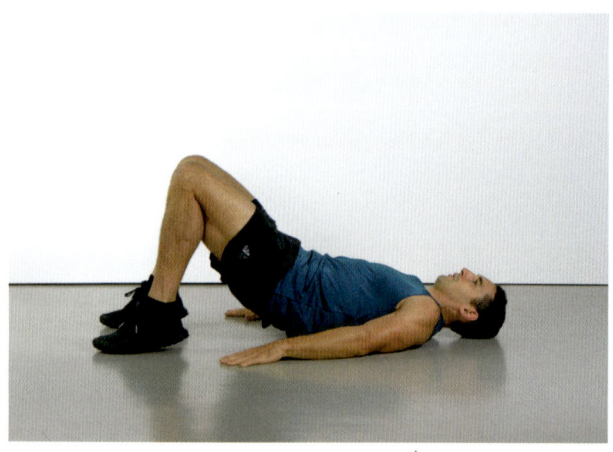

6 Double-glute bridge

Lie on your back with your hands on your hips or with your arms straight or beside your body on the ground and your palms facing down. Bring your heels as close as you can to your butt, raising your hips and pressing down on the balls of your feet. Squeeze your butt cheeks (glutes) before lowering yourself down. Don't allow yourself to collapse – stay tight through your core and make sure your butt doesn't hit the ground.

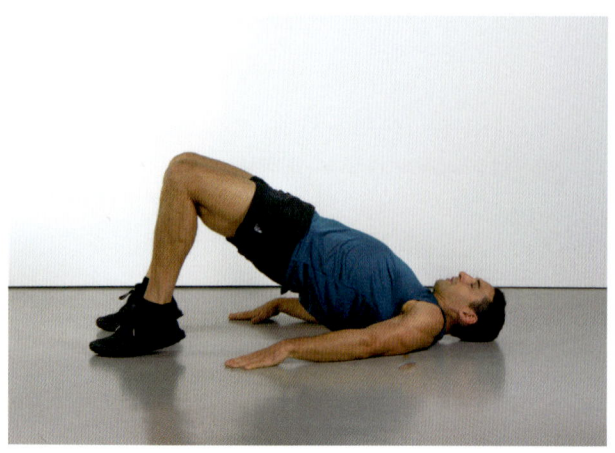

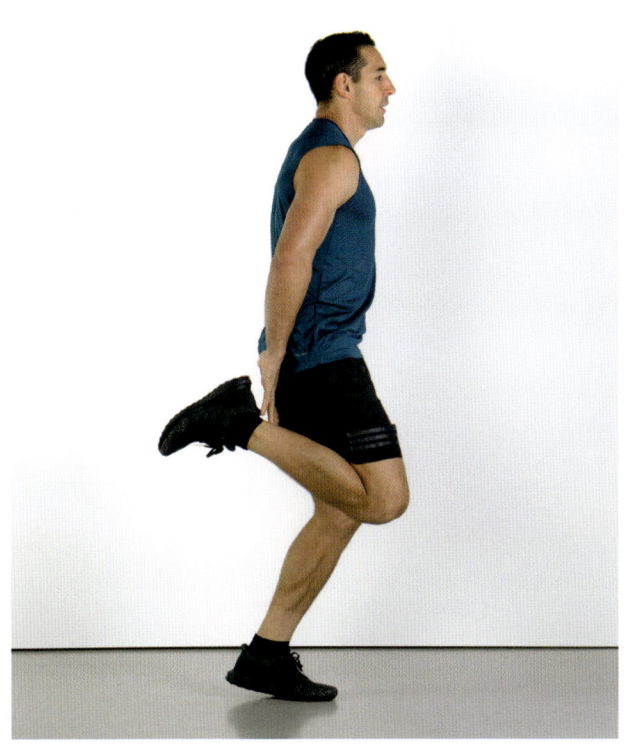

7   **Butt kicks**

Stand with your feet shoulder-width apart and your hands flat behind your back with your palms facing outwards. Bring one heel up to touch your butt, then do the same with the other heel. Try to keep your feet nice and soft and land back on the ball of your foot each time.

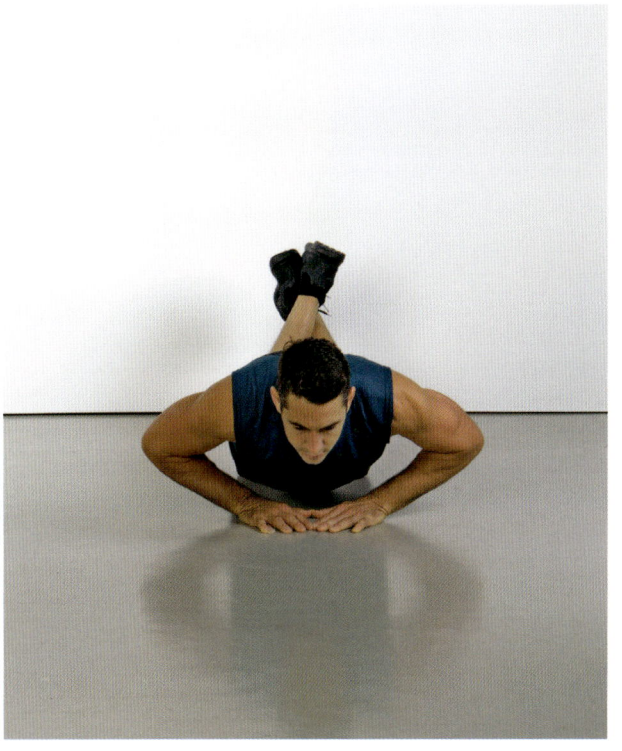

8   **Diamond push-ups**

Kneel on the ground with your ankles crossed, and set your hands so your thumbs and index fingers are touching in line with your chin. From here, lower your body towards the ground and then press back up to the starting position. You should feel this movement in your triceps.

Advanced: Do the exercise in high plank position with your knees off the ground.

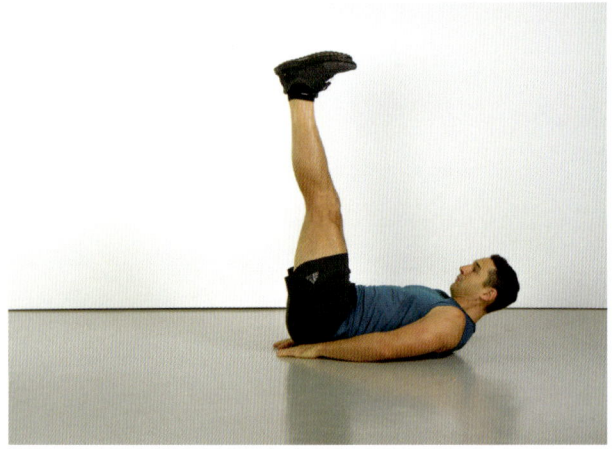

9 Double-leg raises

Lie on your back and tuck both your thumbs under your lower lumbar (base of your back). Raise your legs and then lower them, keeping your heels off the ground.

Advanced: Do the exercise with your arms crossed over your chest.

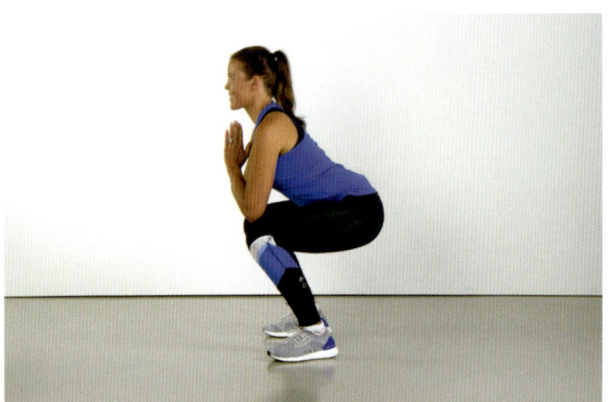

10 Jump squats

Stand with your feet just past shoulder-width apart and your feet slightly pointed outwards so your knees track with your feet. Bending forward at the hips, stick your butt out and bend your knees until they are at a 90-degree angle. Jump up either right or left 90 degrees (or 180 degrees for advanced). Repeat for one full circle going clockwise, and then go anticlockwise for one full circle.

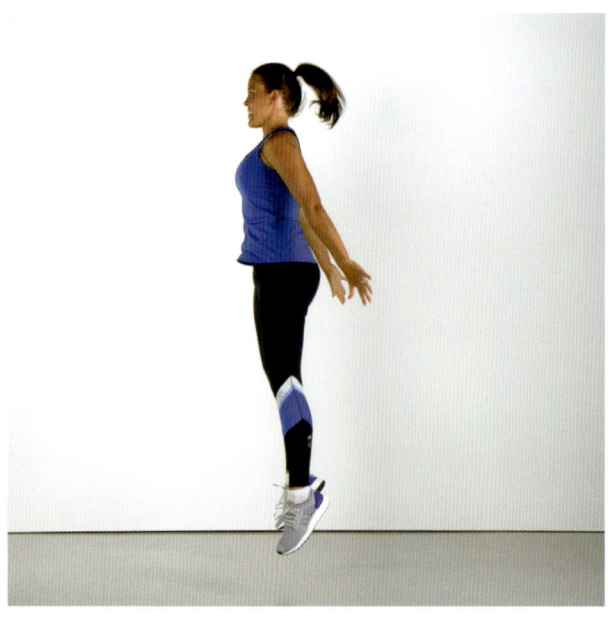

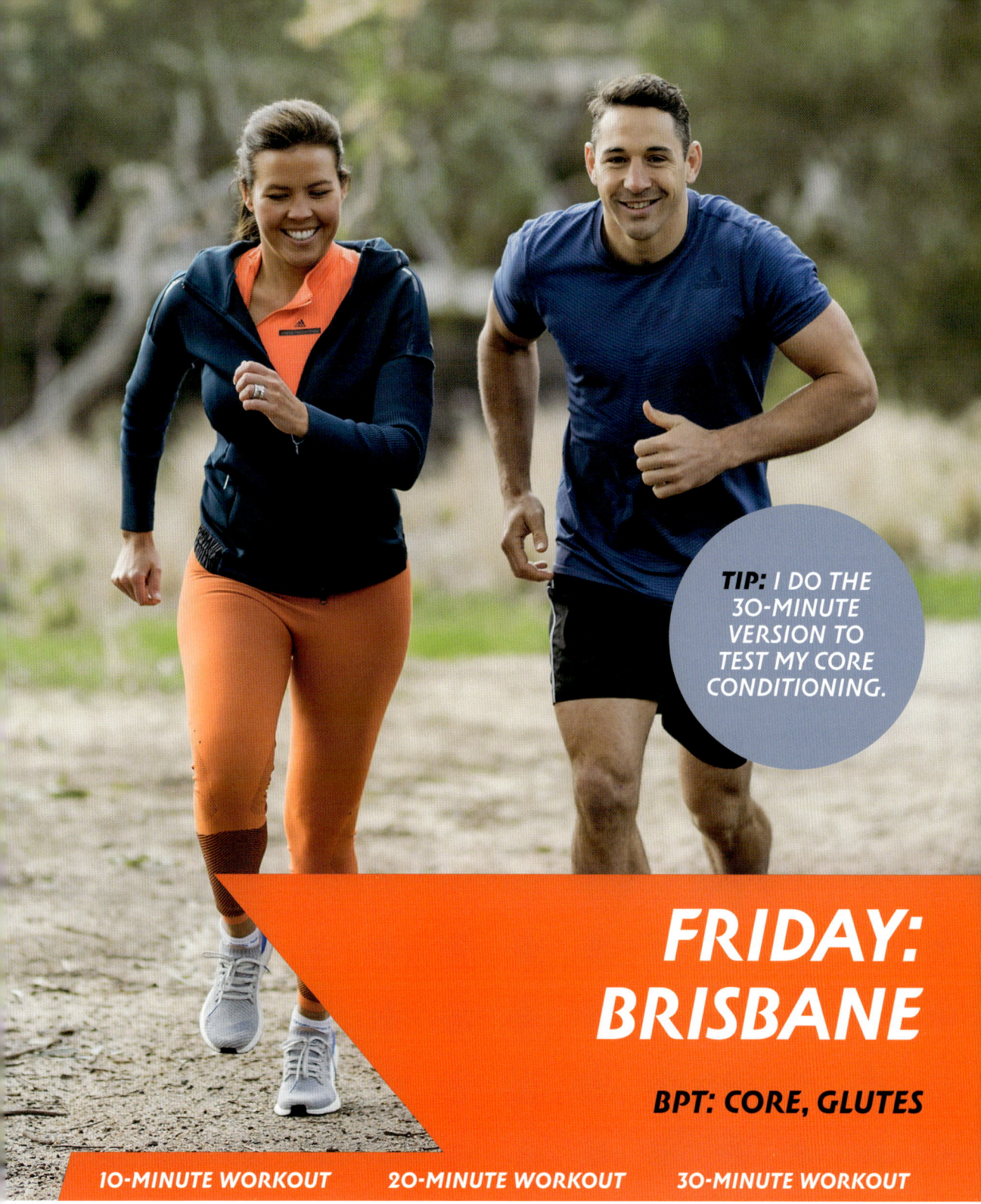

TIP: *I DO THE 30-MINUTE VERSION TO TEST MY CORE CONDITIONING.*

FRIDAY: BRISBANE

BPT: CORE, GLUTES

10-MINUTE WORKOUT	20-MINUTE WORKOUT	30-MINUTE WORKOUT
20 seconds movement / 10 seconds rest 2 sets of each exercise (one lap)	20 seconds movement / 10 seconds rest 2 sets of each exercise (two laps)	20 seconds movement / 10 seconds rest 2 sets of each exercise (three laps)

BLOCK 3: QUEENSLAND

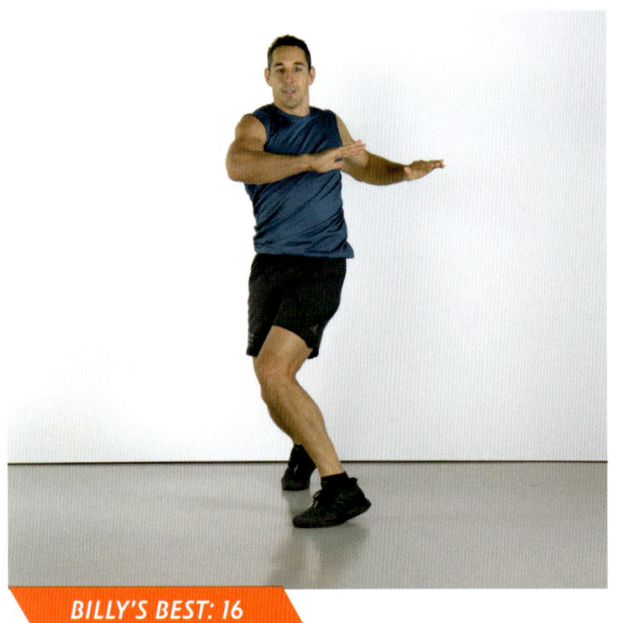

BILLY'S BEST: 16

1. **Torsion twist squats**
   Stand with your feet shoulder-width apart and your arms out nice and wide at shoulder height. Slightly jump to your right, twisting your left hip to your right side and keeping your chest forward. Now come back to the starting position to perform a squat. Stand with your feet shoulder-width apart, slightly tracked out. Holding your hands together, bend forward from the hips and lower your body down, keeping your feet flat on the ground, before pressing back up through your heels to the starting position. Repeat on the other side.

2. **Kick-in/outs**
   Sit on the ground with your hands just behind your butt, your knees bent and your feet just above the ground. Kick your legs out until they are straight and split them before bringing them back together and to the starting position.

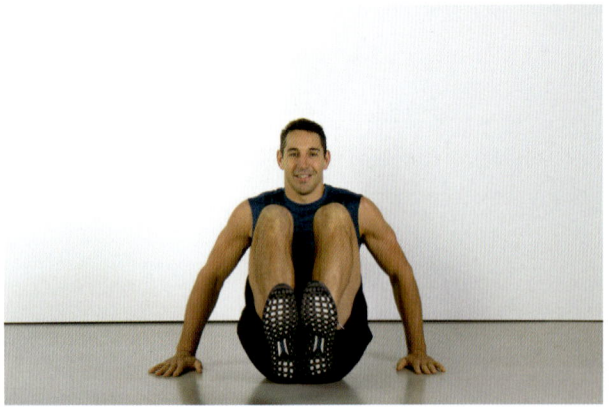

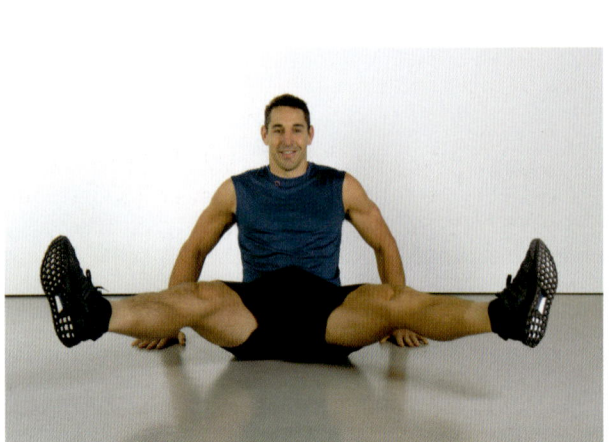

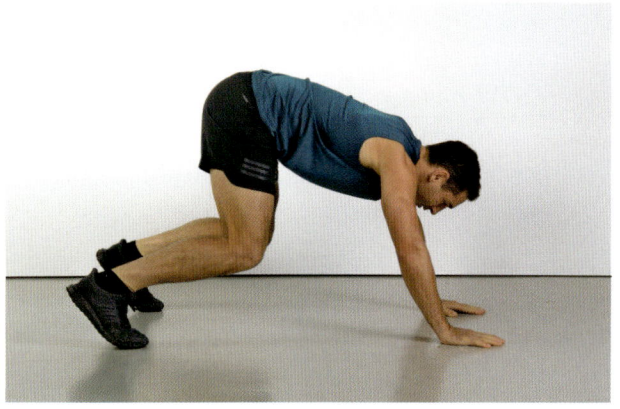

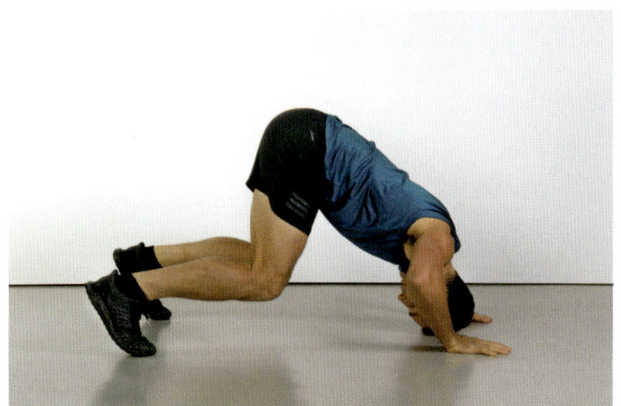

3. **A-frame push-ups**

   Stand with your feet wide apart and slightly tracked out. With your hands shoulder-width apart, and bending at the hips, lean over to touch the ground with your legs straight or bent and your chin slightly tucked. From this starting position, lower yourself down till the top of your head is just off the ground and you're looking through your legs. Your head should be in line with your hands. From here, press back up to the starting position, transferring all the weight into your palms.

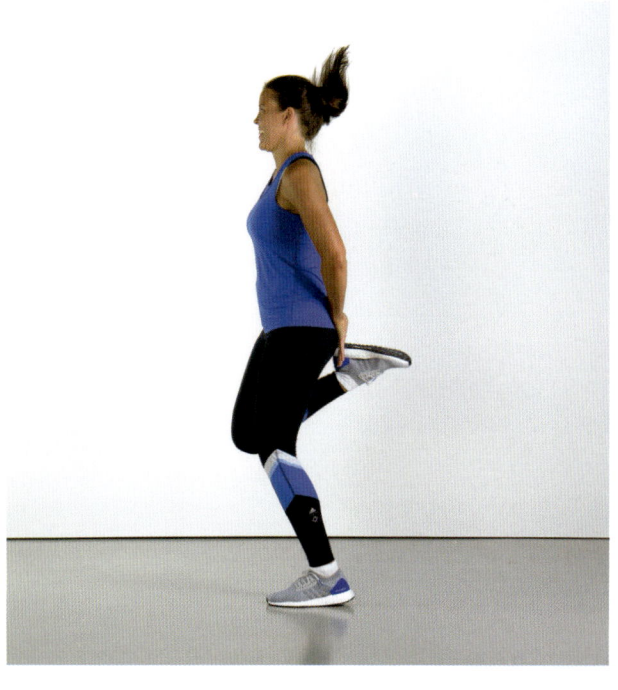

4. **Heel taps**

   Bring your heels towards your butt, then raise your head and, engaging your core, shift your weight so that your right hand touches your right heel. Keeping your core engaged, transfer your weight to the other side so that your left hand touches your left heel.

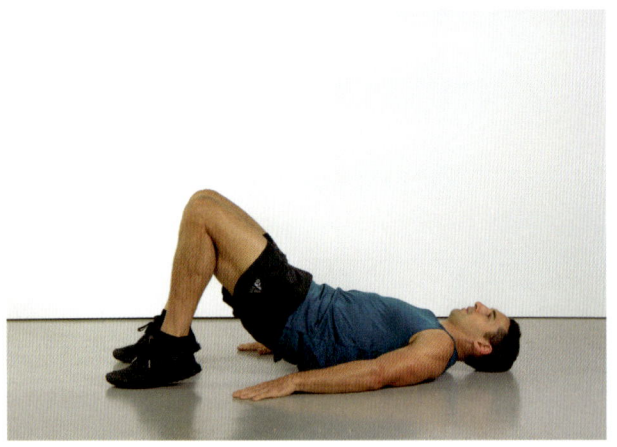

5 Double-glute bridge

Lie on your back with your hands on your hips or with your arms straight on the ground and your palms facing down. Bring your heels as close as you can to your butt, raising your hips and pressing down on the balls of your feet. Squeeze your butt cheeks (glutes) for the allocated time before lowering yourself down. Don't allow yourself to collapse – stay tight through your core and make sure your butt doesn't hit the ground.

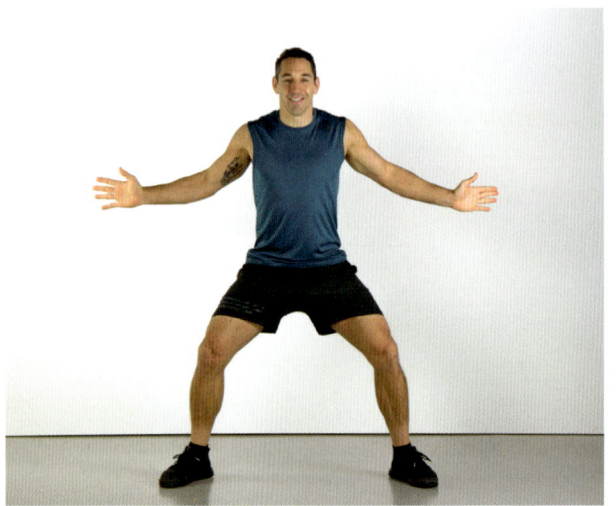

6 Seal jacks

Starting in a relaxed position with your hands touching together in the middle of your chest, jump out so your feet are in a wide stance and your arms split. Bring your feet and hands back together.

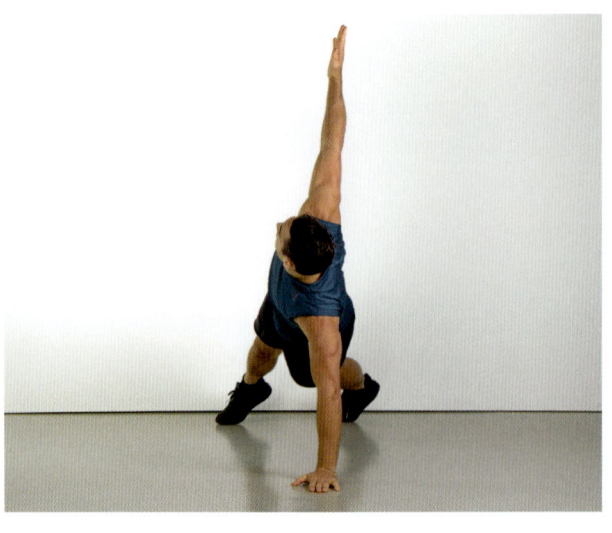

7 Plank rotations

Starting in modified or full plank position, lift one arm off the ground and hold for the allotted time before returning to full plank. Repeat using the other arm.

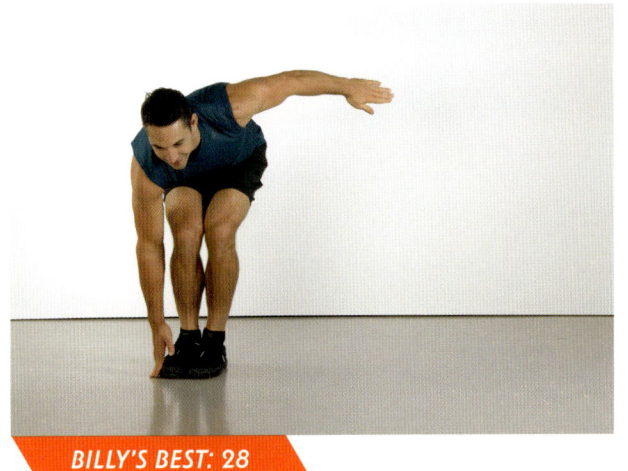

BILLY'S BEST: 28

8 **Slalom taps**
   Start with your feet together, then jump to the left to land on both feet, touching your left hand down next to your left foot. Then jump to the right with both feet, touching your right hand to your right foot.

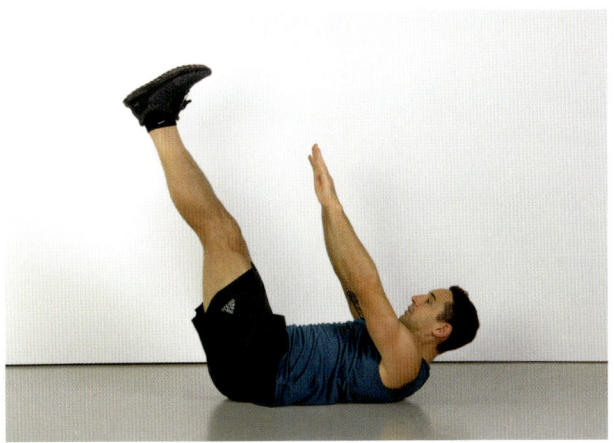

9 **Jackknife**
   Lie on the ground with your legs out straight and your arms above your head. From here, raise your arms and legs until your hands and toes meet. This movement can be done with your knees bent.

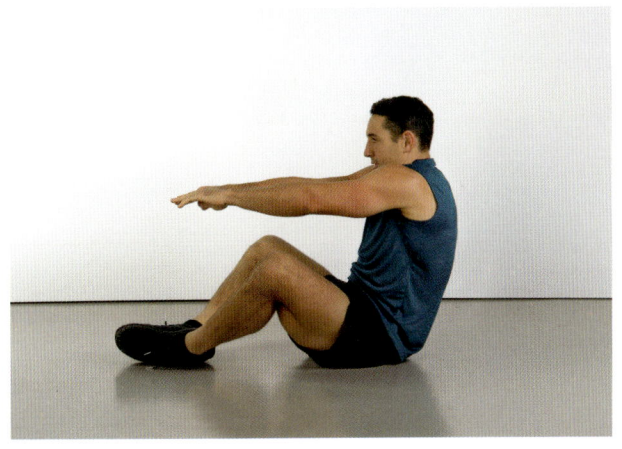

10 **Butterfly sit-ups**
   Sit on the ground with your feet together and as close as possible to your butt, with your knees out wide. From here, lean back until you are lying flat on the ground. Lift your head and then your body back up to the starting position.

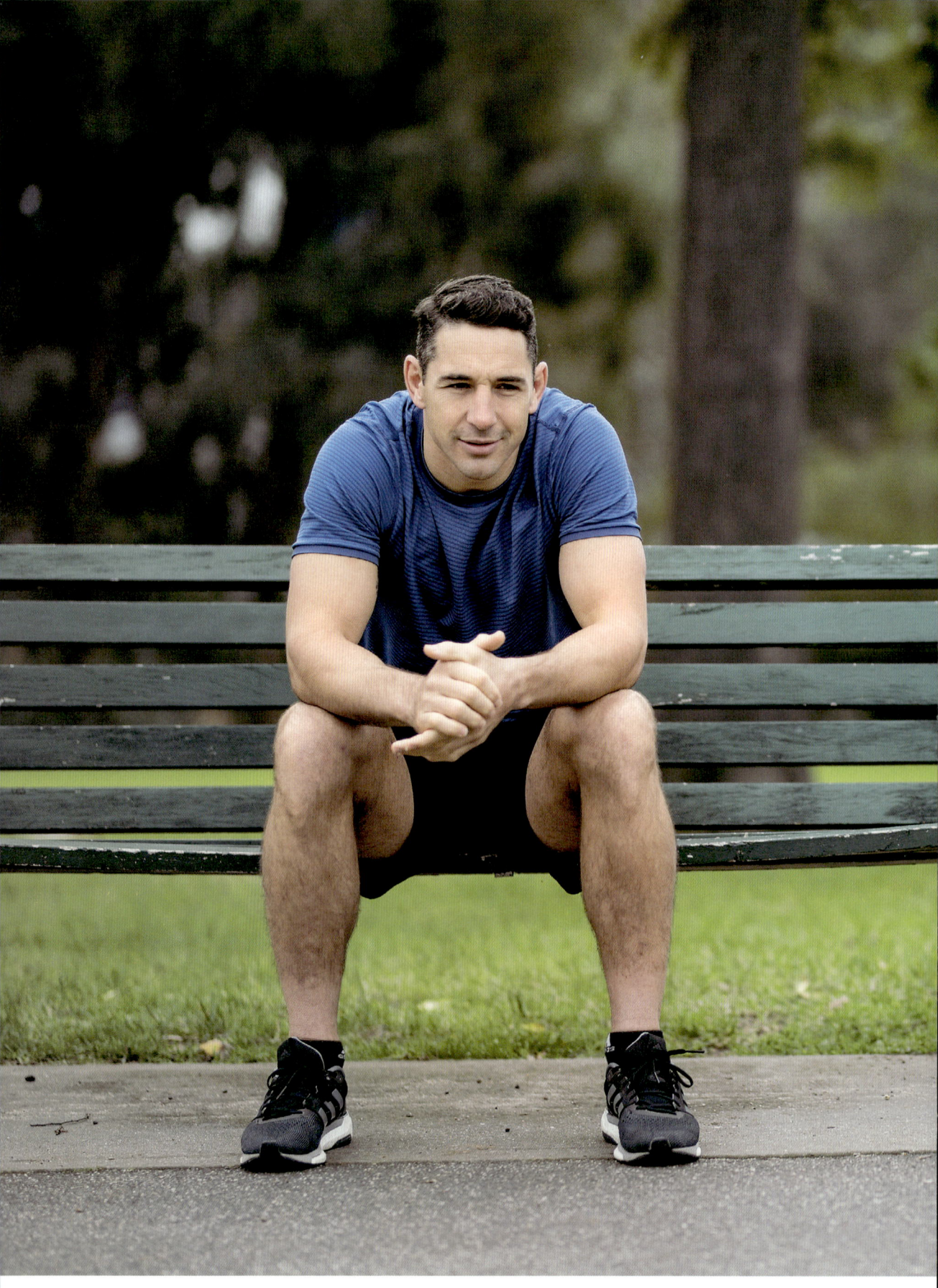

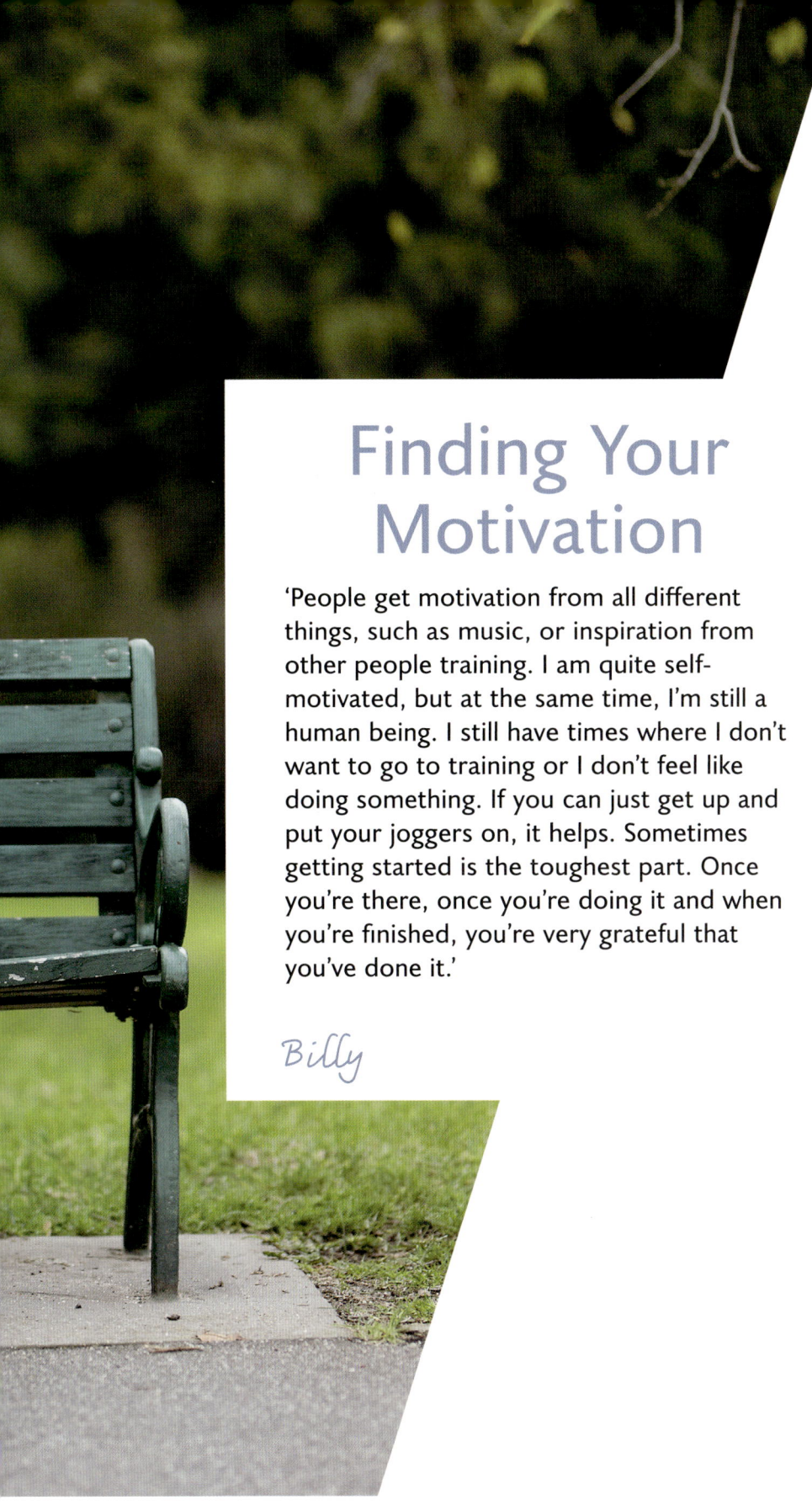

Finding Your Motivation

'People get motivation from all different things, such as music, or inspiration from other people training. I am quite self-motivated, but at the same time, I'm still a human being. I still have times where I don't want to go to training or I don't feel like doing something. If you can just get up and put your joggers on, it helps. Sometimes getting started is the toughest part. Once you're there, once you're doing it and when you're finished, you're very grateful that you've done it.'

Billy

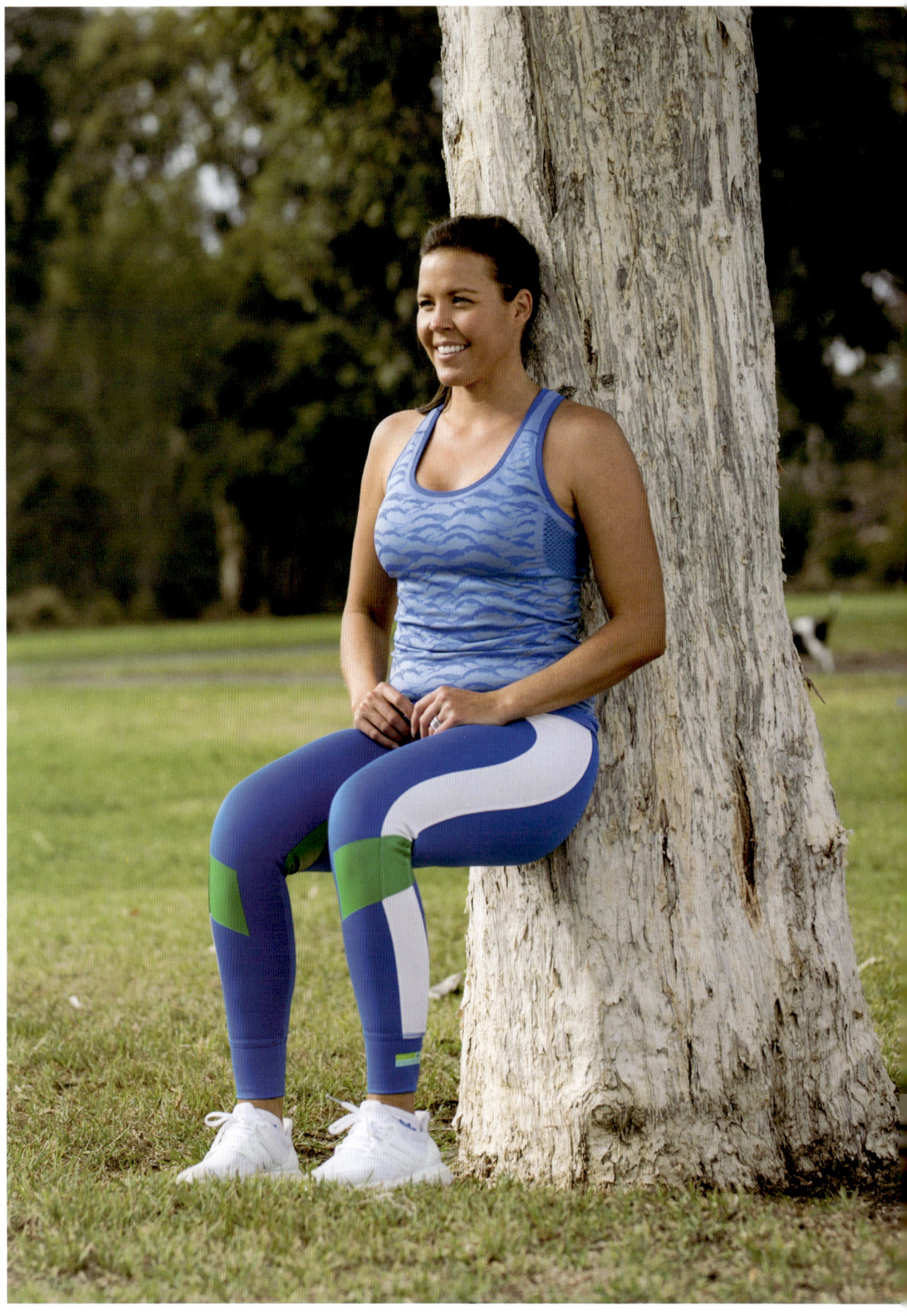

BLOCK 4: SOUTH AUSTRALIA

'I've had the pleasure of playing on the new Adelaide Oval. What a great venue. My travels to Adelaide and surrounding suburbs have always been enjoyable. It's a beautiful city to walk around and take in the fresh air.'

Billy

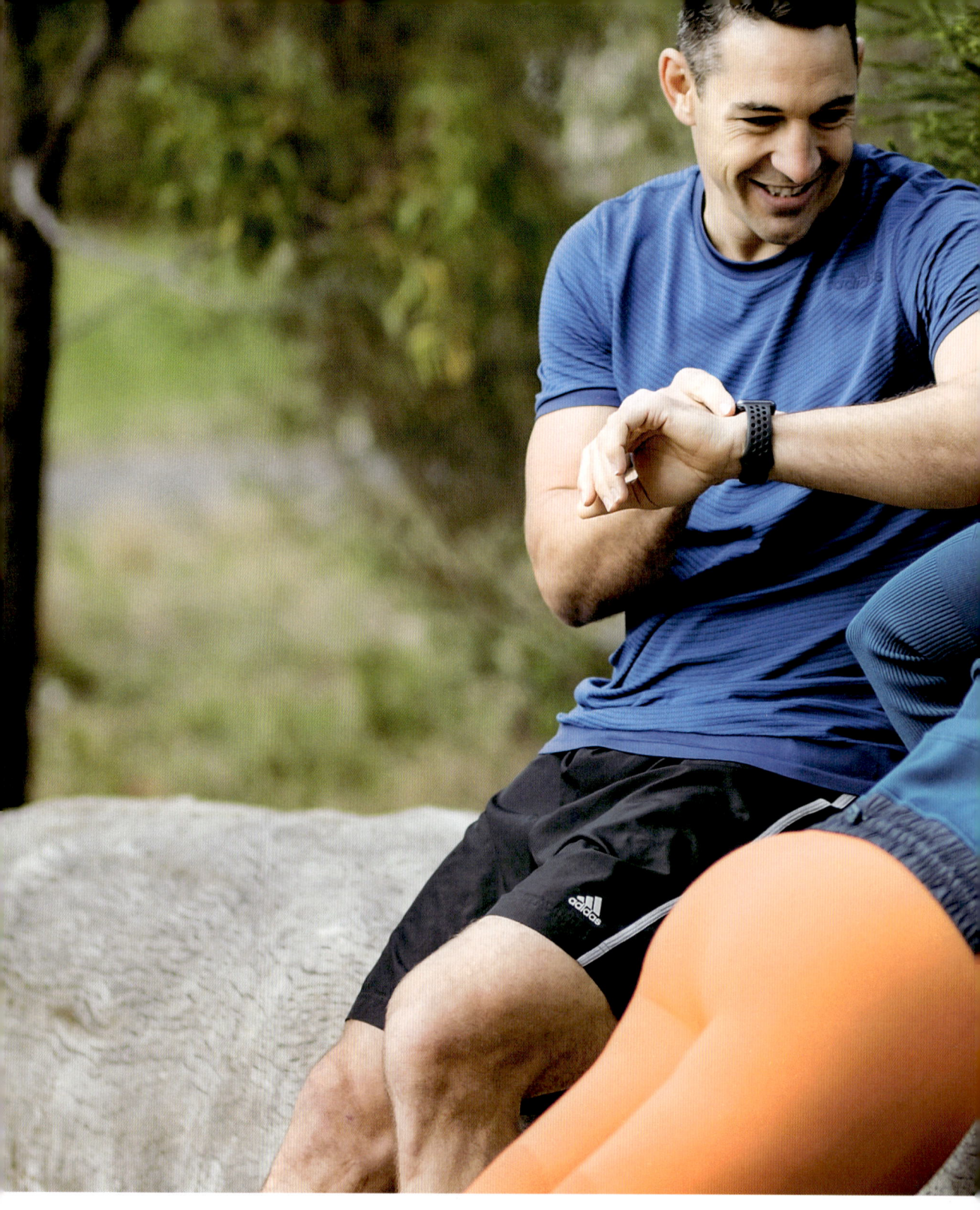

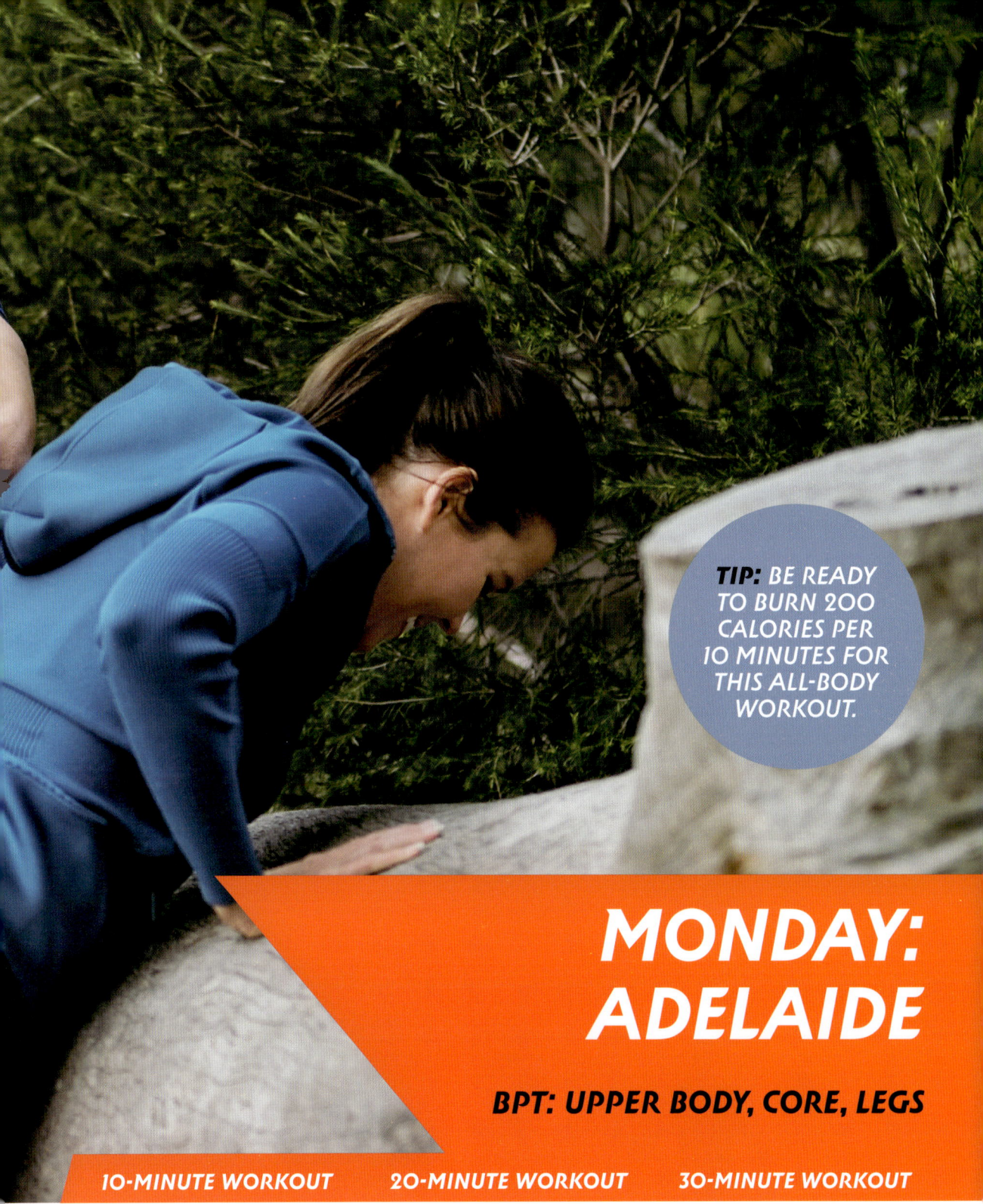

TIP: BE READY TO BURN 200 CALORIES PER 10 MINUTES FOR THIS ALL-BODY WORKOUT.

MONDAY: ADELAIDE

BPT: UPPER BODY, CORE, LEGS

10-MINUTE WORKOUT	20-MINUTE WORKOUT	30-MINUTE WORKOUT
20 seconds movement / 10 seconds rest 2 sets of each exercise (one lap)	20 seconds movement / 10 seconds rest 2 sets of each exercise (two laps)	20 seconds movement / 10 seconds rest 2 sets of each exercise (three laps)

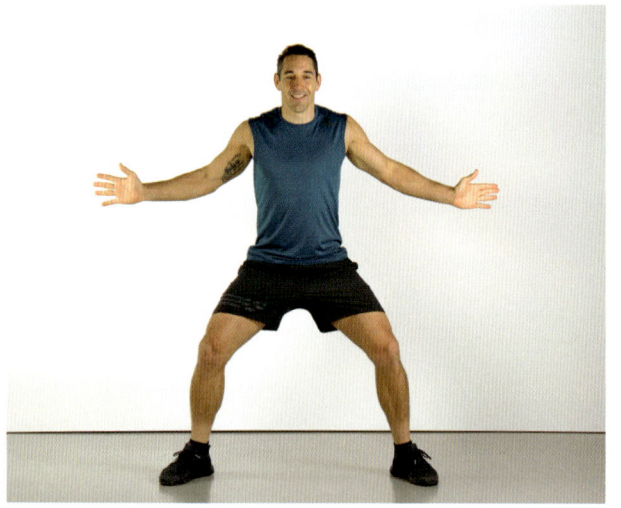

1 Seal jacks

Starting in a relaxed position with your hands touching together in the middle of your chest, jump out so your feet are in a wide stance and your arms split. Bring your feet and hands back together.

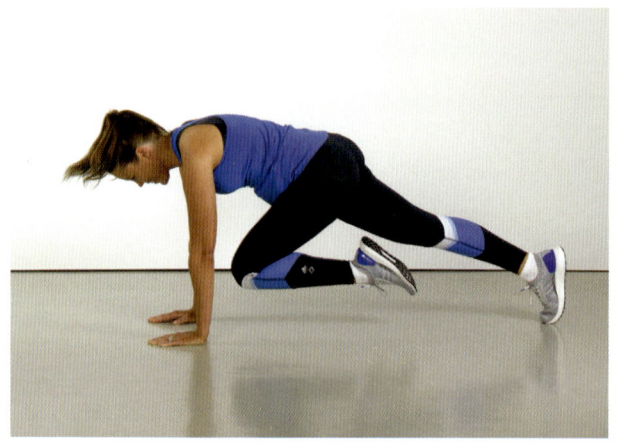

2 Mountain climbers

Start in a high plank position, with your shoulders over your wrists, your feet together and your core engaged. From here, bring one knee up towards your chest and then return it to the starting position. Repeat on the other side.

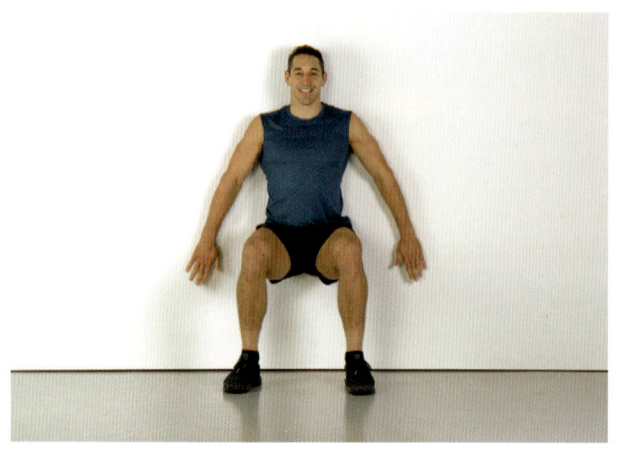

3 Wall sit

Put your back against a wall, feet shoulder-width apart and two steps away from the wall. With your hands firmly against the wall, lower your butt down the wall until your knees are at a 90-degree angle. Hold the position.

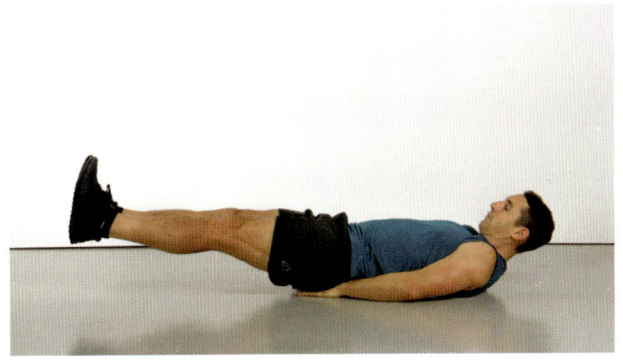

4   **Double-leg raises**

Lie on your back and tuck both your thumbs under your lower lumbar (base of your back). Raise your legs then lower them, keeping your heels off the ground.

Advanced: Do the exercise with your arms crossed over your chest.

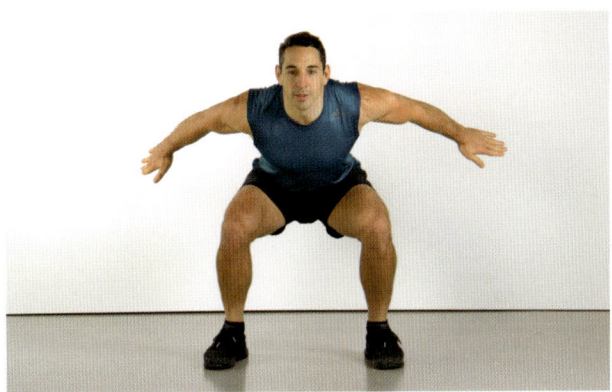

5   **Squat jumps**

Stand with your feet just past shoulder-width apart and slightly pointed outwards so your knees track with your feet. Hinging at the hips, stick your butt out and bend your knees until they are at a 90-degree angle. This is the starting position. With your hands together, drive through your legs and explode up so your feet are off the ground. As you land, lower your body back to the starting position.

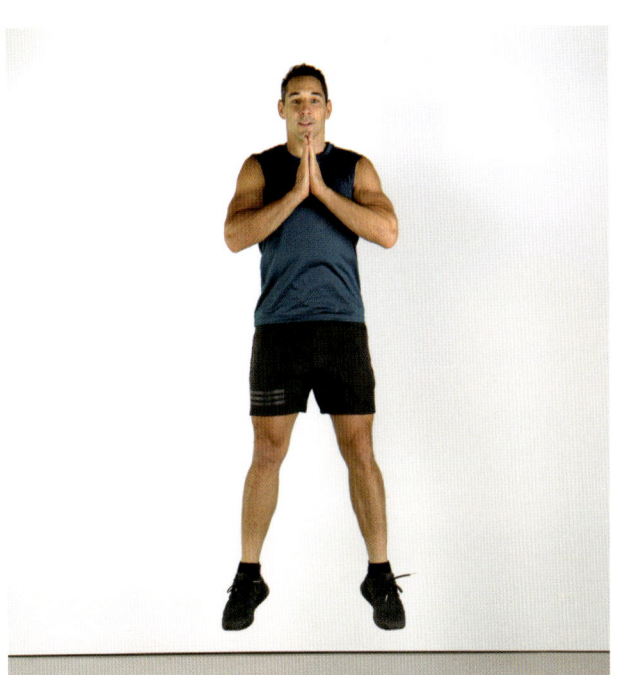

BILLY'S BEST: 22

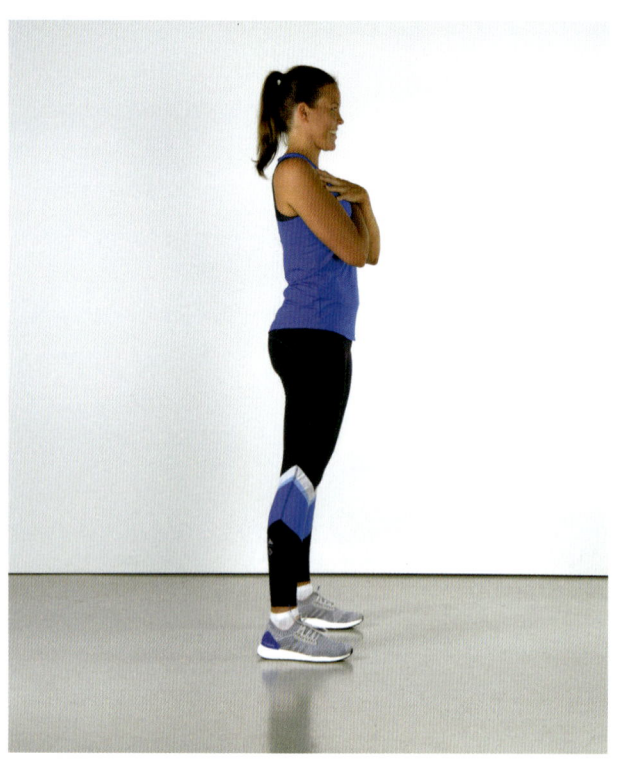

6 Good mornings into squat

Stand with your feet wider than shoulder-width apart, your knees slightly bent and your arms crossed over your chest. Sticking your butt out, lean forward, keeping your knees slightly bent. Once you feel this movement in your hamstrings, bend your knees into a squat so your elbows touch your knees before standing back up to the starting position.

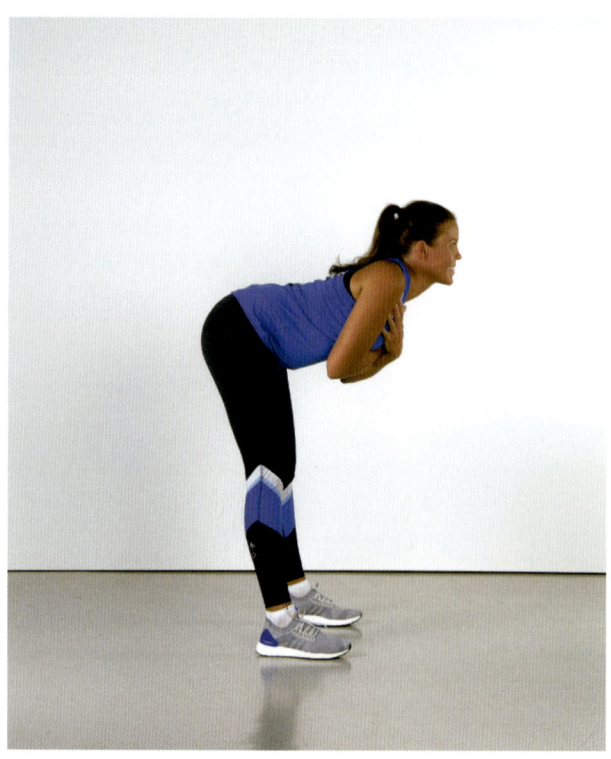

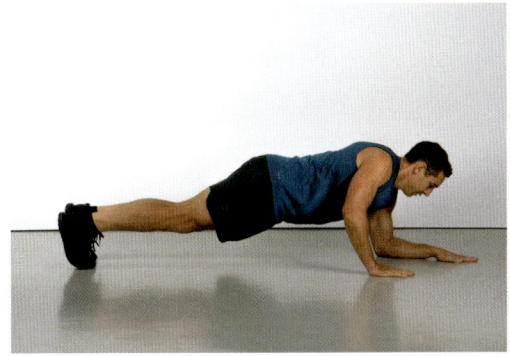

7 Moving plank

Lie with your forearms on the ground, your knees off the ground and your feet together. From here, with your toes touching the ground, lean slightly forward to engage your core, lifting yourself up into the high plank position. Keep alternating between the high and low plank positions. (Note: Your back should not be sagging or bent.)

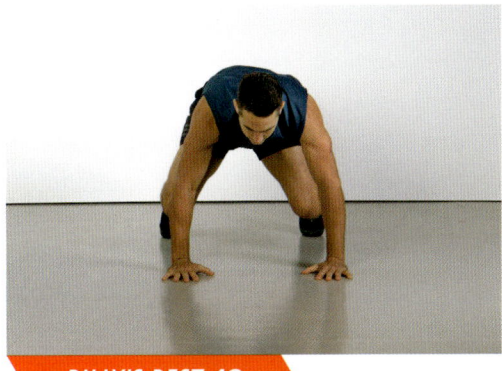

8 Lateral shoot-throughs

Start in high plank position with your hands firmly on the ground and your shoulders above your wrists. Bend your knees at a 90-degree angle and have your toes firmly on the ground and your knees off the ground. This is the starting position. Now turn your left foot so it is flat on the ground. Kick your right foot in front of your left foot and out to the side, so your right leg is now straight and your left foot is firmly on the ground. Now pull your right leg back to the starting position. Repeat on the other side.

BILLY'S BEST: 10

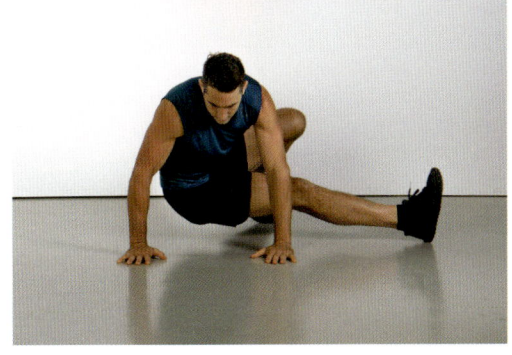

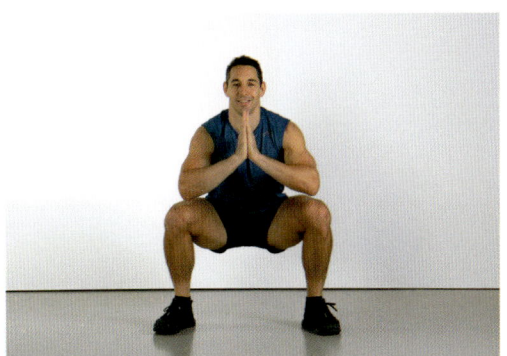

9 Pulse squats

Stand with your feet just past shoulder-width apart and slightly tracked out. Squat with your hips back and your legs at a 90-degree angle, then pulse up and down.

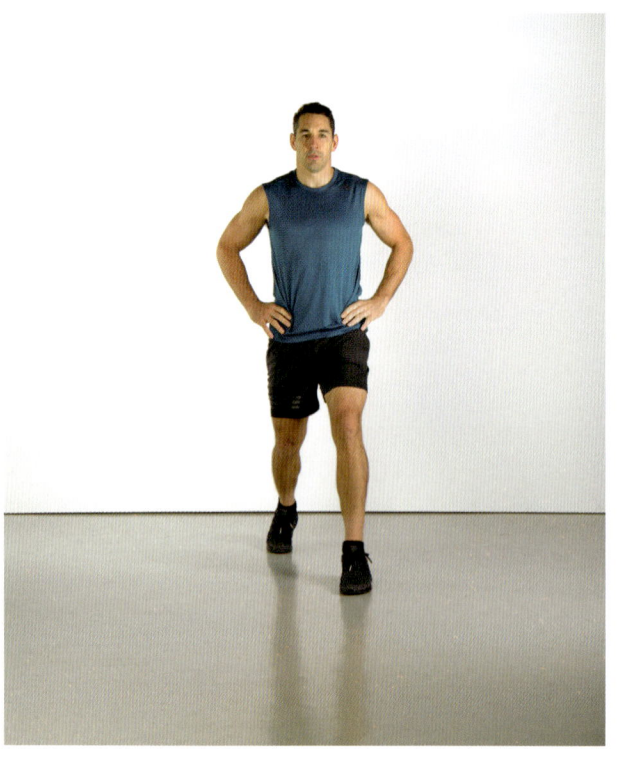

10 Plyometric split lunges

10.1 Start with your feet shoulder-width apart and your hands on your hips. Split your legs before dropping your back knee down in line with the heel of your leading foot – both legs should be at a 90-degree angle – then push up and repeat on the other side.

10.2 Alternatively, stand with your feet shoulder-width apart and your hands on your hips. Step one leg back and then lower it until it is 90 degrees to the ground. Step forward to the starting position. Repeat on the other side to complete the movement.

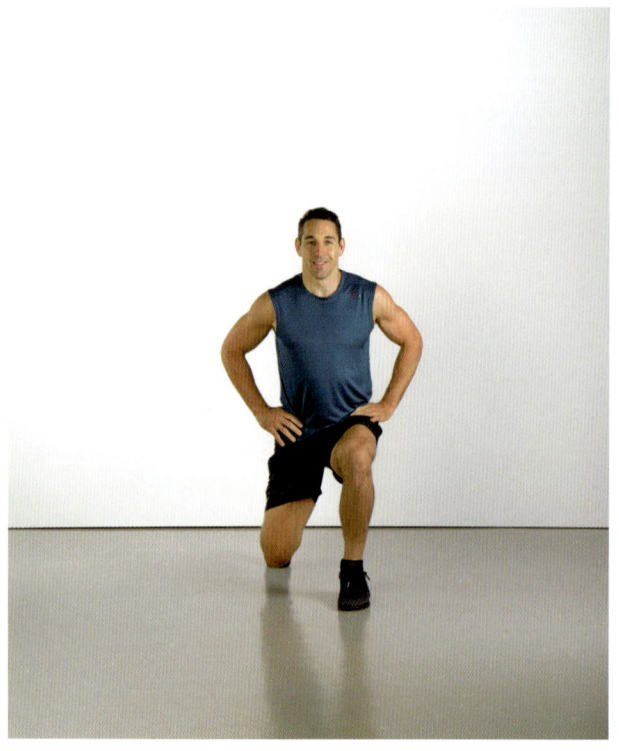

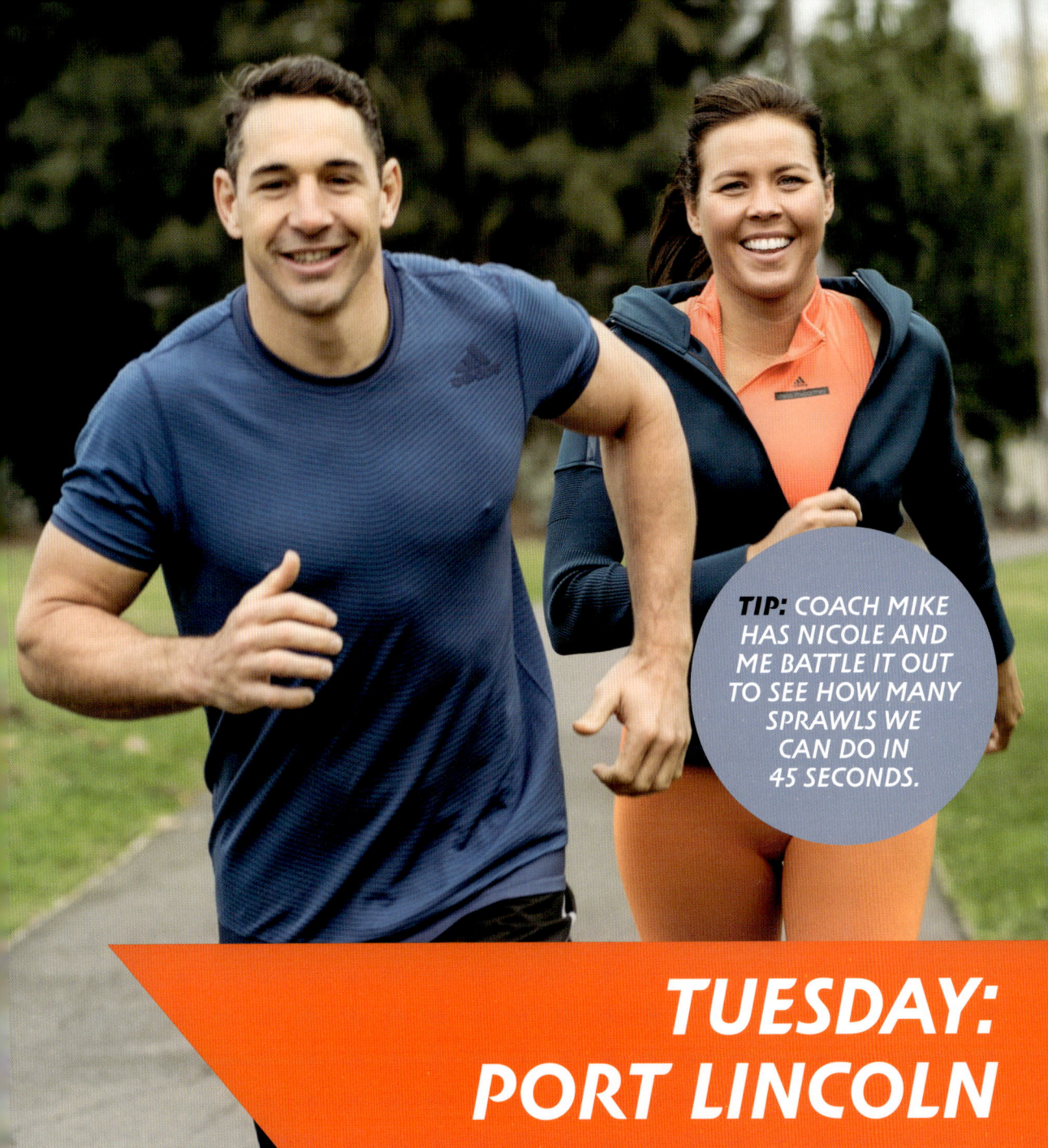

TIP: COACH MIKE HAS NICOLE AND ME BATTLE IT OUT TO SEE HOW MANY SPRAWLS WE CAN DO IN 45 SECONDS.

TUESDAY: PORT LINCOLN

BPT: BICEPS, SHOULDERS, LEGS, CARDIO

10-MINUTE WORKOUT

20 seconds movement /
10 seconds rest
2 sets of each exercise
(one lap)

20-MINUTE WORKOUT

20 seconds movement /
10 seconds rest
2 sets of each exercise
(two laps)

30-MINUTE WORKOUT

20 seconds movement /
10 seconds rest
2 sets of each exercise
(three laps)

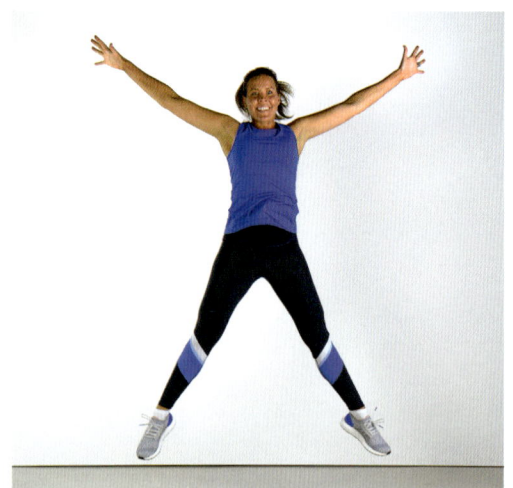

1. **Star jumps**

   Begin in a relaxed stance with your arms close to your body. Jump your feet out wide past shoulder-width and raise both your arms above your head, then land back in the starting position.

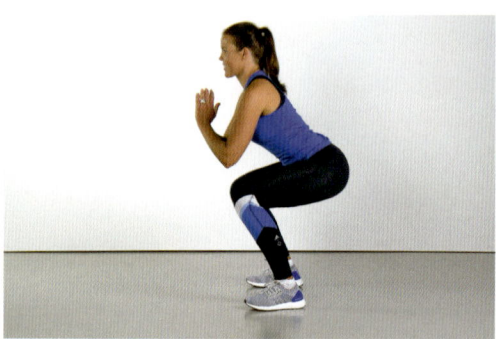
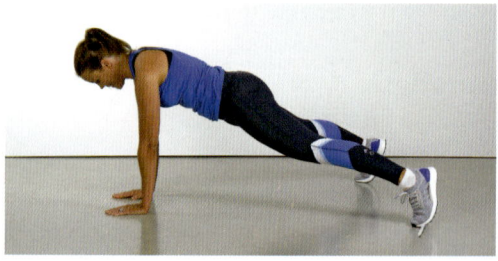

2. **Sprawls**

   Stand with your feet shoulder-width apart, then squat until both your hands and both your feet are firmly on the ground. From this position transfer your weight into your shoulders and shoot your feet back so that your legs are out wide, then jump your feet back up and stand up into the starting position.

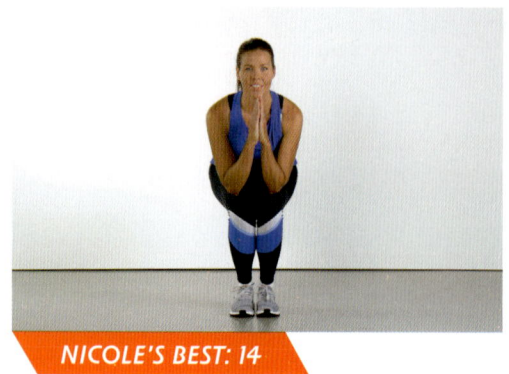

3. **Close-feet squats**

   Stand near a wall with your feet together and your hands on your hips. Bend at the hips, stick your butt out to the wall and lower yourself down as far as you can go with all your weight in the back of your heels. From here, drive through your heels back up to the starting position.

NICOLE'S BEST: 14

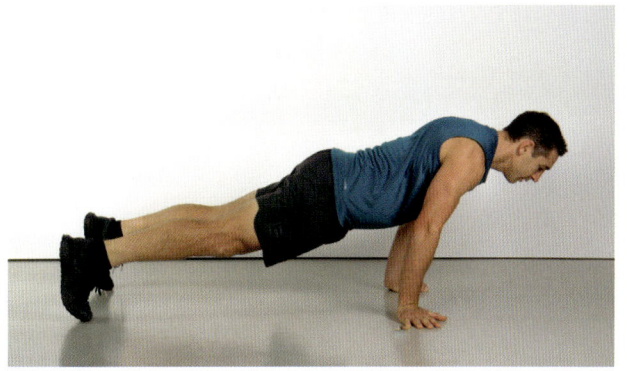

4 Pseudo planche hold

Start in the high plank position with your arms and hands slightly tracked out and your arms straight. From here, tilt forward slightly, squeezing your core, until you are on your toes. Keep your arms straight and lean as far forward as possible without collapsing. Hold this position. You should feel this movement in your biceps, core and shoulders.

5 Plyometric split lunges

5.1 Start with your feet shoulder-width apart and your hands on your hips. Split your legs before dropping your back knee down in line with the heel of your leading foot – both legs should be at a 90-degree angle – then push up and repeat on the other side.

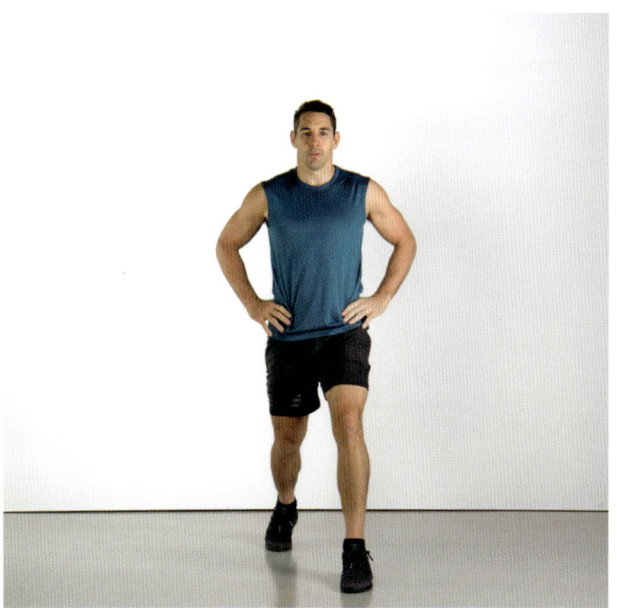

5.2 Alternatively, stand with your feet shoulder-width apart and your hands on your hips. Step one leg back and then lower it until it is 90 degrees to the ground. Step forward to the starting position. Repeat on the other side to complete the movement.

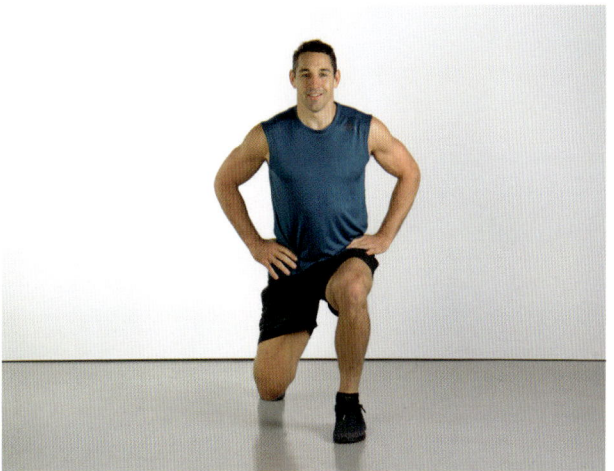

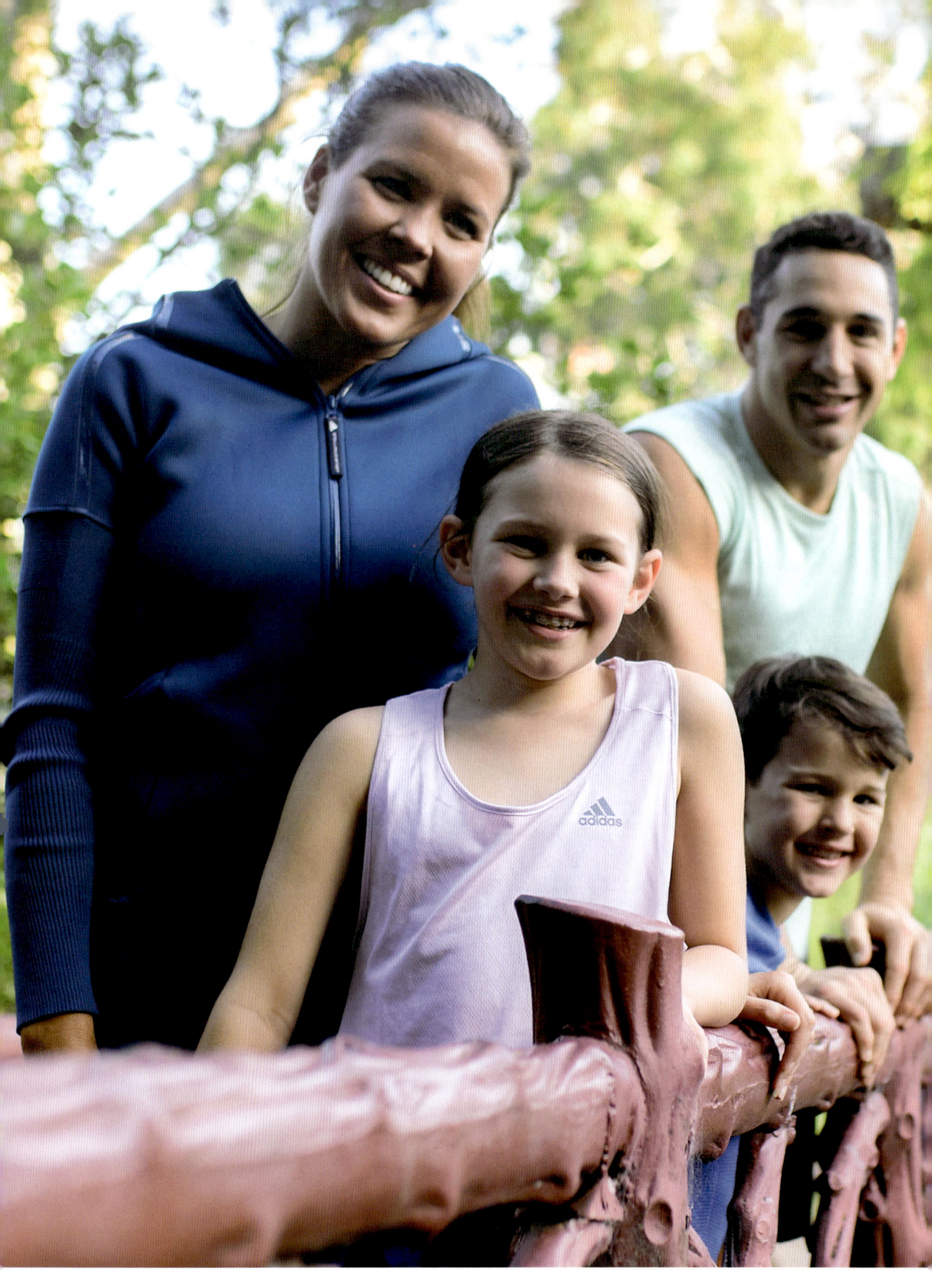

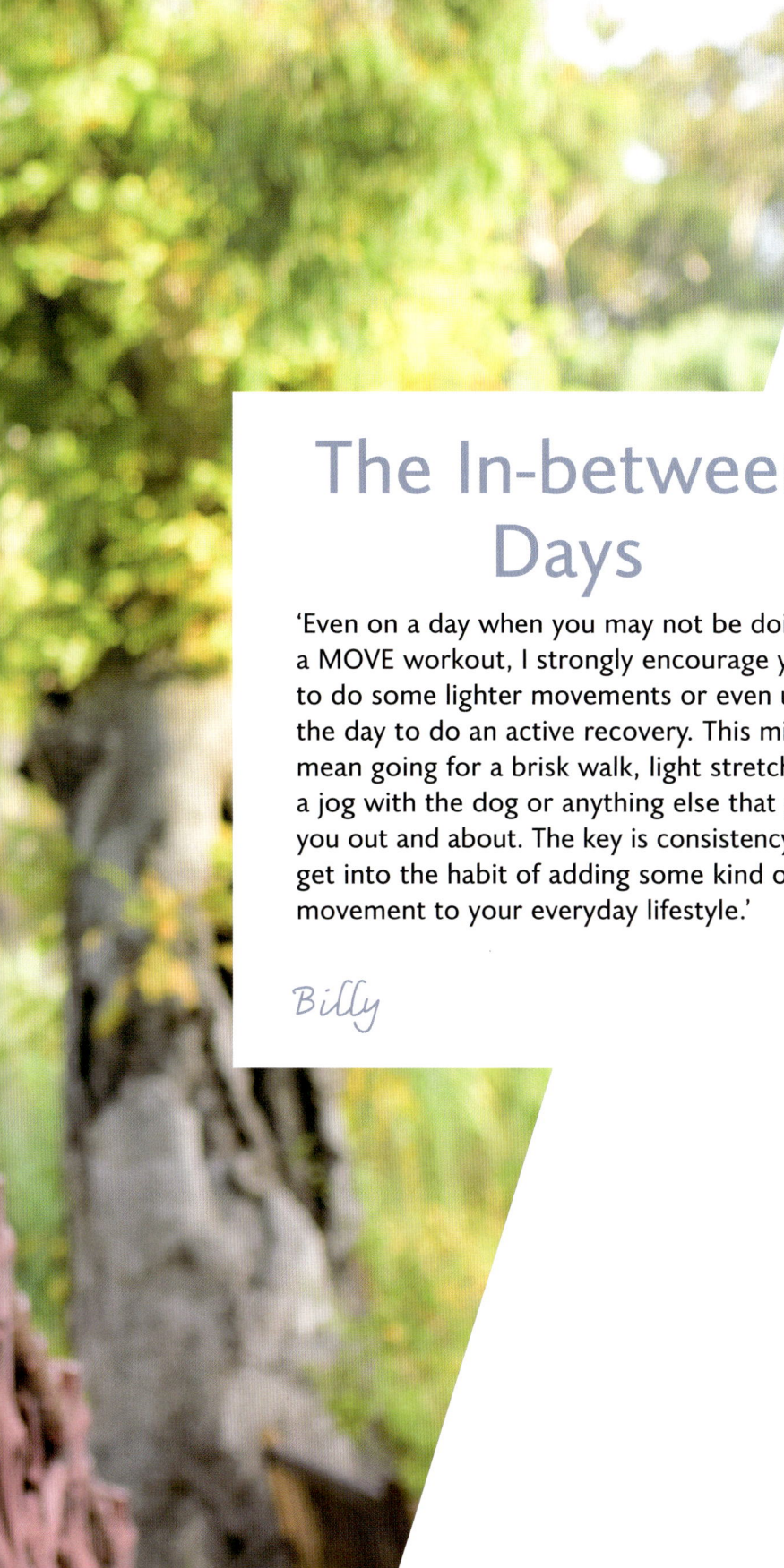

The In-between Days

'Even on a day when you may not be doing a MOVE workout, I strongly encourage you to do some lighter movements or even use the day to do an active recovery. This might mean going for a brisk walk, light stretching, a jog with the dog or anything else that gets you out and about. The key is consistency – get into the habit of adding some kind of movement to your everyday lifestyle.'

Billy

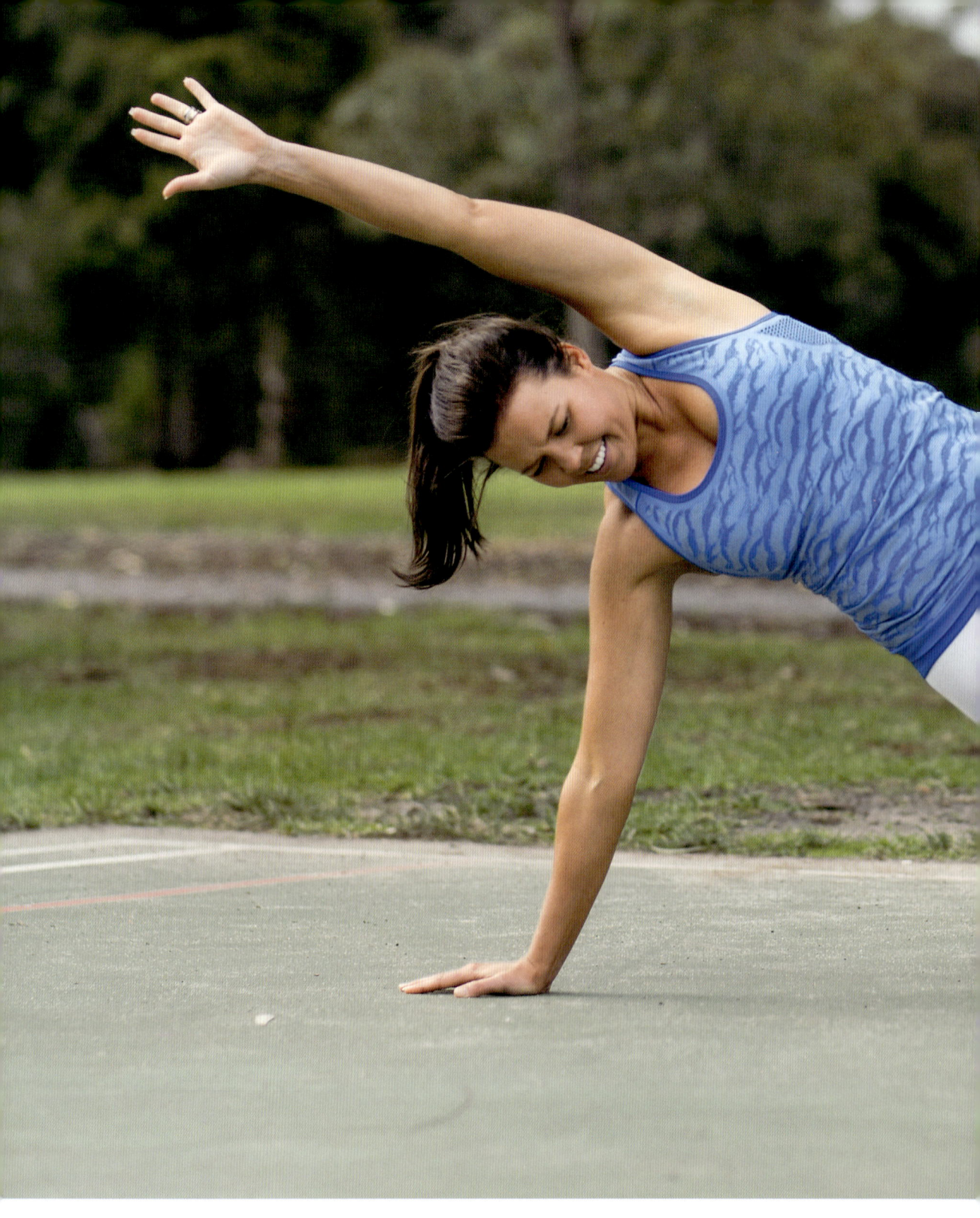

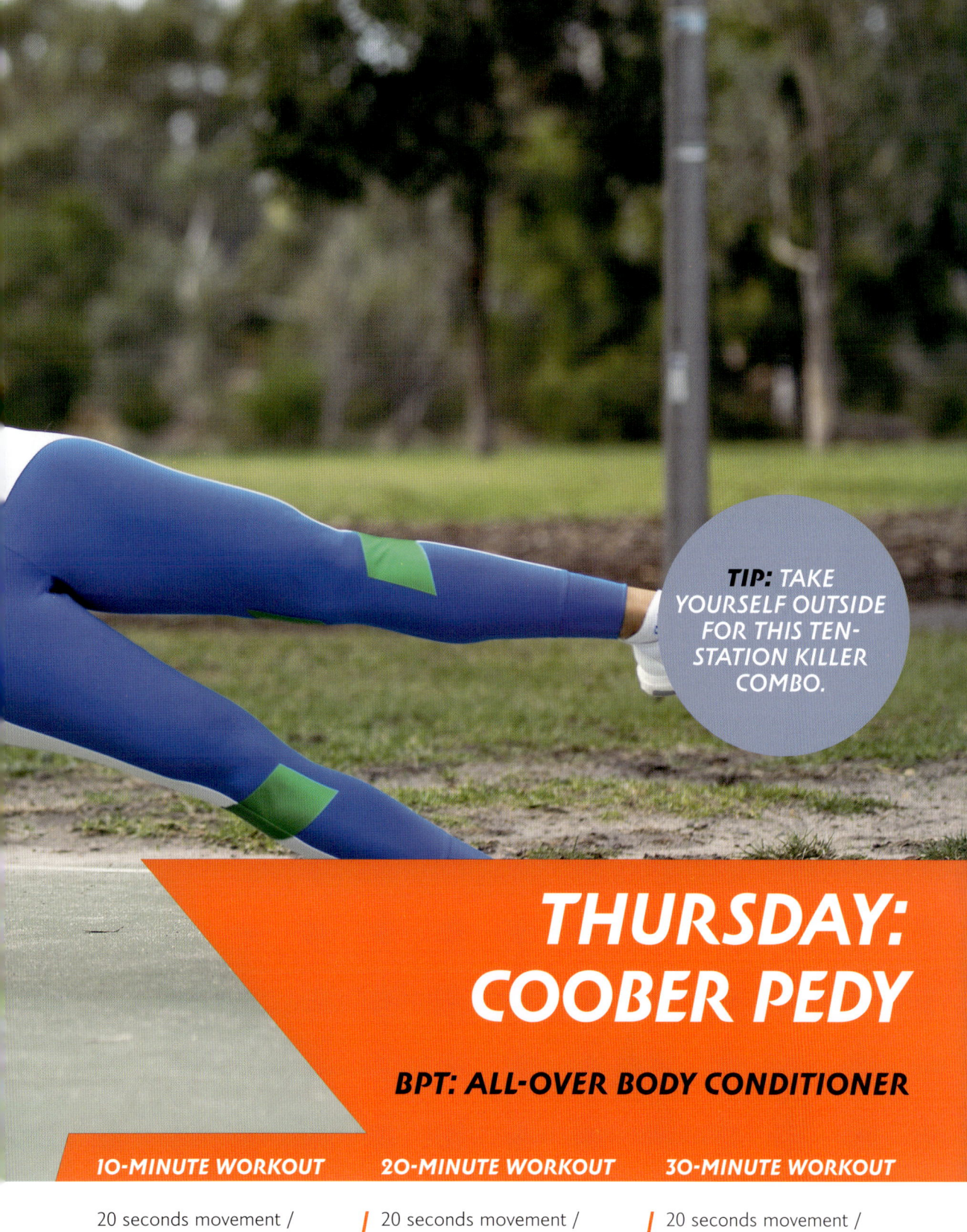

TIP: TAKE YOURSELF OUTSIDE FOR THIS TEN-STATION KILLER COMBO.

THURSDAY: COOBER PEDY

BPT: ALL-OVER BODY CONDITIONER

10-MINUTE WORKOUT

20 seconds movement /
10 seconds rest
2 sets of each exercise
(one lap)

20-MINUTE WORKOUT

20 seconds movement /
10 seconds rest
2 sets of each exercise
(two laps)

30-MINUTE WORKOUT

20 seconds movement /
10 seconds rest
2 sets of each exercise
(three laps)

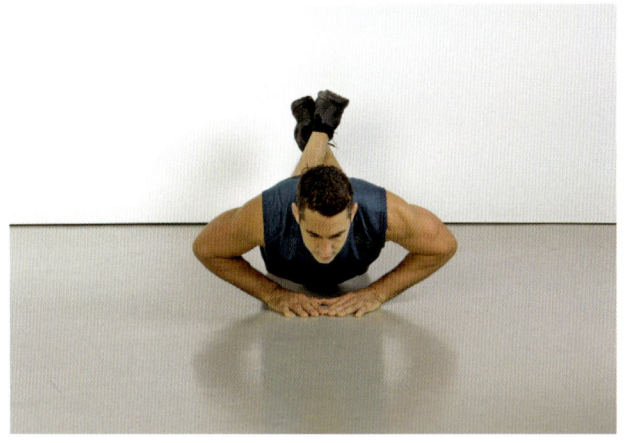

1. **Diamond push-ups**

   Kneel on the ground with your ankles crossed, and set your hands so your thumbs and index fingers are touching in line with your chin. From here, lower your body towards the ground and then press back up to the starting position. You should feel this movement in your triceps.

   Advanced: Do the exercise in high plank position with your knees off the ground.

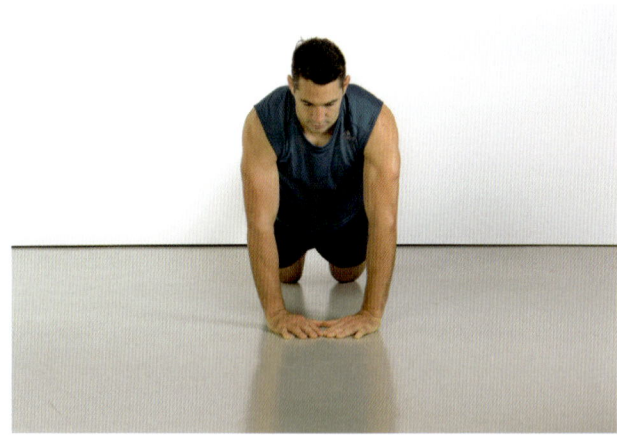

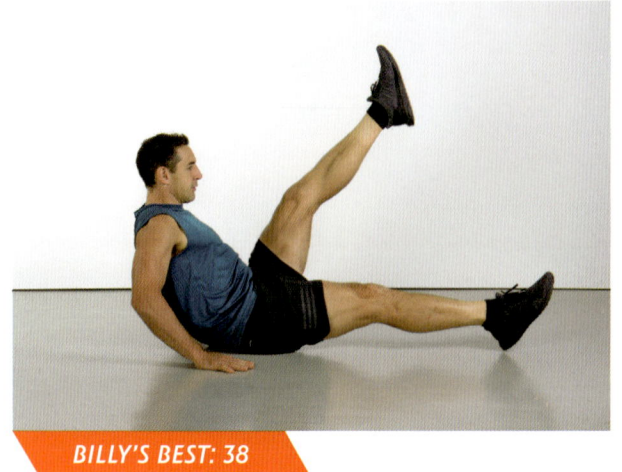

2. **Scissor kicks**

   Sit on the ground with your legs extended in front and lean back with your hands in a comfortable position by your side. Raise one leg as high as you can, keeping it straight, then return it to the ground. Repeat with the other leg.

   BILLY'S BEST: 38

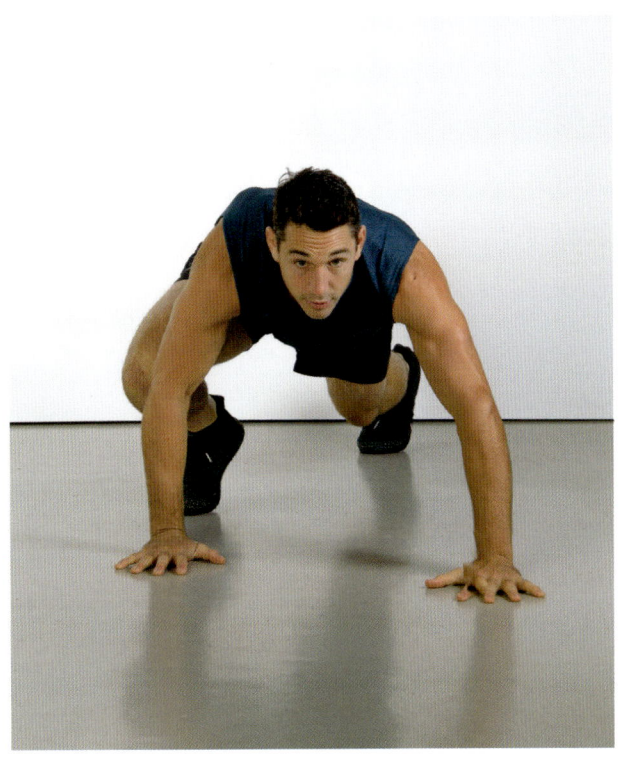

3 Bear crawl

Start in the push-up position with your knees bent at a 90-degree angle and positioned directly under your hips. Engage your core and do not raise or round your back. This is your starting position. Walk your right hand and your left foot forward, and then your left hand and your right foot forward. Continue for 5 metres. Now, keeping your hips down and your core engaged, reverse the movement by walking your left arm and your right foot back, and then your right arm and your left leg back. Continue until you have returned to your starting position.

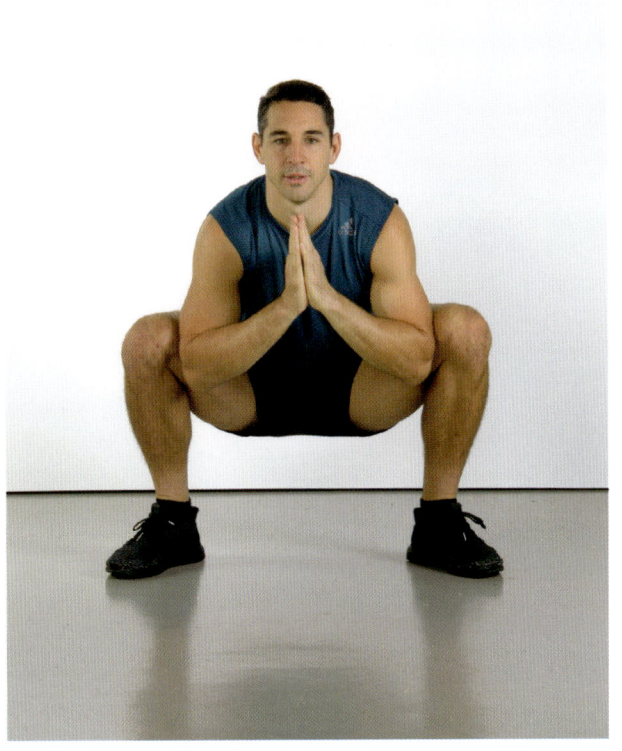

4 Frog squats

Stand with your feet shoulder-width apart and your feet slightly tracked out. Bend down to full squat position with your elbows tucked inside your legs. This is the starting position. From here, raise your hips and then lower them back to the starting position.

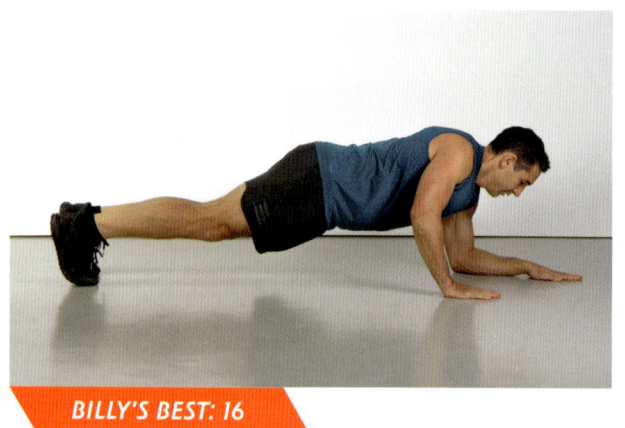

BILLY'S BEST: 16

5 **Moving plank**
Lie with your forearms on the ground, your knees off the ground and your feet together. From here, with your toes touching the ground, lean slightly forward to engage your core, lifting yourself up into the high plank position. Keep alternating between the high and low plank positions. (Note: Your back should not be sagging or bent.)

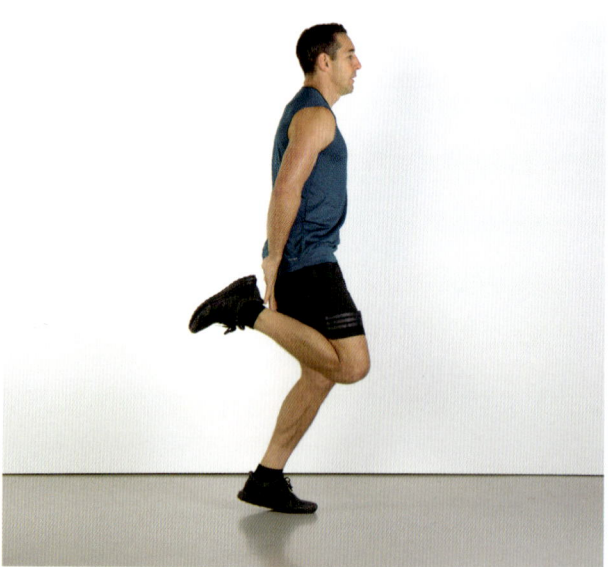

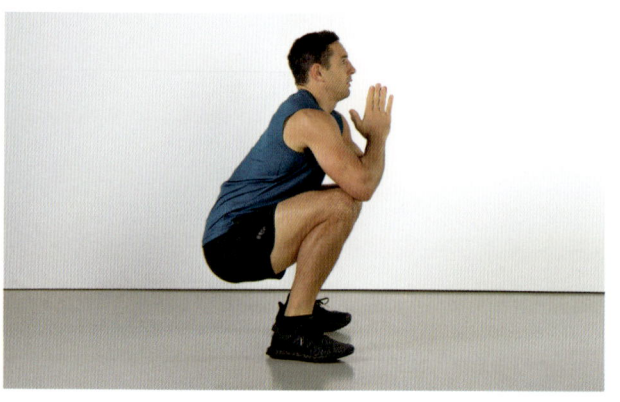

6 **4 x butt kicks, 2 x deep squats**
For the butt kicks, stand with your feet shoulder-width apart and your hands flat behind your back with your palms facing outwards. Bring one heel up to touch your butt, then do the same with the other heel. Try to keep your feet nice and soft and land back on the ball of your foot each time.

For the deep squats, stand with your feet shoulder-width apart, slightly tracked out. Holding your hands clasped together, bend at your hips and lower your body down, keeping your feet flat on the ground and going as low as you can before pressing back up through your heels to the starting position.

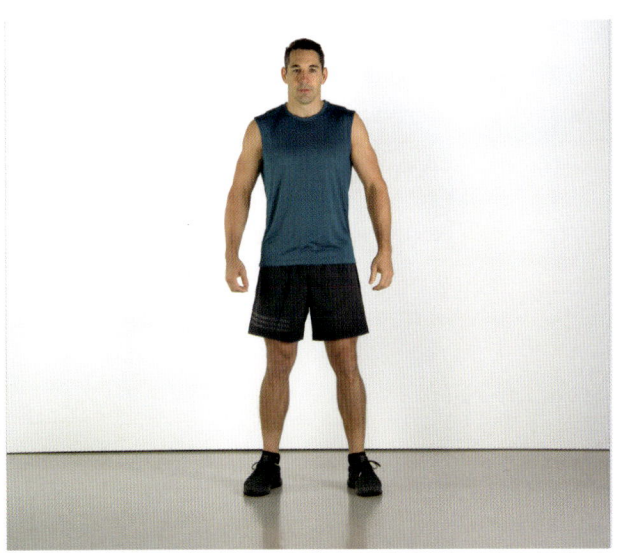

7 **Burpees**

Stand in a relaxed position with your feet shoulder-width apart. Squat and place your hands firmly on the ground with your feet back. Shoot your legs back so you are in a high plank position, then lower your body so your torso is just touching the ground. Release your hands and then, placing your hands back on the ground, raise your torso and jump your feet back so both hands and both feet are on the ground. Stand back up, then jump up and raise your hands above your head.

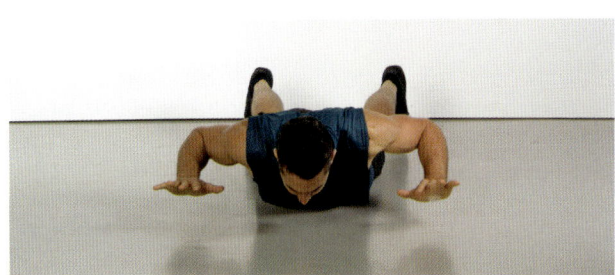

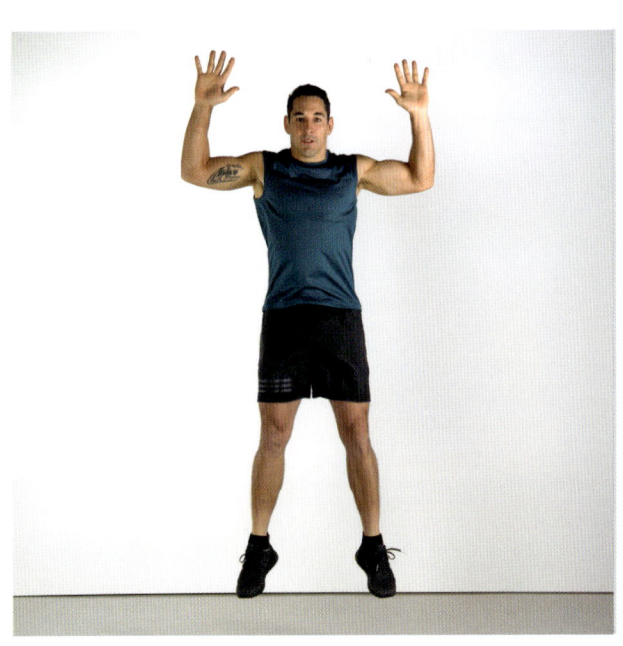

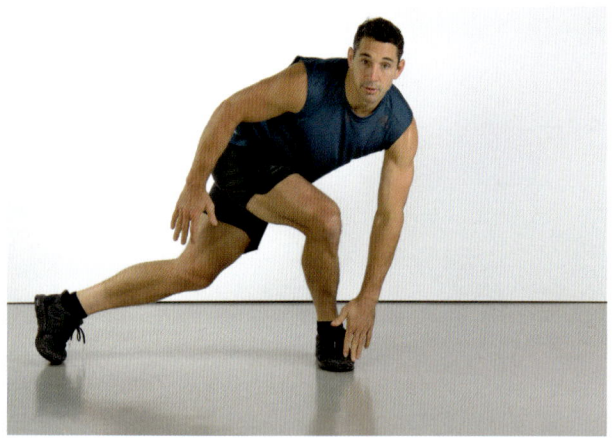

8 Ice skaters

Start with your feet shoulder-width apart. Step half a foot to your left, swing your right leg behind your left leg, and with your right hand touch your left toe. From here, step to your right, swing your left leg behind your right leg, and with your left hand touch your right toe.

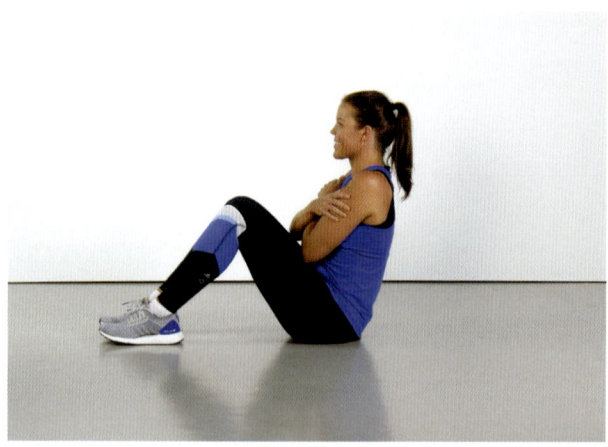

9 Sit-ups

Lie on your back, bend your legs and place your feet firmly on the ground to stabilise your lower body. Cross your arms over your chest, then curl your upper body all the way up to touch your knees. Slowly lower yourself down to return to the starting point.

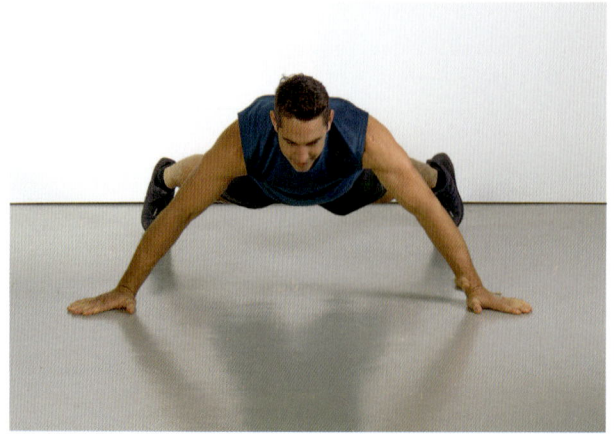

10 Spider-Man holds

Start in a high plank position but with your hands out nice and wide and your legs as wide as your hands. From here, raise your knees and lean forward slightly, engaging your core and squeezing your glutes. You should also feel this movement in your biceps and shoulders.

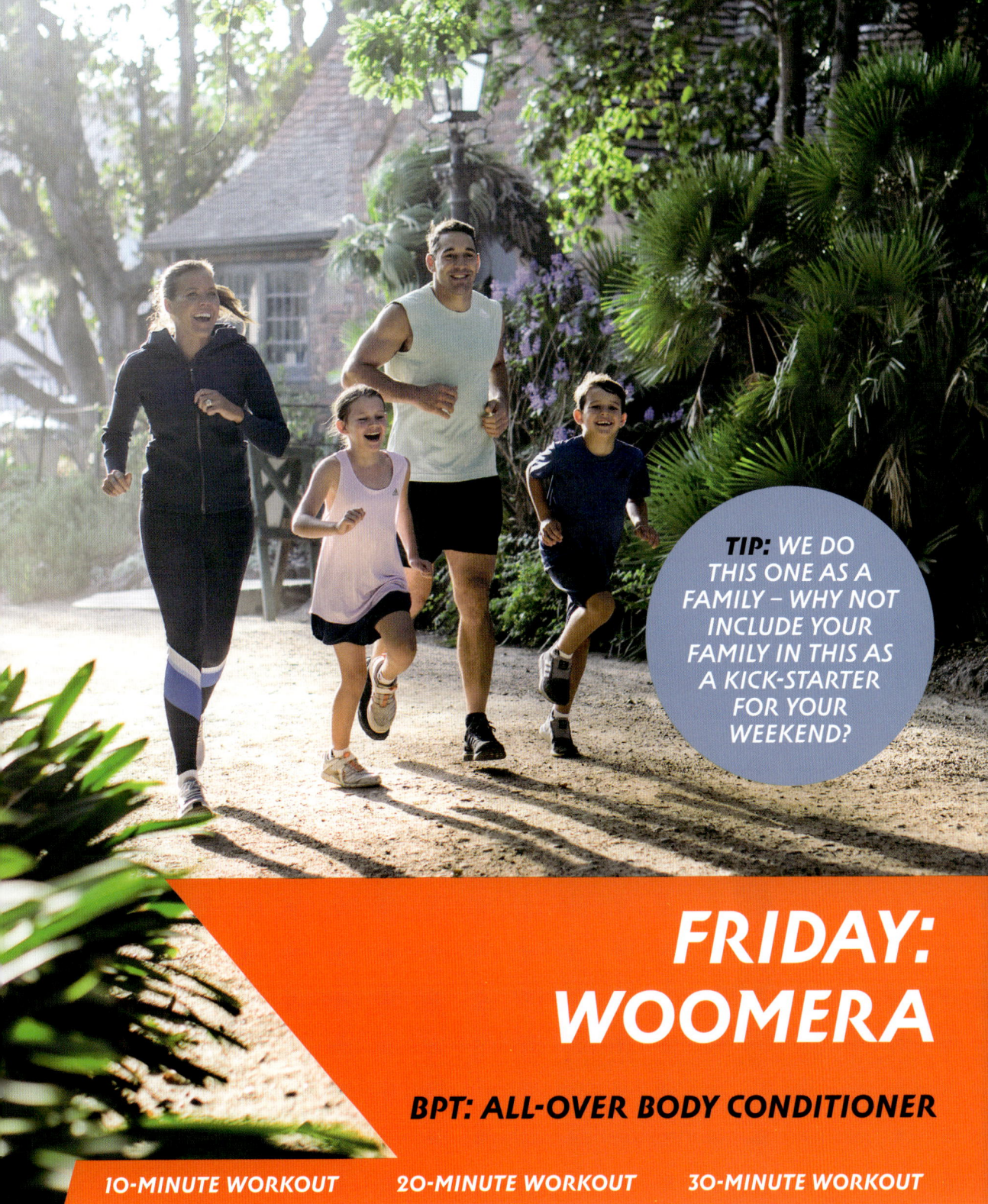

TIP: WE DO THIS ONE AS A FAMILY – WHY NOT INCLUDE YOUR FAMILY IN THIS AS A KICK-STARTER FOR YOUR WEEKEND?

FRIDAY: WOOMERA

BPT: ALL-OVER BODY CONDITIONER

10-MINUTE WORKOUT

20 seconds movement /
10 seconds rest
2 sets of each exercise
(one lap)

20-MINUTE WORKOUT

20 seconds movement /
10 seconds rest
2 sets of each exercise
(two laps)

30-MINUTE WORKOUT

20 seconds movement /
10 seconds rest
2 sets of each exercise
(three laps)

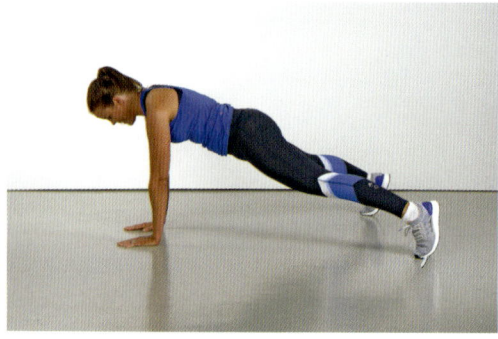

1 **Sprawls**
Stand with your feet shoulder-width apart, then squat until both your hands and both your feet are firmly on the ground. From this position transfer your weight into your shoulders and shoot your feet back so that your legs are out wide, then jump your feet back up and stand up into the starting position.

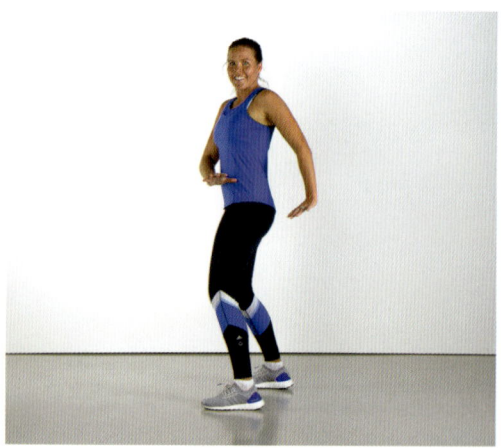

2 **Toe touches**
Lie on your back with your legs up in the air and your toes flexed. Run your hands up your shins as far as you can go towards your toes, then release back to the starting position.

3 **2 x torsion twists, 1 x deep squat**
For the torsion twists, stand with your feet shoulder-width apart and your arms out nice and wide at shoulder height. Slightly jump to your right, twisting your left hip to your right side and keeping your chest forward. Now come back to the starting position. Repeat on the other side.

For the deep squat, stand with your feet shoulder-width apart, slightly tracked out. Holding your hands together, bend forward at the hips and lower your body down, keeping your feet flat on the ground and going as low as you can before pressing back up through your heels to the starting position.

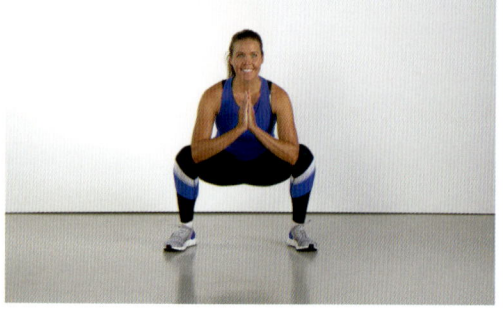

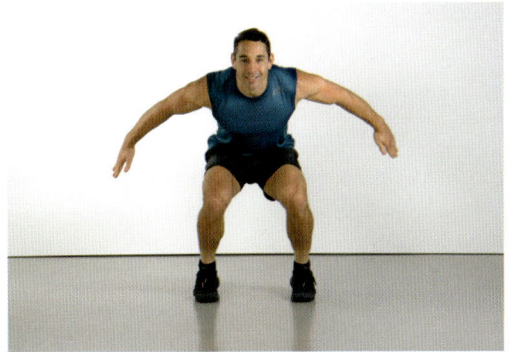

4 **Tuck jumps**

Stand with your feet shoulder-width apart and your knees slightly bent. Raise your hands above your head and jump both knees off the ground towards your chest, landing with your feet shoulder-width apart.

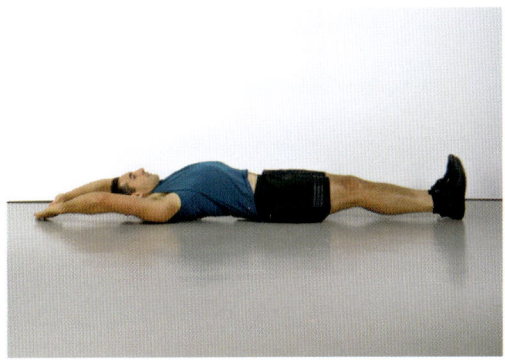

5 **Elbow to knee**

Lie on your back with your arms stretched out above your head. Bring your right knee up towards your chest and your right elbow towards your knee. Go as far as you can before returning to the starting position. Repeat with your left knee and elbow.

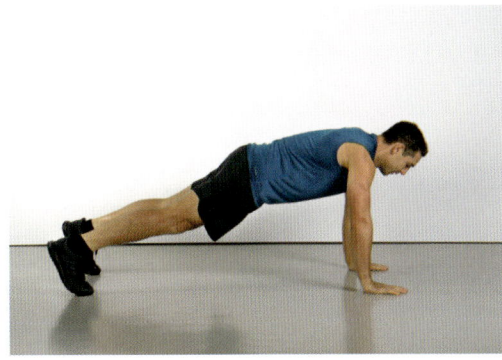

6 **Burpees**

Stand in a relaxed position with your feet shoulder-width apart. Squat and place your hands firmly on the ground with your feet back. Shoot your legs back so you are in a high plank position, then lower your body so your torso is just touching the ground. Release your hands and then, placing your hands back on the ground, raise your torso and jump your feet back so both hands and both feet are on the ground. Stand back up, then jump up and raise your hands above your head.

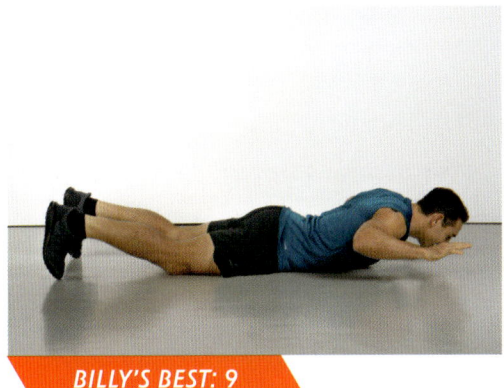

BILLY'S BEST: 9

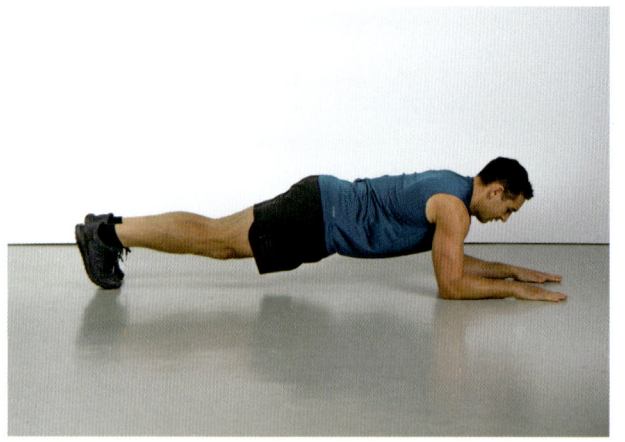

7 Plank hold

Lie on the ground in a forearm plank position, your knees off the ground and your feet together. From here, with your toes touching the ground, lean slightly forward to engage your core. Hold the position for the duration of time. (Note: Your back should not be sagging or bent.)

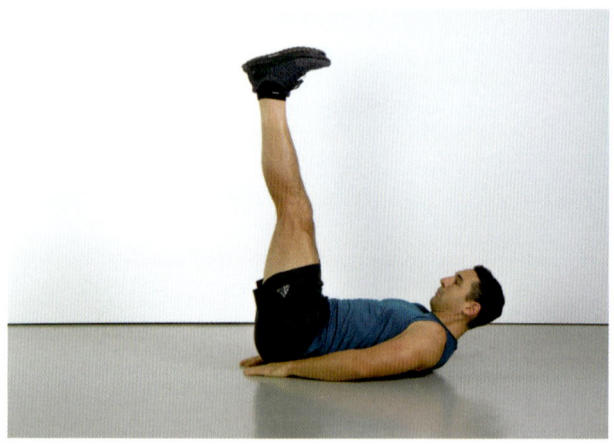

8 Double-leg raises

Lie on your back and tuck both your thumbs under your lower lumbar (base of your back). Raise your legs then lower them, keeping your heels off the ground.

Advanced: Do the exercise with your arms crossed over your chest.

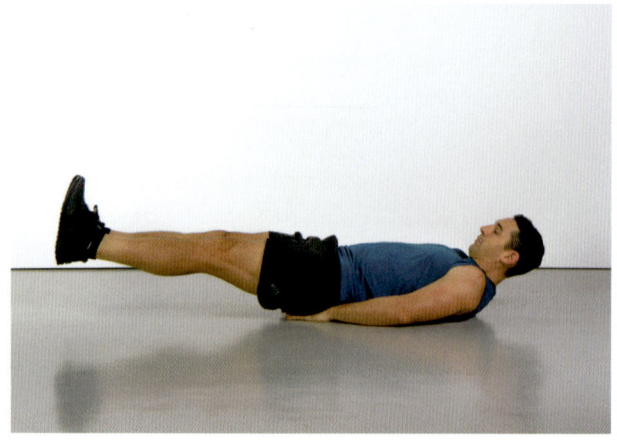

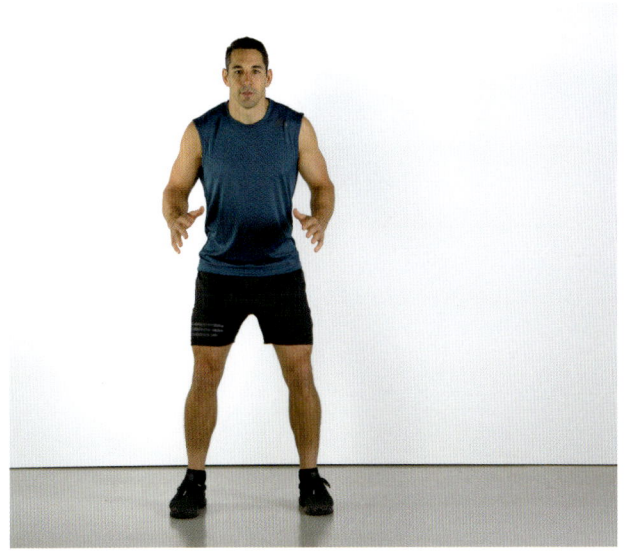

9 Ice skaters

Start with your feet shoulder-width apart. Take a step to your left, swing your right leg behind your left leg, and with your right hand touch your left toe. From here, step to your right, swing your left leg behind your right leg, and with your left hand touch your right toe.

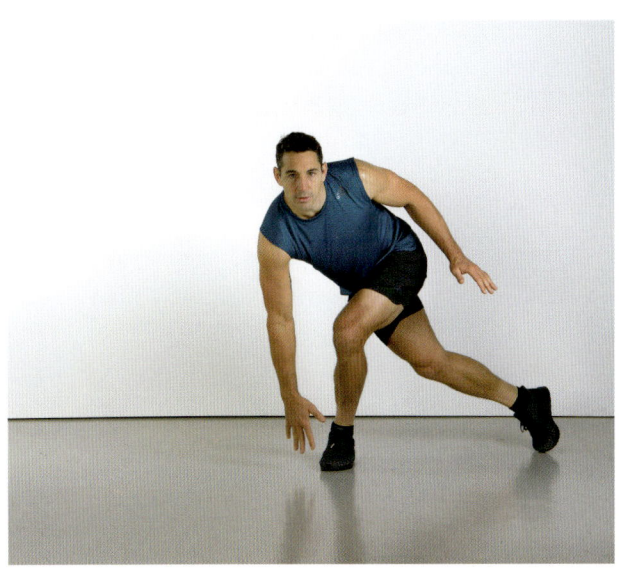

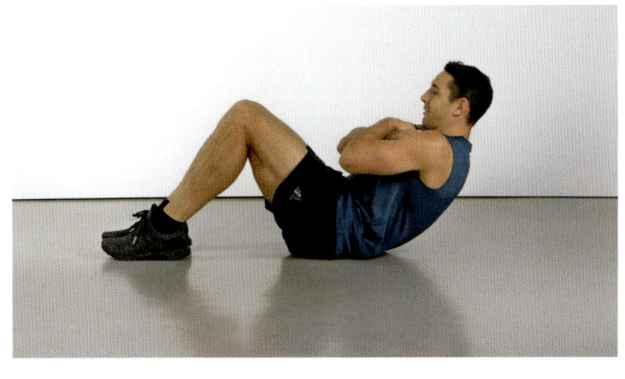

10 Sit-ups

Lie on your back, bend your legs and place your feet firmly on the ground to stabilise your lower body. Cross your arms over your chest, then curl your upper body all the way up to touch your knees. Slowly lower yourself down to return to the starting point.

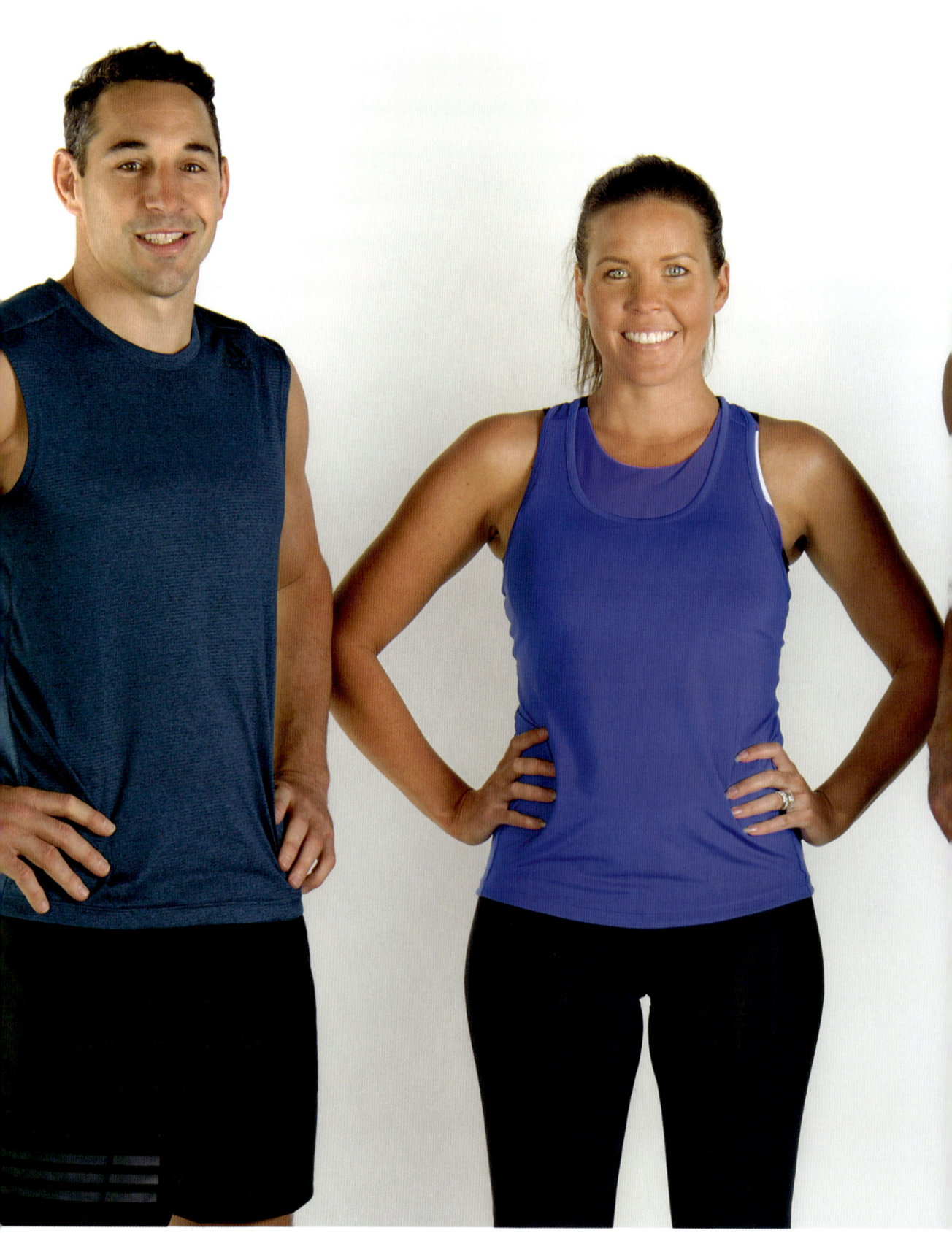

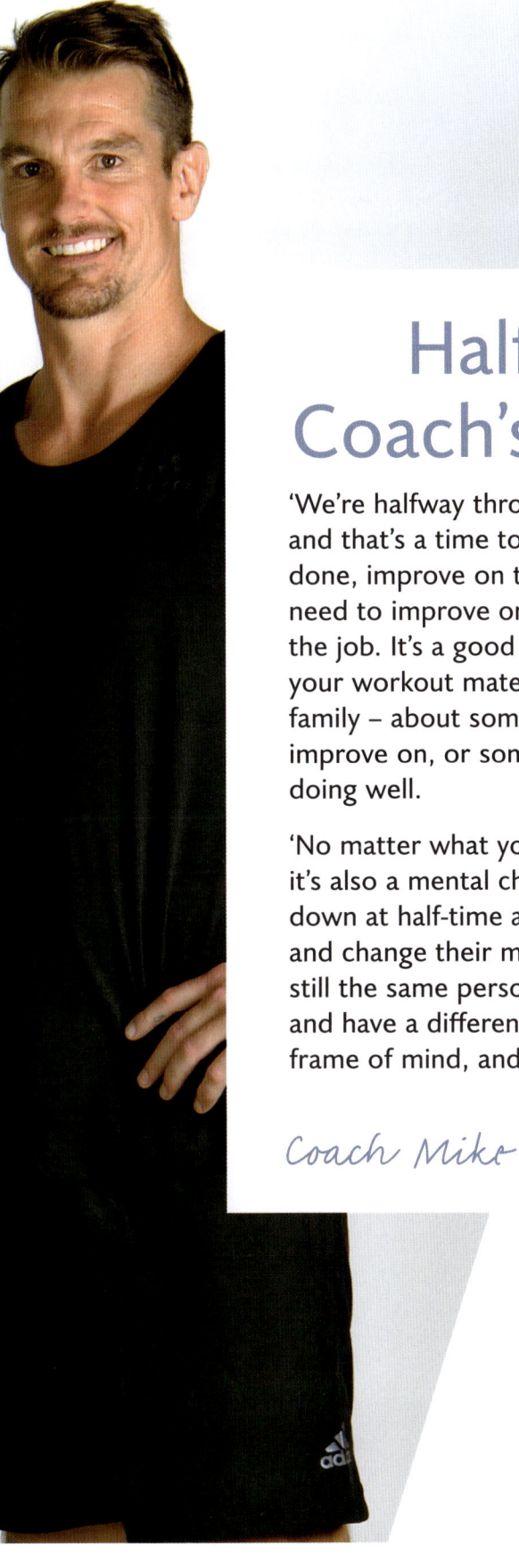

Half-Time Coach's Pep Talk

'We're halfway through the book now, and that's a time to reflect on what you've done, improve on the things that you need to improve on, and go out and finish the job. It's a good opportunity to talk to your workout mates – be they friends or family – about some things that you can improve on, or some things that you're doing well.

'No matter what you're doing physically, it's also a mental challenge. People can sit down at half-time and think about things and change their mindset. Physically you're still the same person, but you can go out and have a different attitude and a different frame of mind, and things can change.'

Coach Mike

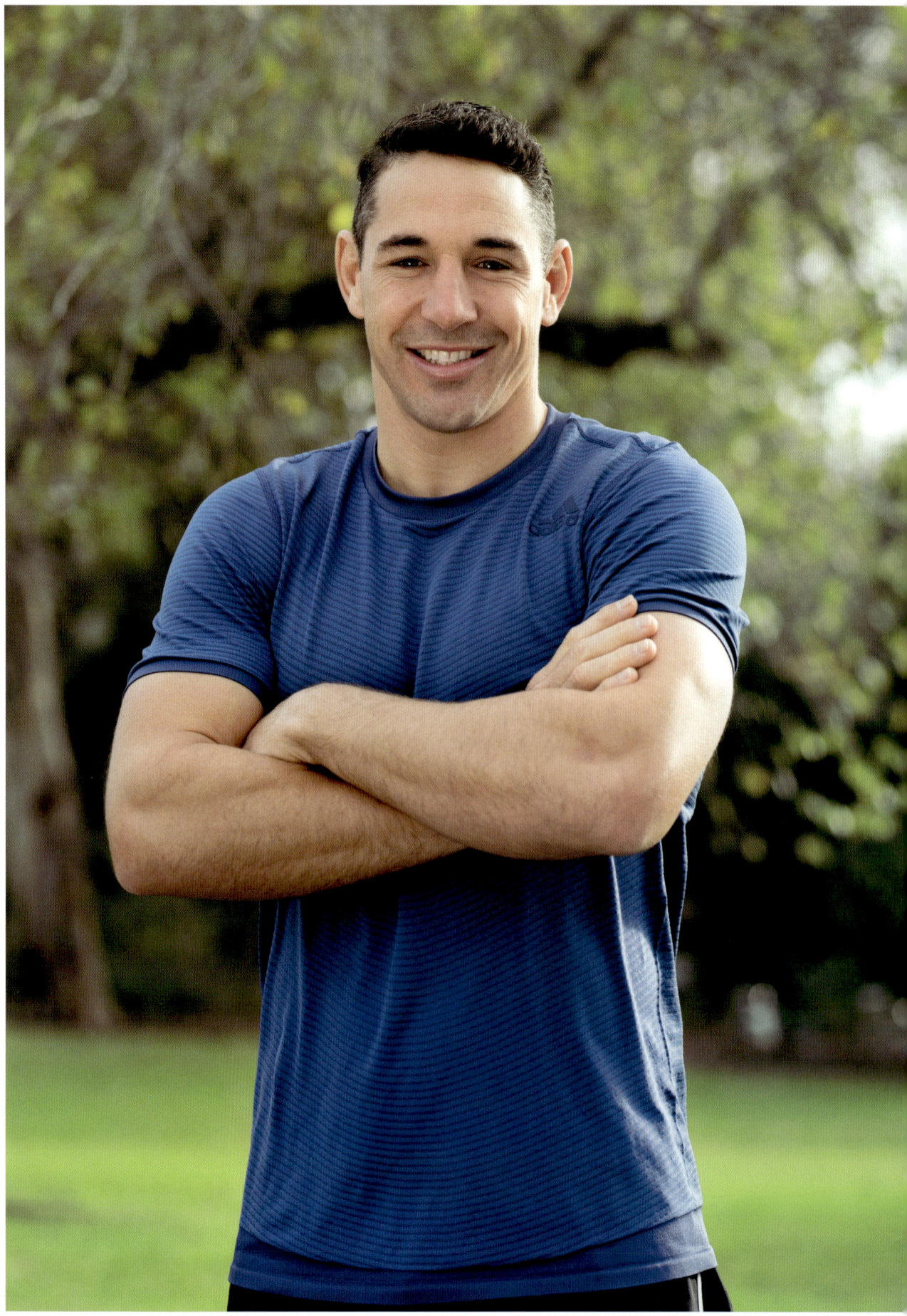

BLOCK 5: AUSTRALIAN CAPITAL TERRITORY

'The nation's capital is pretty often a tough road-trip for us Queenslanders. The weather is usually a lot colder than we're used to. In the cooler months, it's a great idea to keep your body moving indoors: a couple of push-ups, sit-ups and planks. Warmer yet?'

Billy

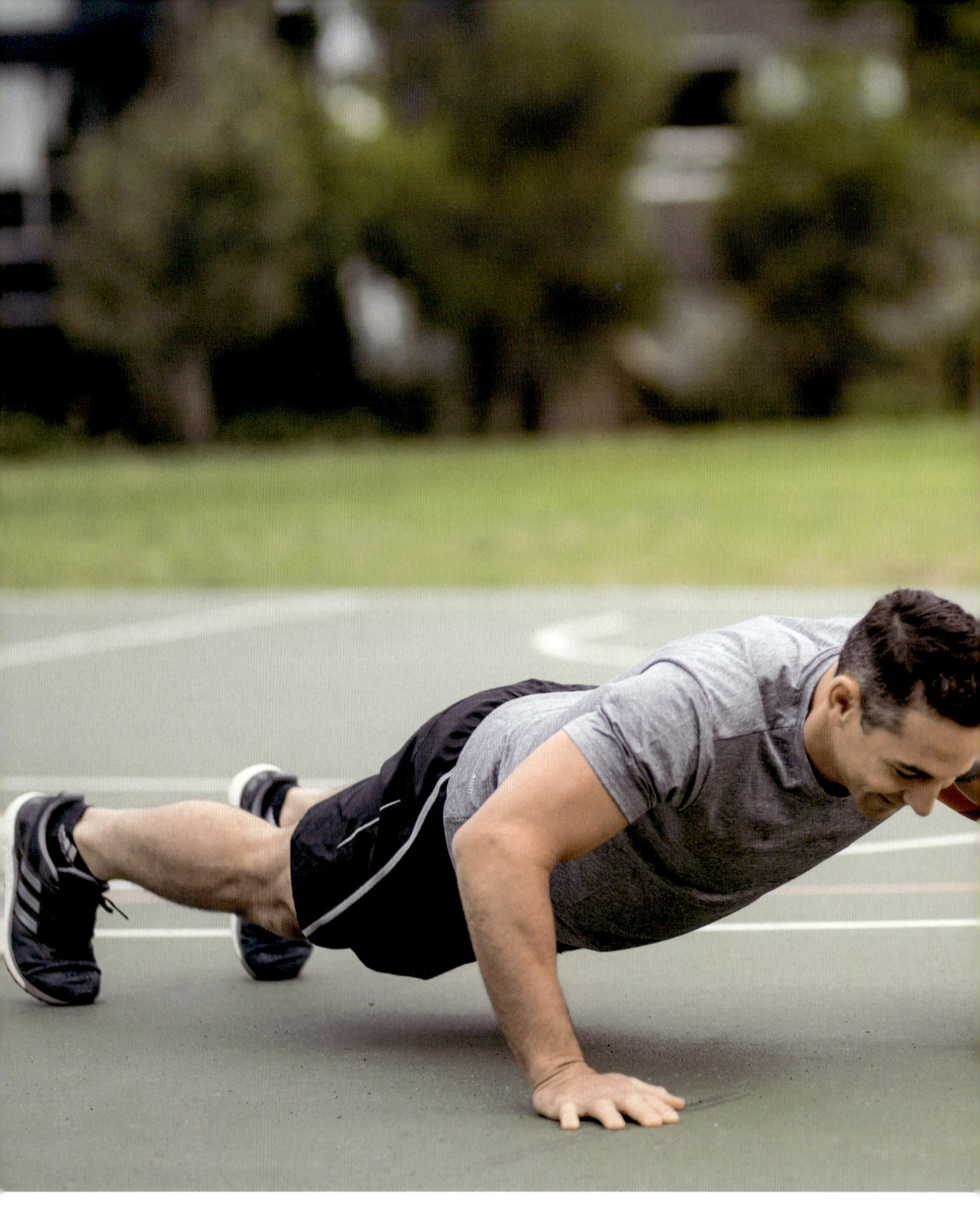

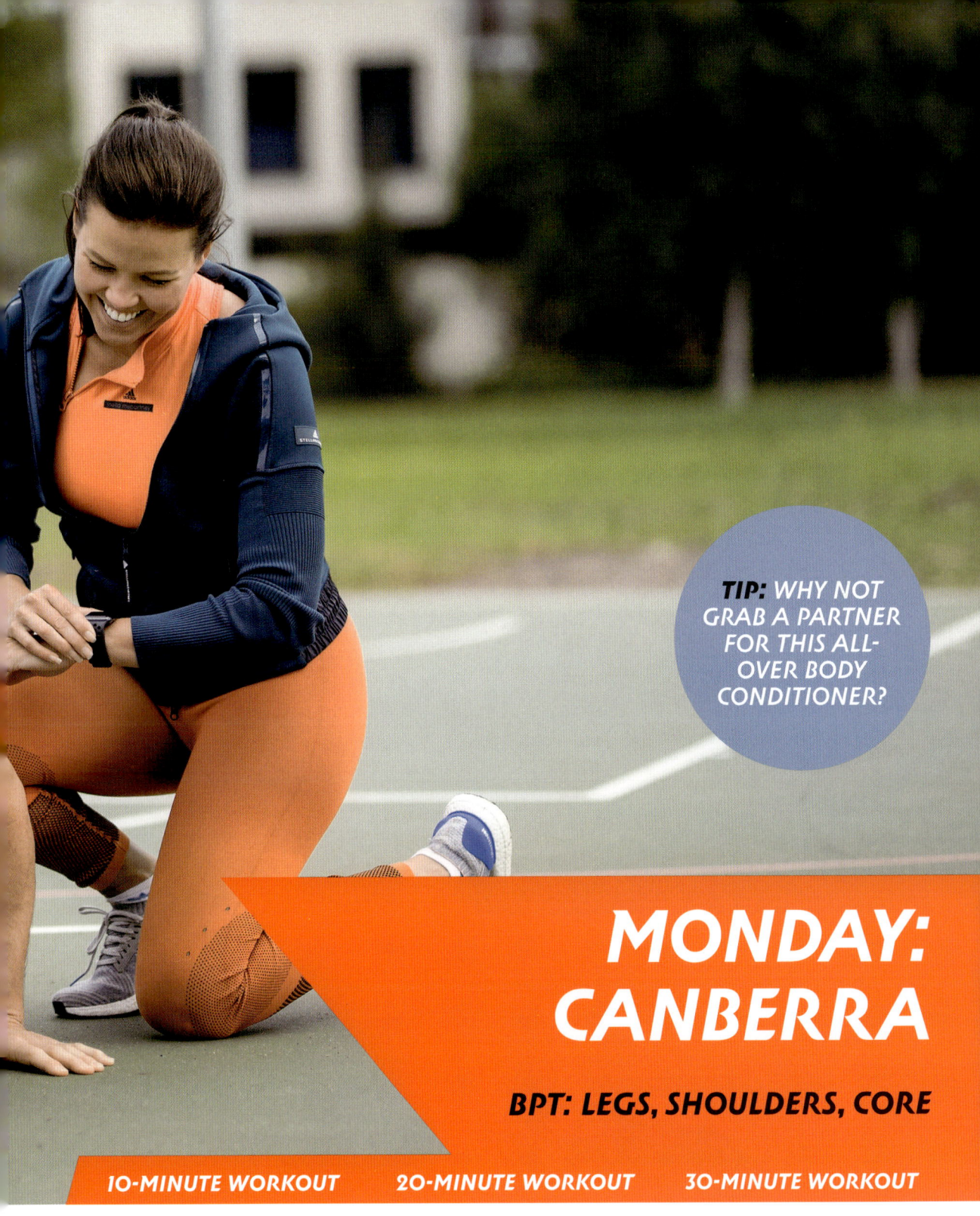

TIP: WHY NOT GRAB A PARTNER FOR THIS ALL-OVER BODY CONDITIONER?

MONDAY: CANBERRA

BPT: LEGS, SHOULDERS, CORE

10-MINUTE WORKOUT	20-MINUTE WORKOUT	30-MINUTE WORKOUT
20 seconds movement / 10 seconds rest 2 sets of each exercise (one lap)	20 seconds movement / 10 seconds rest 2 sets of each exercise (two laps)	20 seconds movement / 10 seconds rest 2 sets of each exercise (three laps)

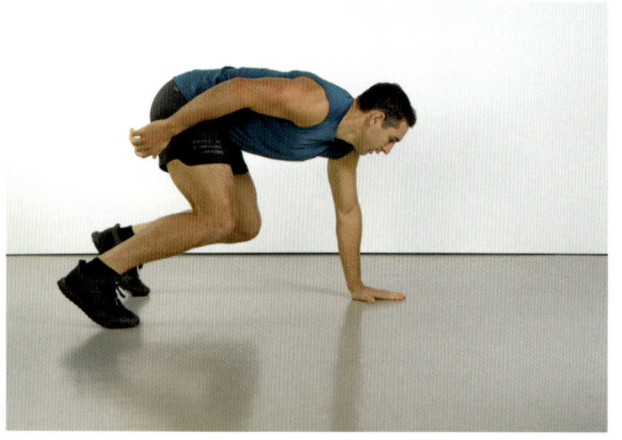

1 Inchworms

Stand with your feet just wide enough apart that when you bend forward to touch the ground your legs remain straight. From the bent position, walk your hands out until you are in a high plank position. Engage your core and squeeze your glutes. Now walk your hands back, keeping your legs straight, before engaging your core to stand up into the starting position.

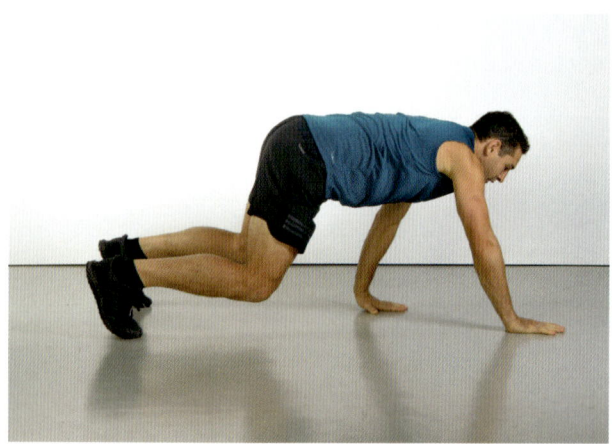

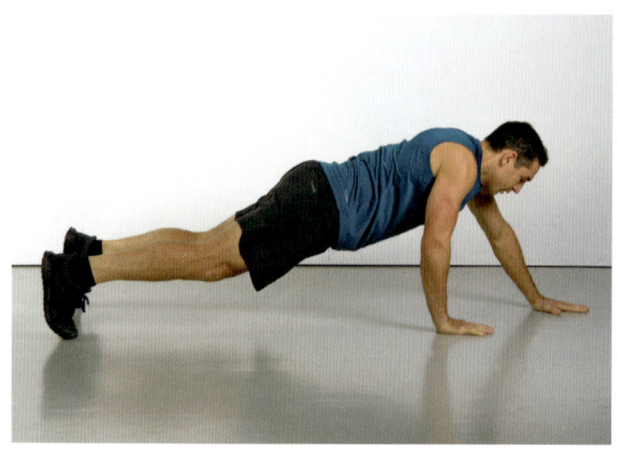

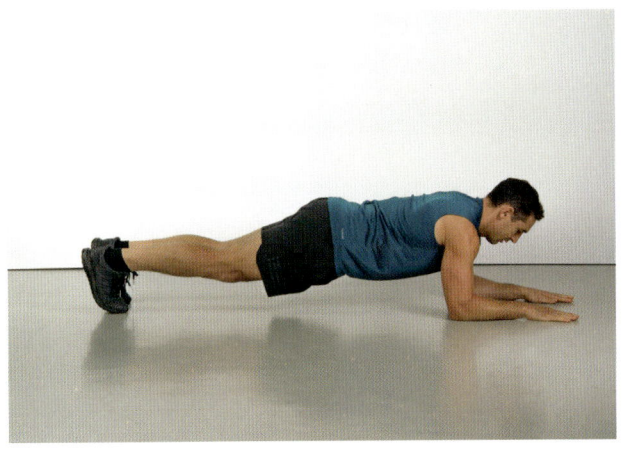

2   **Plank**

Place your forearms on the ground and lift your knees off the ground with your feet together and your toes touching the ground. From here, lean slightly forward to engage your core. Hold the position for the duration of time. (Note: Your back should not be sagging or bent.)

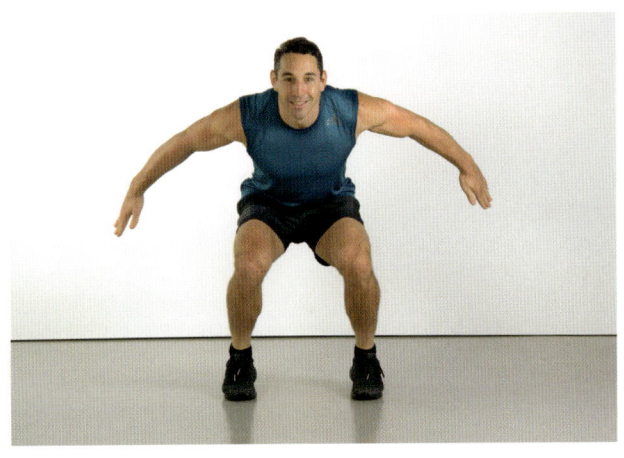

3   **Tuck jumps**

Stand with your feet shoulder-width apart and your knees slightly bent. Raise your hands above your head and jump both knees off the ground towards your chest, landing with your feet shoulder-width apart.

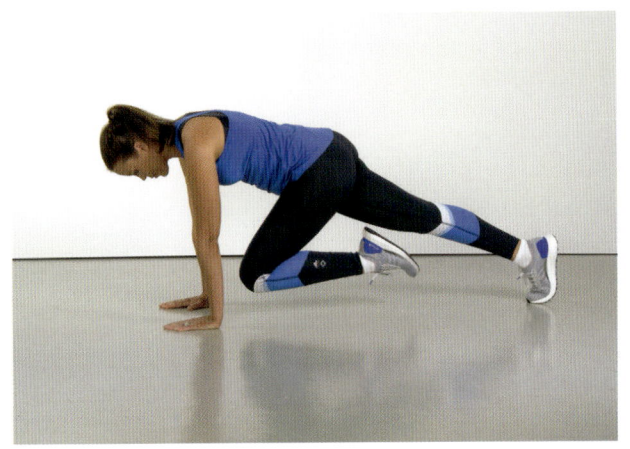

4   **Mountain climbers**

Start in a high plank position, with your shoulders over your wrists, your feet together and your core engaged. From here, bring one knee up towards your chest and then return it to the starting position. Repeat on the other side.

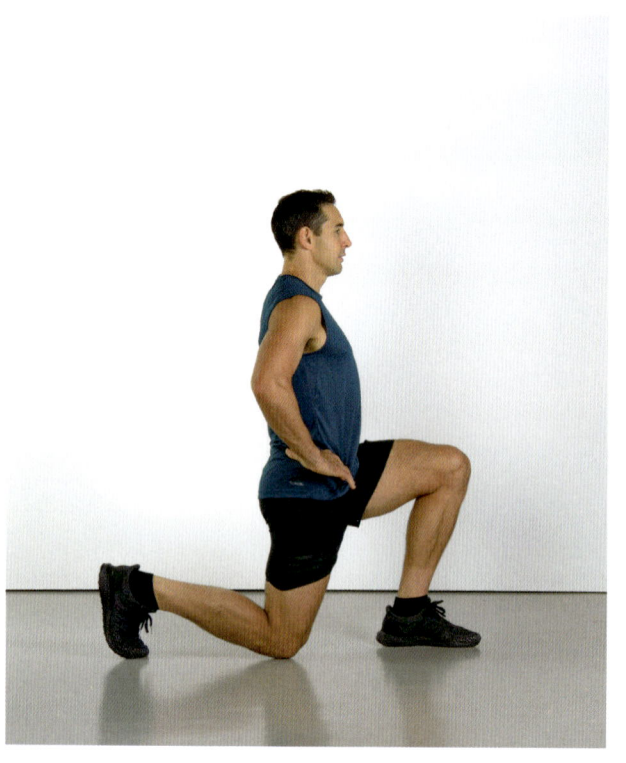

5 Reverse lunges

Stand with your feet shoulder-width apart and your hands on your hips. Step one leg back and then lower it until it is 90 degrees to the ground. Step forward to the starting position. Repeat on the other side to complete the movement.

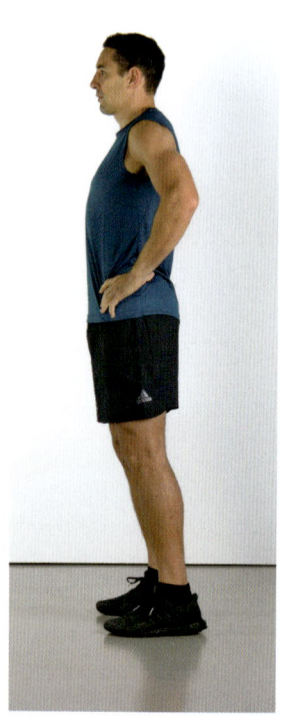 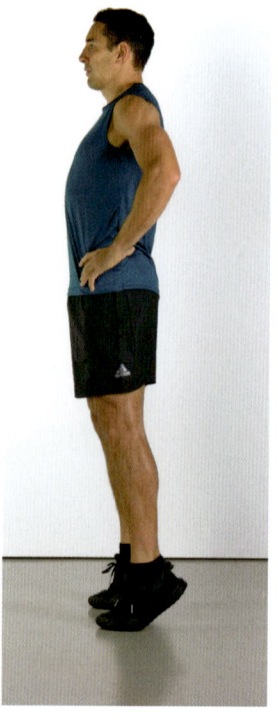

6 Calf raises

Stand with your feet shoulder-width apart and your hands on your hips. From here, slightly transfer your weight forward, taking your heels off the ground until you are on the balls of your feet. Lower yourself back down so your feet are flat on the ground.

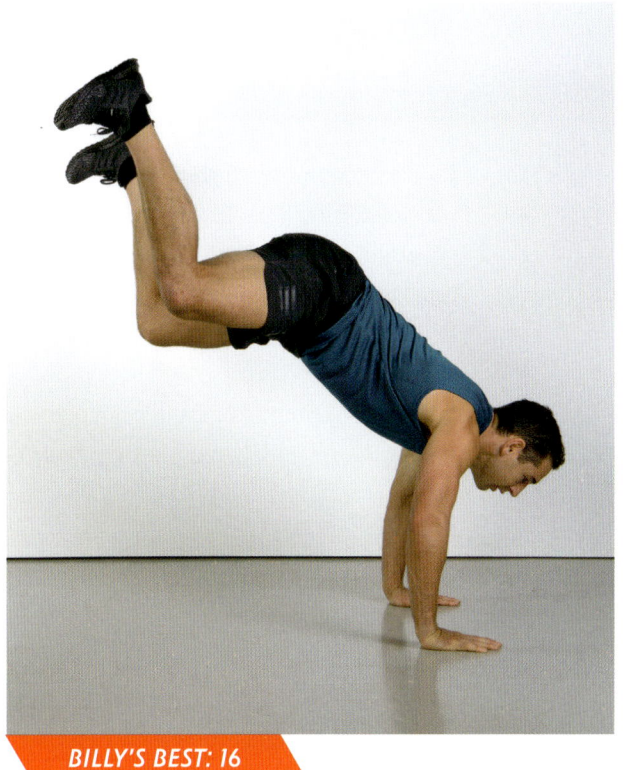

BILLY'S BEST: 16

7 Donkey kicks

Bend over and place your hands on the ground with your shoulders over your wrists. From here, bend your knees at a 90-degree angle and lean forward. Take your feet off the ground and then kick out your legs to a comfortable distance before returning to the starting position.

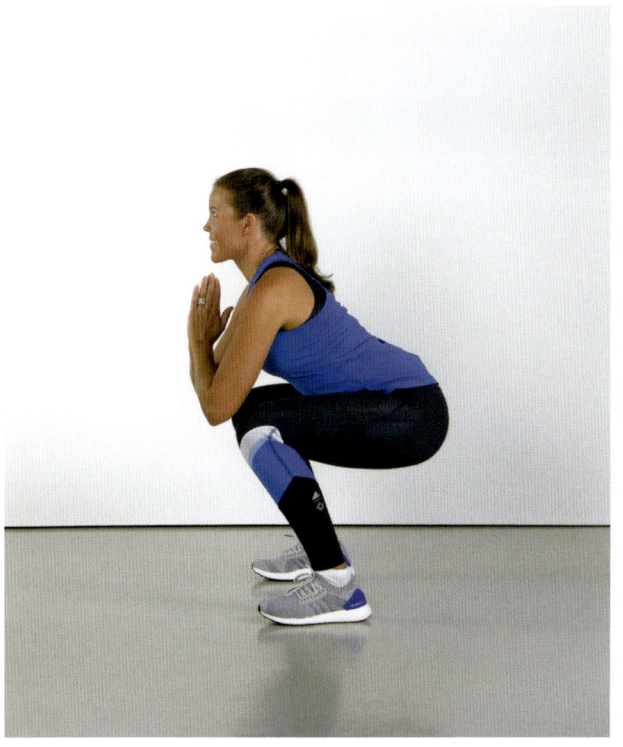

8 Squats

Stand with your feet just past shoulder-width apart and your feet slightly pointed outwards so your knees track with your feet. Bend at the hips, stick your butt out and bend your knees until they are at a 90-degree angle. Return to starting position.

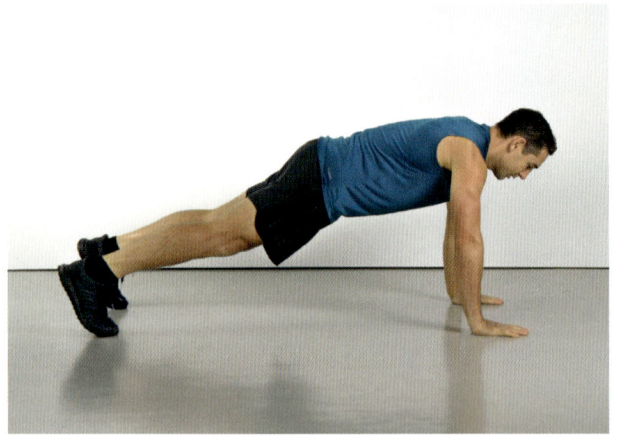

9 Burpees

Stand in a relaxed position with your feet shoulder-width apart. Squat and place your hands firmly on the ground with your feet back. Shoot your legs back so you are in a high plank position, then lower your body so your torso is just touching the ground. Release your hands and then, placing your hands back on the ground, raise your torso and jump your feet back so both hands and both feet are on the ground. Stand back up, then jump up and raise your hands above your head.

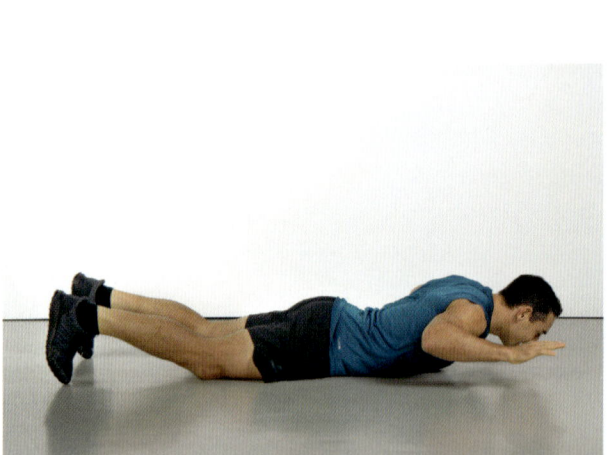

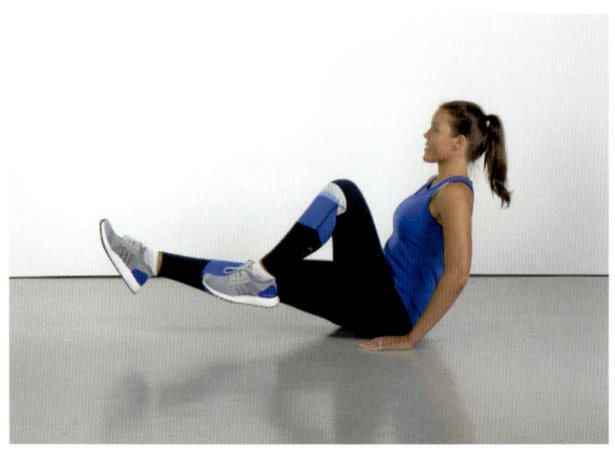

10 Bicycle kicks

Starting position is sitting on the ground with your hands slightly behind your butt. Raise both legs and move them in a cycling motion throughout the time allocated.

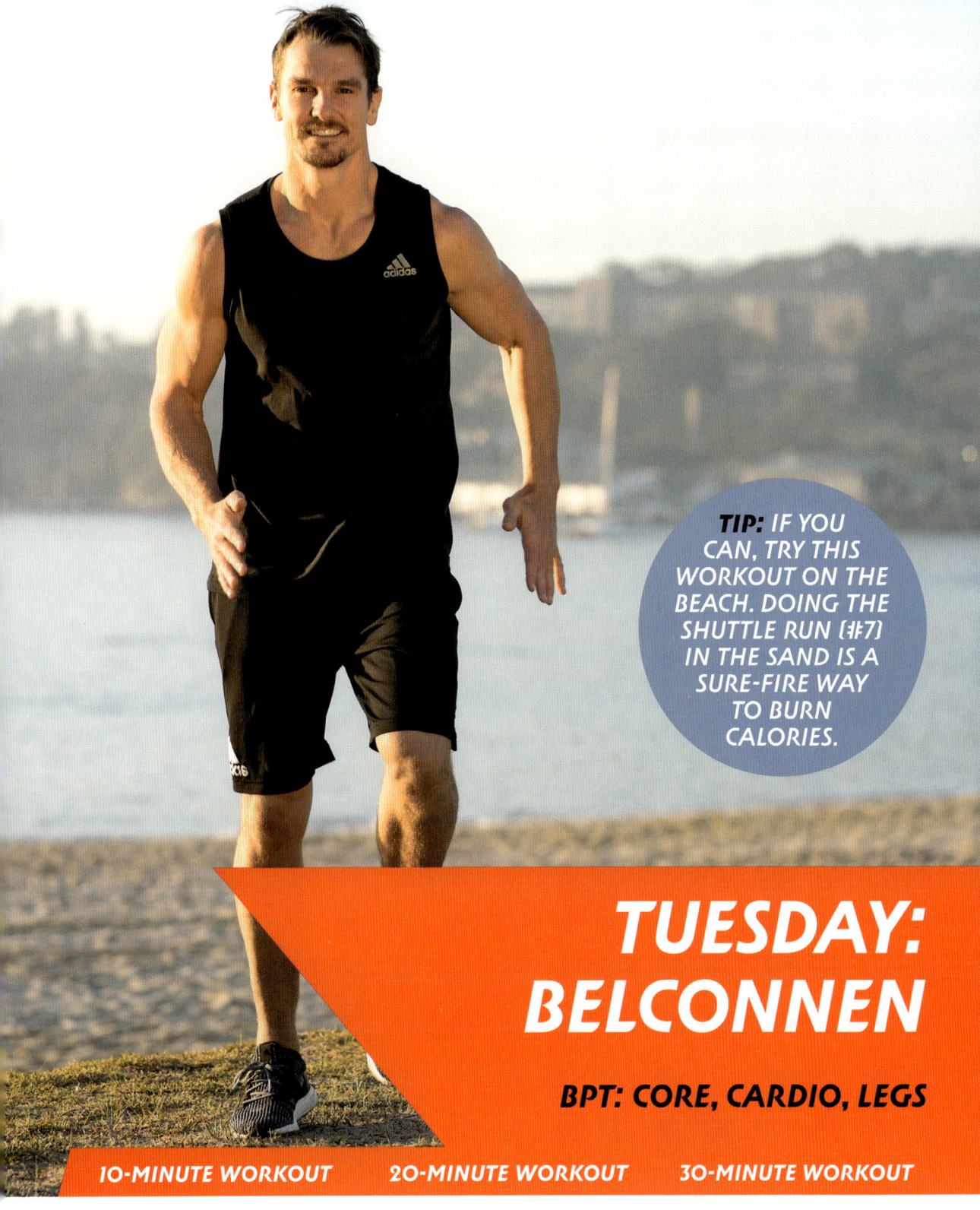

TIP: *IF YOU CAN, TRY THIS WORKOUT ON THE BEACH. DOING THE SHUTTLE RUN (#7) IN THE SAND IS A SURE-FIRE WAY TO BURN CALORIES.*

TUESDAY: BELCONNEN

BPT: CORE, CARDIO, LEGS

10-MINUTE WORKOUT	20-MINUTE WORKOUT	30-MINUTE WORKOUT
20 seconds movement / 10 seconds rest 2 sets of each exercise (one lap)	20 seconds movement / 10 seconds rest 2 sets of each exercise (two laps)	20 seconds movement / 10 seconds rest 2 sets of each exercise (three laps)

BLOCK 5: AUSTRALIAN CAPITAL TERRITORY

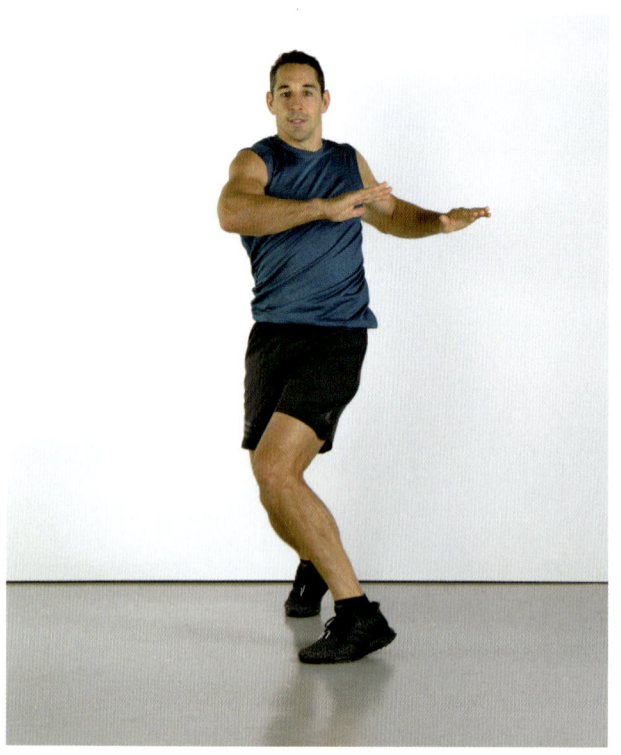

1   2 x torsion twists, 1 x jump squat

For the torsion twists, stand with your feet shoulder-width apart and your arms out nice and wide at shoulder height. Slightly jump to your right, twisting your left hip to your right side and keeping your chest forward. Now come back to the starting position. Repeat on the other side.

For the squat, stand with your feet just past shoulder-width apart and your feet slightly pointed outwards so your knees track with your feet. Hinging at the hips, stick your butt out and bend your knees until they are at a 90-degree angle. Jump up either right or left 90 degrees (or 180 degrees for advanced). Repeat for one full circle going clockwise, and then go anticlockwise for one full circle.

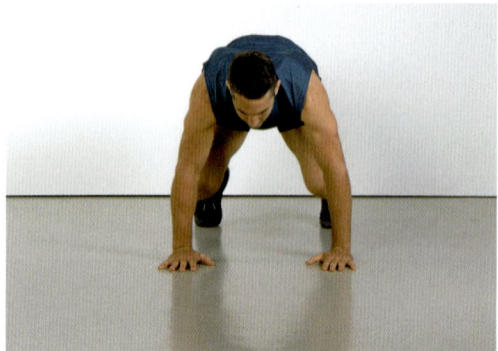

2   Lateral shoot-throughs

Start in high plank position with your hands firmly on the ground and your shoulders above your wrists. Bend your knees at a 90-degree angle and have your toes firmly on the ground and your knees off the ground. This is the starting position. Now turn your left foot so it is flat on the ground. Kick your right foot in front of your left foot and out to the side, so your right leg is now straight and your left foot is firmly on the ground. Now pull your right leg back to the starting position. Repeat on the other side.

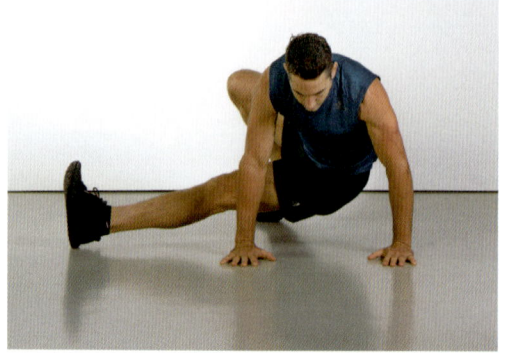

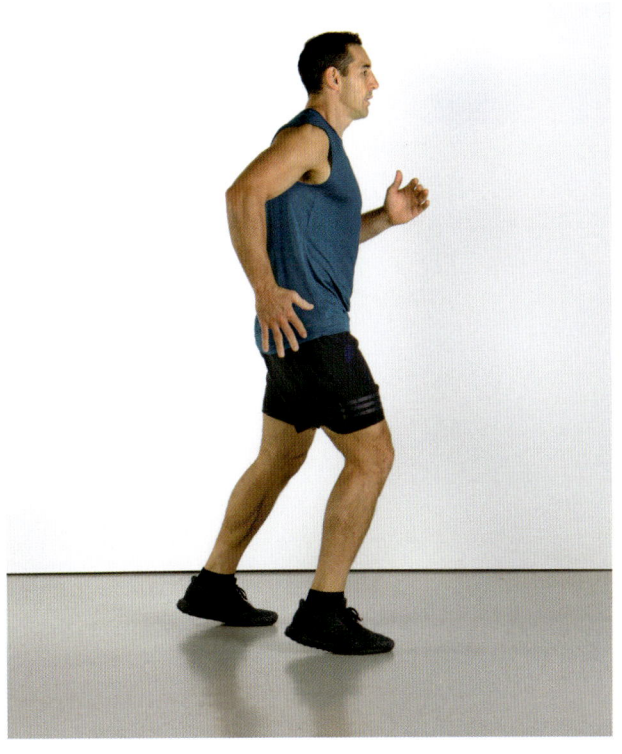

3 **4 x shuffles, 2 x plyometric split lunges**

For the shuffles, stand with your feet shoulder-width apart and your hands on your hips. Split your feet so your back toe is in line with your front heel. Alternate four times.

3.1 For the plyometric split lunges, start with your feet shoulder-width apart and your hands on your hips. Split your legs before dropping your back knee down in line with the heel of your leading foot – both legs should be at a 90-degree angle – then push up and repeat on the other side.

3.2 Alternatively, stand with your feet shoulder-width apart and your hands on your hips. Step one leg back and then lower it until it is 90 degrees to the ground. Step forward to the starting position. Repeat on the other side to complete the movement.

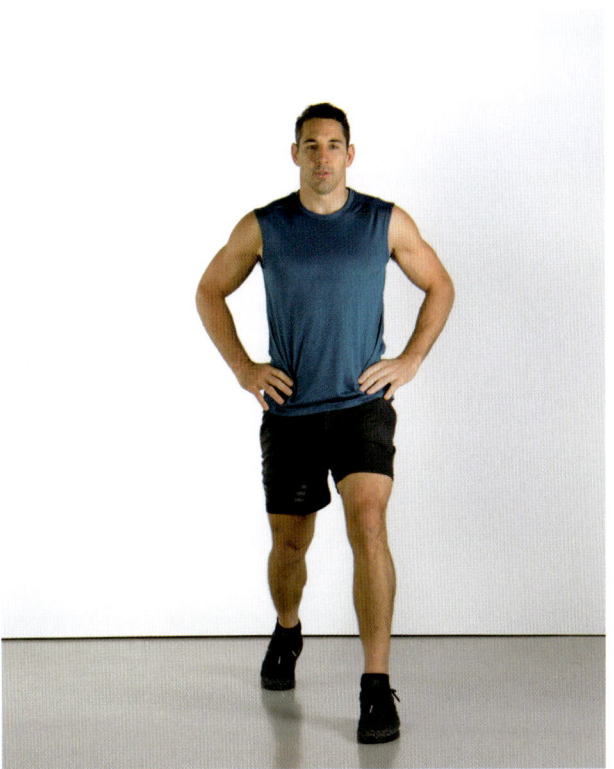

4 **Duck walks**

Stand with your feet just past shoulder-width apart and slightly tracked out. Bend at the hips, squat as low as you can go. From here, take two steps forward and two steps back.

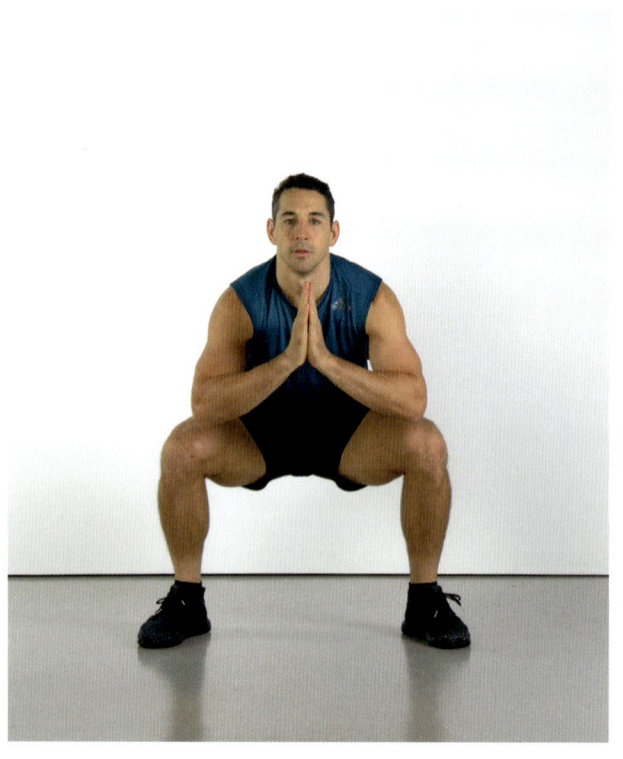

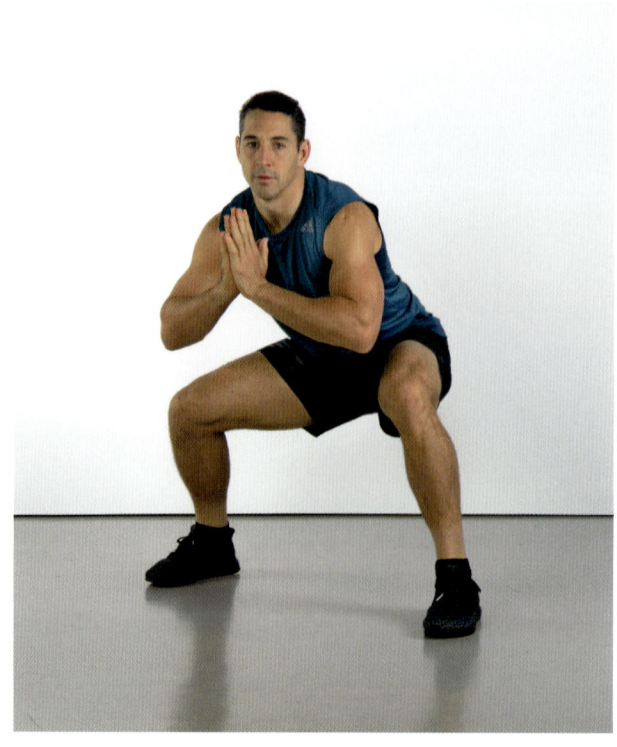

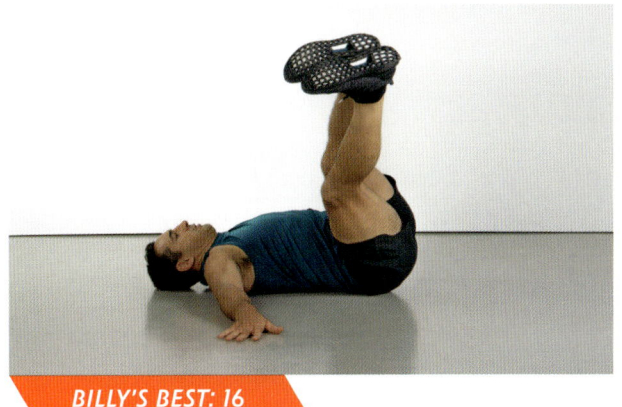

BILLY'S BEST: 16

5   **Windscreen wipers**

Starting position is lying on the ground with your legs raised up straight and your arms by your sides. Rotate your hips and bring your legs down to one side without letting your shoulders lift off the ground. Squeezing your core, bring your legs back to the starting position. Repeat on the other side.

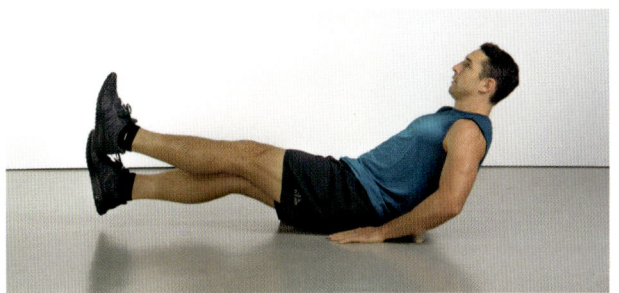

6   **Flutter kicks**

Starting position is lying on your back with your thumbs tucked under your lower lumbar (base of your back) on either side of your body. Raise your legs and kick them up and down in a small fluttering motion, engaging your core.

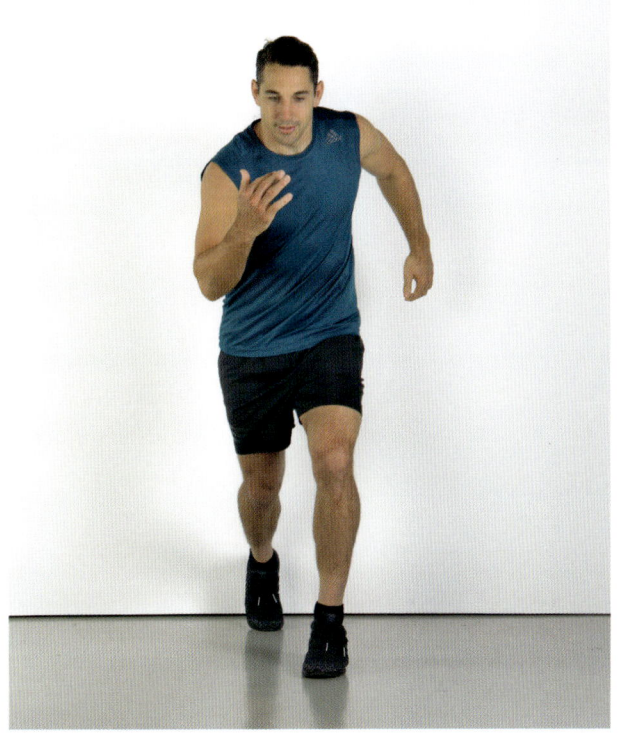

7   **Shuttle run**

Picking a distance that suits your environment, run up and back for the duration of time.

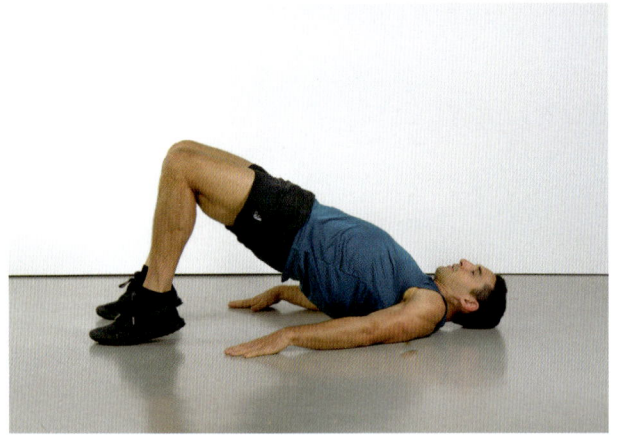

8   Double-glute bridge

Lie on your back with your hands on your hips or with your arms straight on the ground and your palms facing down. Bring your heels as close as you can to your butt, raising your hips and pressing down on the balls of your feet. Squeeze your butt cheeks (glutes) for the allocated time before lowering yourself down. Don't allow yourself to collapse – stay tight through your core and make sure your butt doesn't hit the ground.

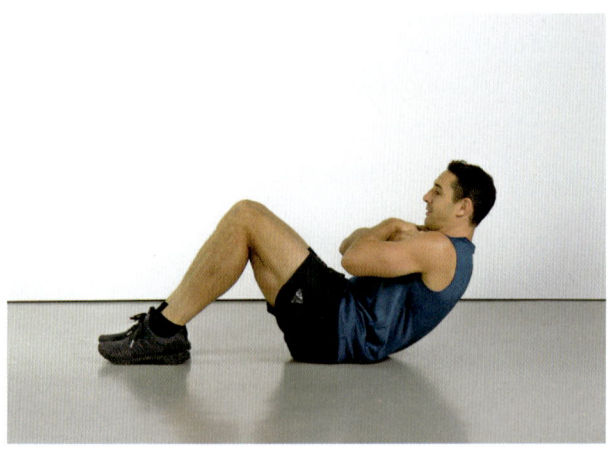

9   Sit-ups

Lie on your back, bend your legs and place your feet firmly on the ground to stabilise your lower body. Cross your arms over your chest, then curl your upper body all the way up to touch your knees. Slowly lower yourself down to return to the starting point.

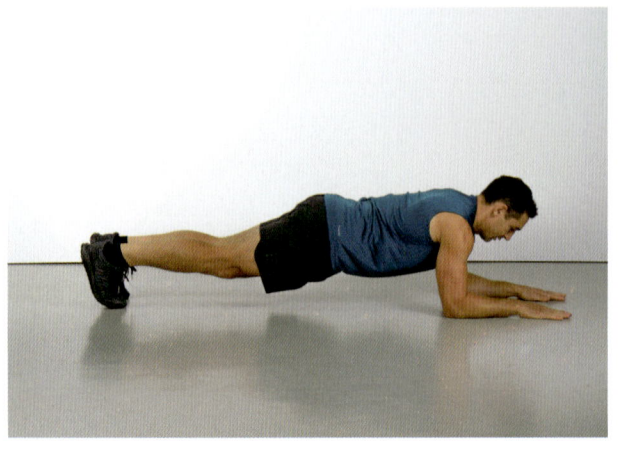

10   Plank hold

Lie with your forearms on the ground, your knees off the ground and your feet together with your toes touching the ground. From here, lean slightly forward to engage your core. Hold the position for the duration of time. (Note: Your back should not be sagging or bent.)

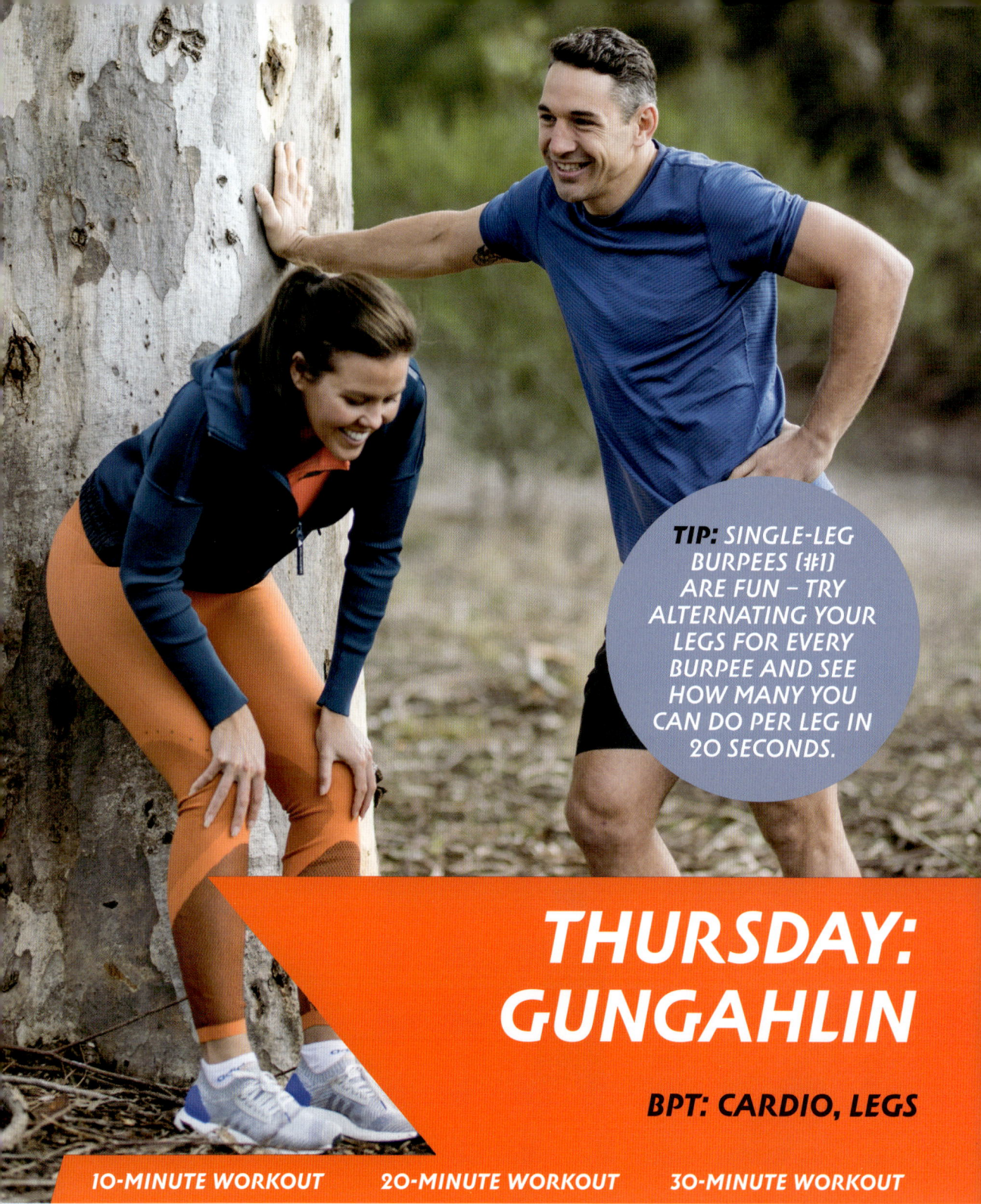

TIP: SINGLE-LEG BURPEES (#1) ARE FUN – TRY ALTERNATING YOUR LEGS FOR EVERY BURPEE AND SEE HOW MANY YOU CAN DO PER LEG IN 20 SECONDS.

THURSDAY: GUNGAHLIN

BPT: CARDIO, LEGS

10-MINUTE WORKOUT	20-MINUTE WORKOUT	30-MINUTE WORKOUT
20 seconds movement / 10 seconds rest 2 sets of each exercise (one lap)	20 seconds movement / 10 seconds rest 2 sets of each exercise (two laps)	20 seconds movement / 10 seconds rest 2 sets of each exercise (three laps)

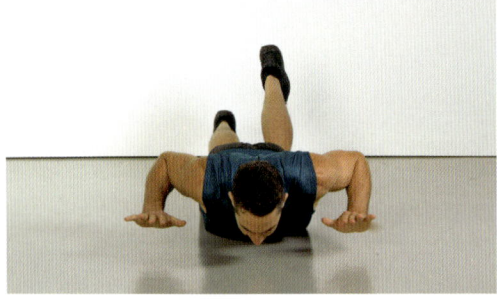

1. Single-leg burpees

Stand in a relaxed position with your feet shoulder-width apart. Squat and place your hands firmly on the ground with your feet back. Shoot your legs back so you are in a high plank position with one leg off the ground, then lower your body so your torso is just touching the ground. Release your hands and then, placing your hands back on the ground, raise your torso and jump your feet forward, keeping the one leg off the ground throughout the whole movement. Stand back up, then jump up and raise your hands above your head.

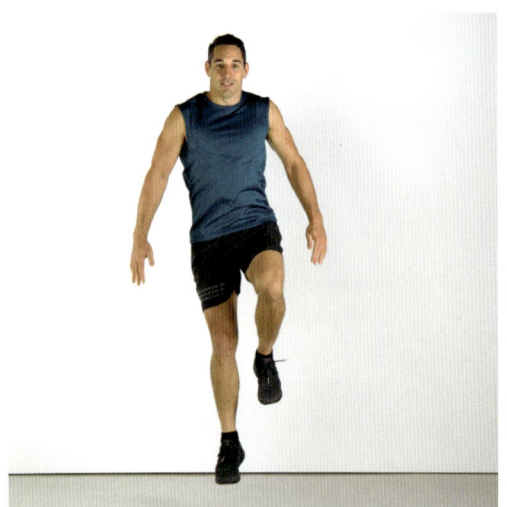

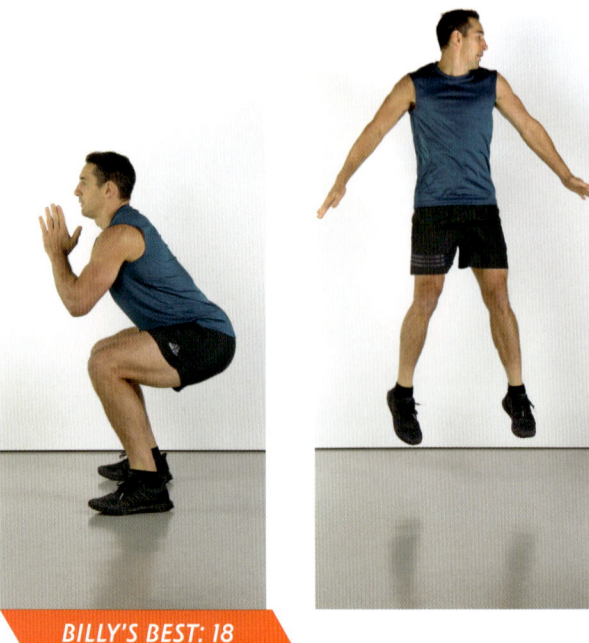

2. 180-degree jump squats

Stand with your feet just past shoulder-width apart and your feet pointed slightly outwards so your knees track with your feet. Bend at the hips, stick your butt out and bend your knees until they are at a 90-degree angle. Jump up either right or left 180 degrees. Repeat for one full circle going clockwise, and then go anticlockwise for one full circle.

BILLY'S BEST: 18

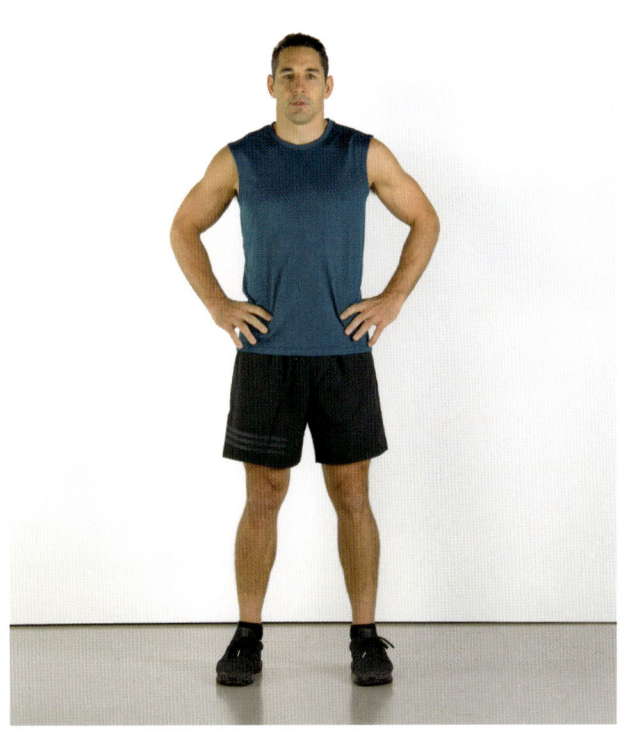

3 Forward lunges

Stand with your feet shoulder-width apart and your hands on your hips. Step one leg forward and lower your back leg to a 90-degree position so your knee is in line with the heel of your leading foot. Step back to the starting position and then repeat on the other side to complete the movement.

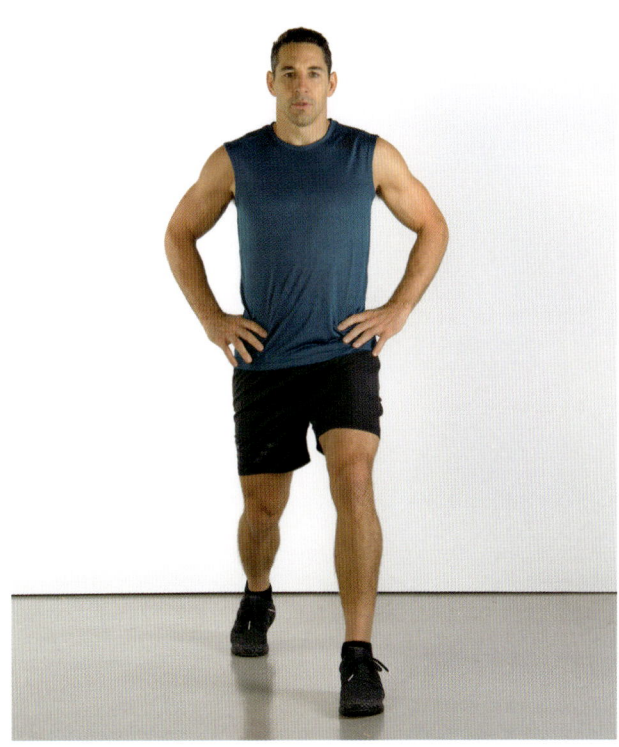

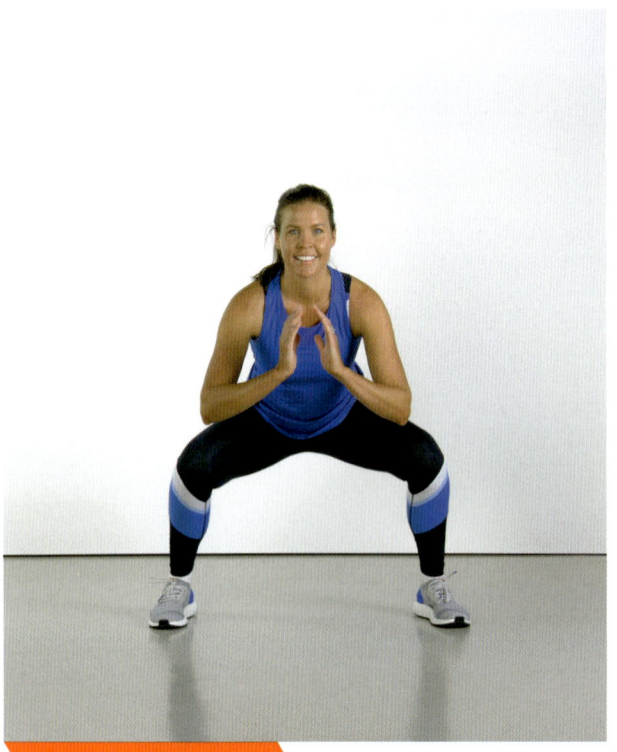

4 **In/out jump squats**

Stand with your feet just past shoulder-width apart and your hands touching in front of your chest. Squat so your knees are bent and arms are straight and out to the side. Then explode up, bringing your feet together and your arms out to your sides before returning to the starting position.

NICOLE'S BEST: 14

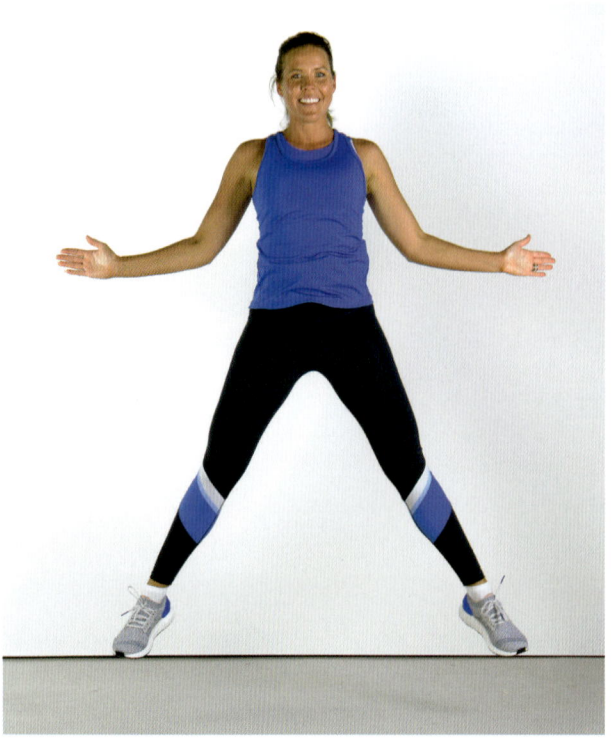

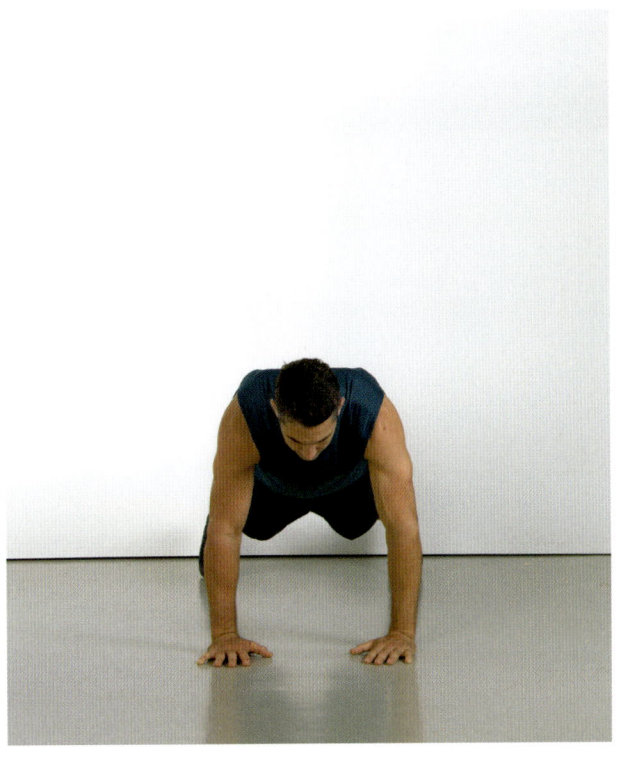

5 Plank rotations

Starting in modified or full plank position, lift one arm off the ground and hold for the allotted time before returning to full plank. Repeat using the other arm.

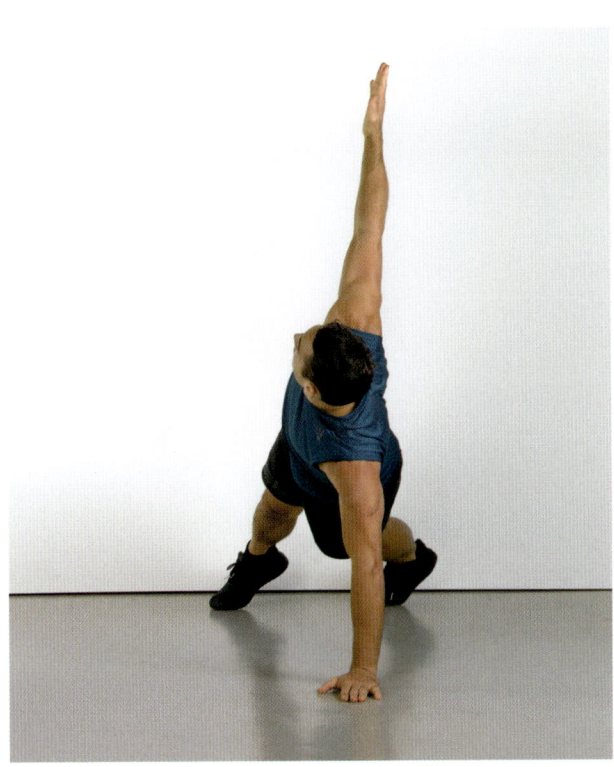

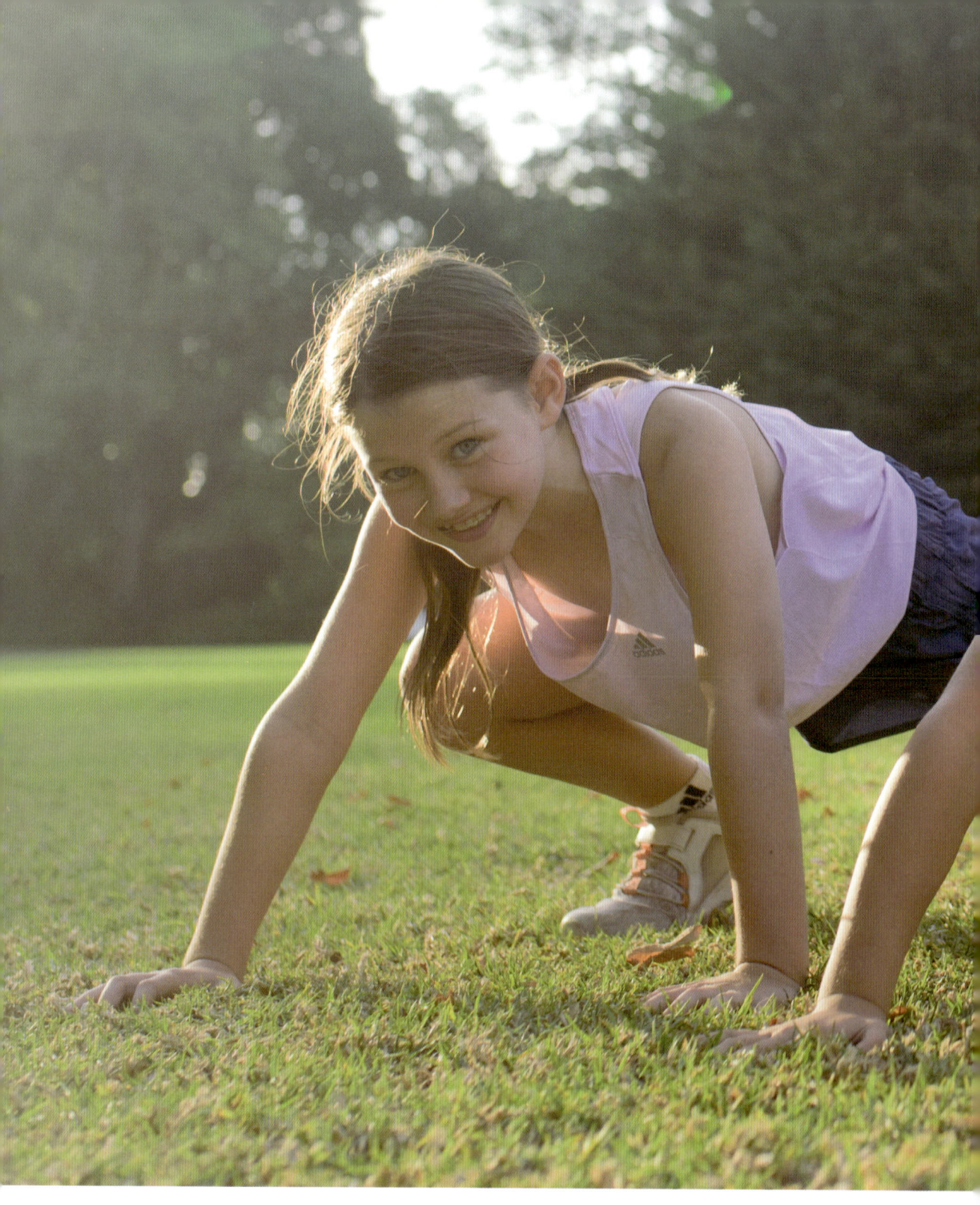

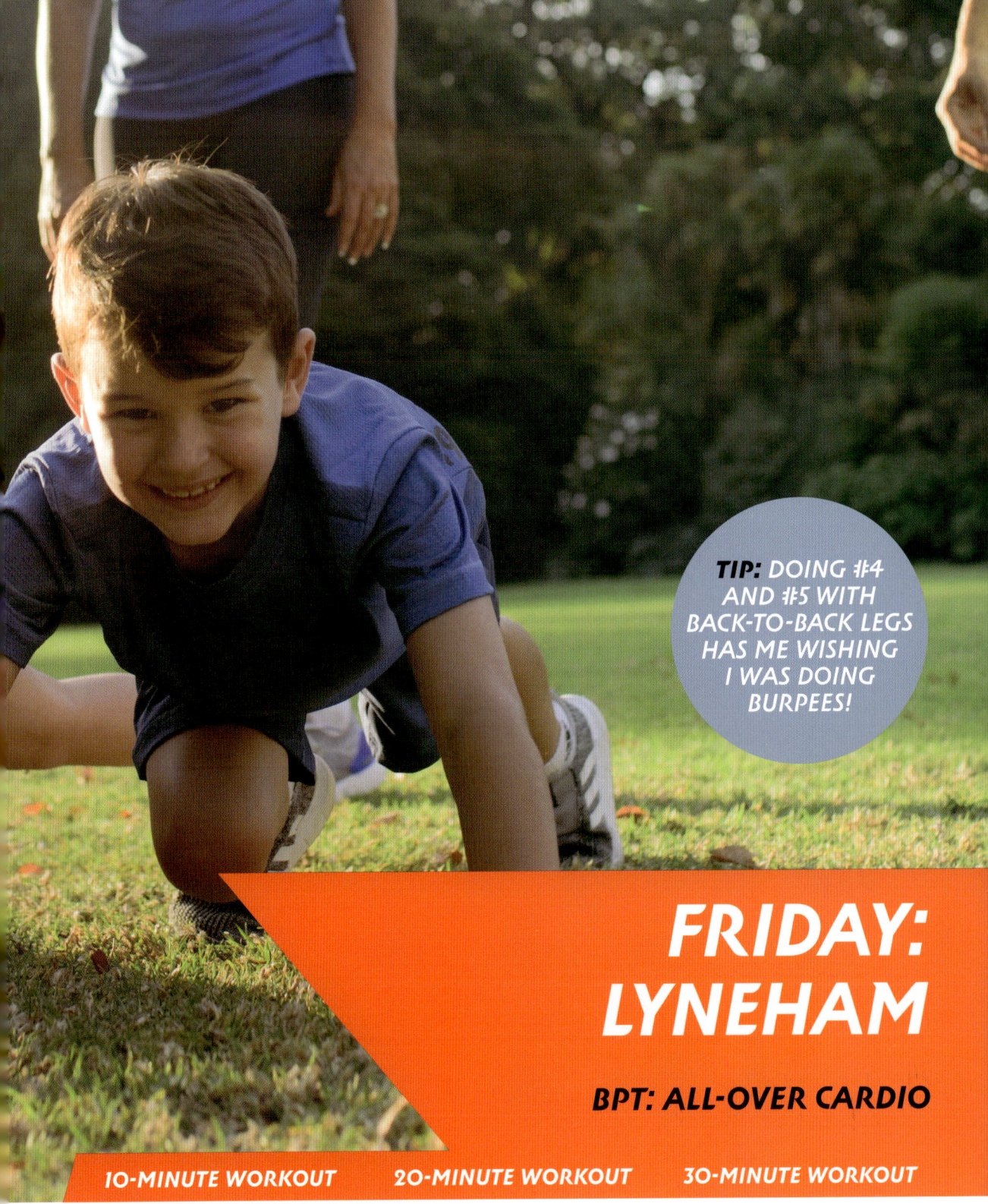

TIP: DOING #4 AND #5 WITH BACK-TO-BACK LEGS HAS ME WISHING I WAS DOING BURPEES!

FRIDAY: LYNEHAM

BPT: ALL-OVER CARDIO

10-MINUTE WORKOUT

20 seconds movement /
10 seconds rest
2 sets of each exercise
(one lap)

20-MINUTE WORKOUT

20 seconds movement /
10 seconds rest
2 sets of each exercise
(two laps)

30-MINUTE WORKOUT

20 seconds movement /
10 seconds rest
2 sets of each exercise
(three laps)

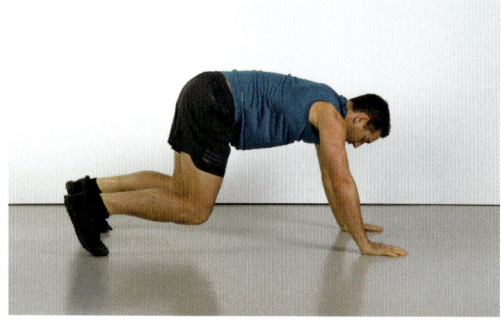

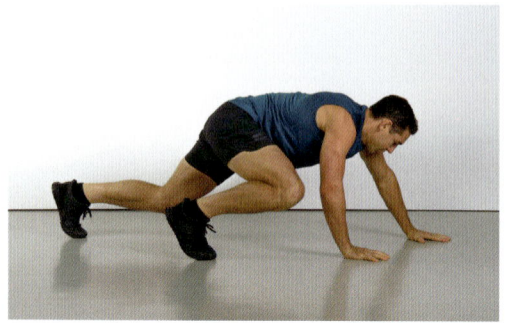

1 Bear crawl

Start in the push-up position with your knees bent at a 90-degree angle and positioned directly under your hips. Engage your core and do not raise or round your back. This is your starting position. Walk your right hand and your left foot forward, and then your left hand and your right foot forward. Continue until you reach 5 metres. Now, keeping your hips down and your core engaged, reverse the movement by walking your left arm and your right foot back, and then your right arm and your left leg back. Continue until you have returned to your starting position.

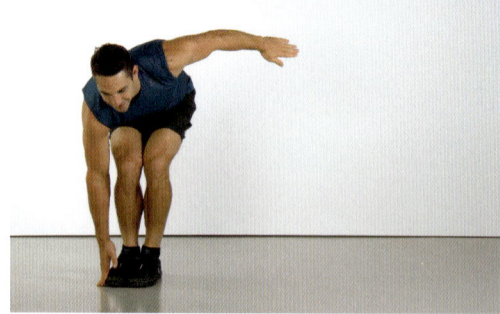

2 Slalom taps

Start with your feet together, then jump to the left to land on both feet, touching your left hand down next to your left foot. Then jump to the right with both feet, touching your right hand to your right foot.

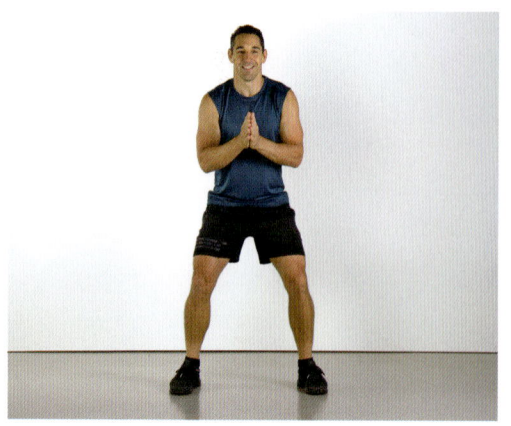

3 Seal jacks

Starting in a relaxed position with your hands touching together in the middle of your chest, jump out so your feet are in a wide stance and your arms split. Bring your feet and hands back together.

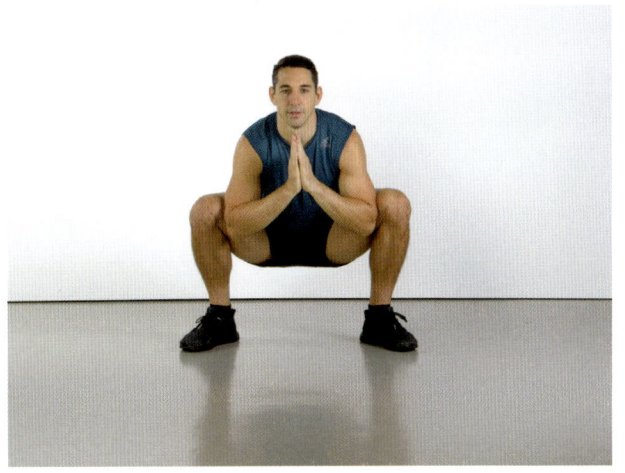

4 Frog squats

Stand with your feet shoulder-width apart and your feet slightly tracked out. Bend down to full squat position with your elbows tucked inside your legs. This is the starting position. From here, raise your hips and then lower them back to the starting position.

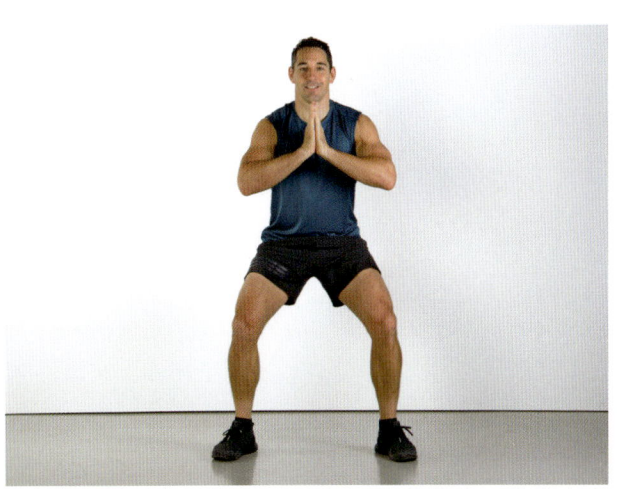

5 Pulse squats

Stand with your feet just past shoulder-width apart and slightly tracked out. Squat with your hips back and your legs at a 90-degree angle, then pulse up and down.

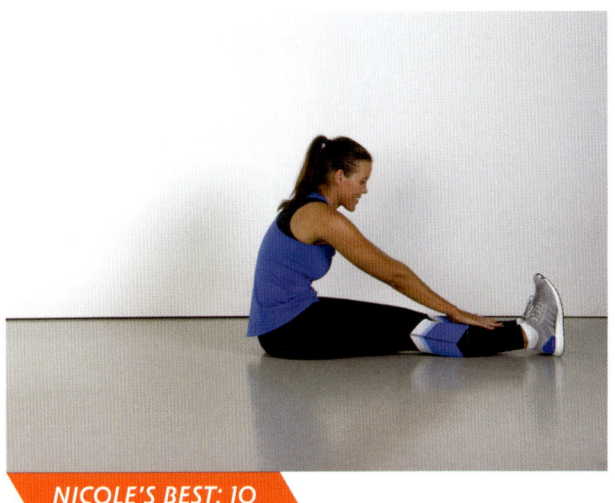

6 Straight-leg sit-ups

Lie flat on the ground with your arms by your sides. Lifting your head up and engaging your core, reach towards your toes, keeping your arms and legs straight. Return to the starting position.

NICOLE'S BEST: 10

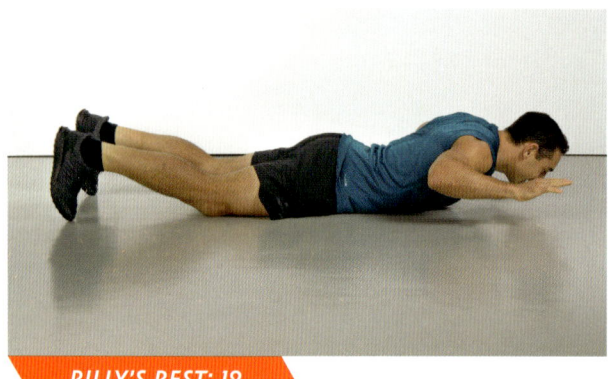

BILLY'S BEST: 12

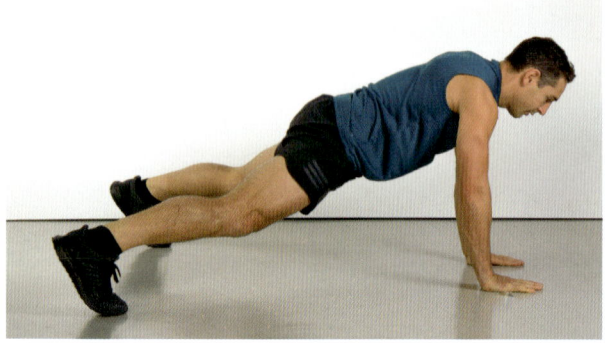

7 **Burpees**

Stand in a relaxed position with your feet shoulder-width apart. Squat and place your hands firmly on the ground with your feet back. Shoot your legs back so you are in a high plank position, then lower your body so your torso is just touching the ground. Release your hands and then, placing your hands back on the ground, raise your torso and jump your feet back so both hands and both feet are on the ground. Stand back up, then jump up and raise your hands above your head.

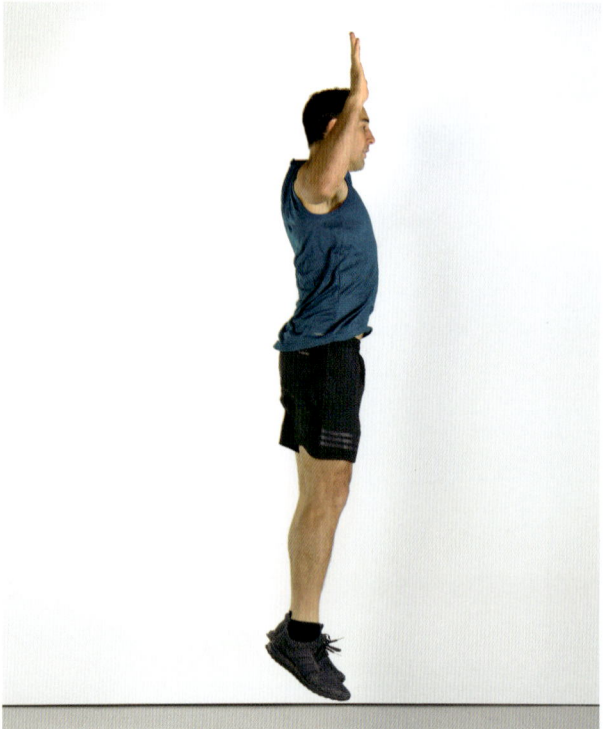

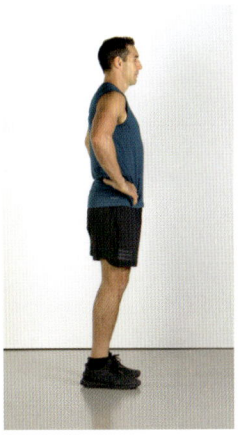 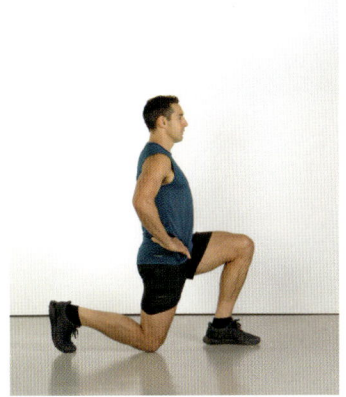

8   1 x squat, 2 x reverse lunges

For the squat, stand with your feet just past shoulder-width apart and your feet slightly pointed outwards so your knees track with your feet. Hinging at the hips, stick your butt out and bend your knees until they are at a 90-degree angle.

For the reverse lunges, stand with your feet shoulder-width apart and your hands on your hips. Step one leg back and then lower it until it is 90 degrees to the ground. Step forward to the starting position. Repeat on the other side to complete the movement.

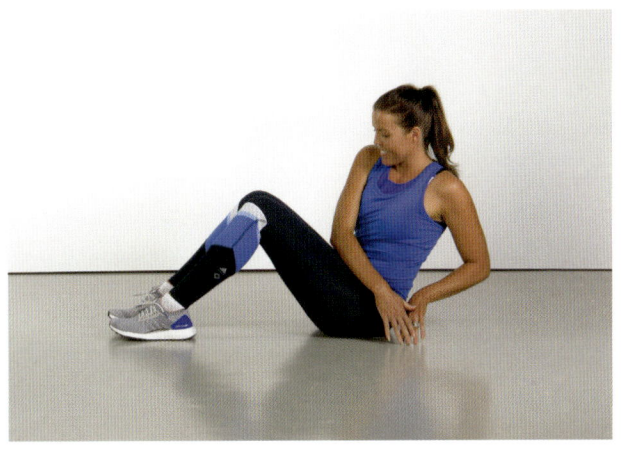

9   Russian twists

Sit on the ground with your knees bent and your feet flat on the ground. Clasping your hands in front of your chest, twist your torso to one side and touch the ground, engaging your core. Then shift your weight and twist your torso to touch the ground on the other side.

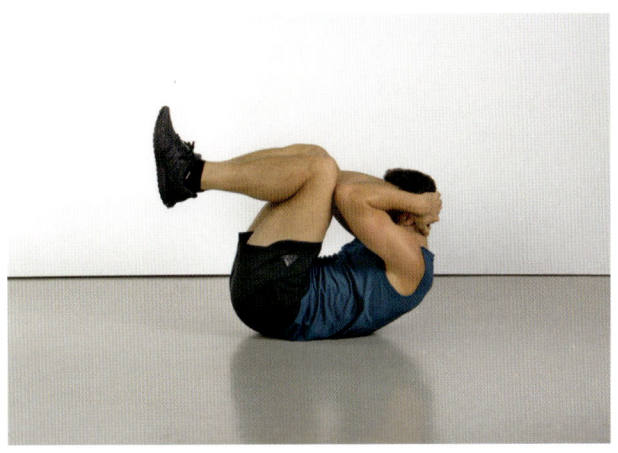

10   Crunches

Lie on your back with your legs off the ground, with knees bent at a 90-degree angle to your body. With your hands crossed behind your head, bring your elbows in next to your ears. Bring your elbows up to your knees and then return to the starting position.

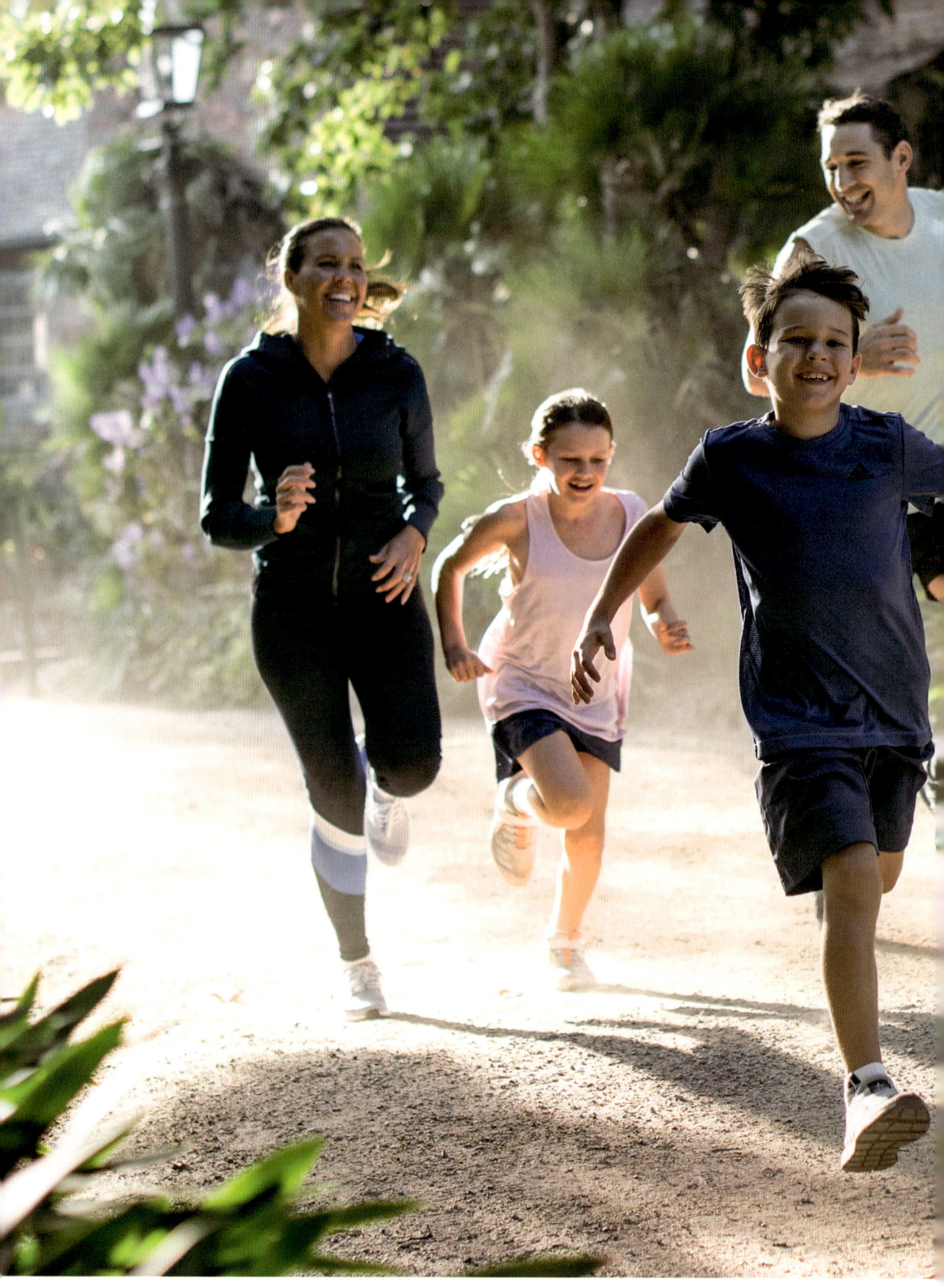

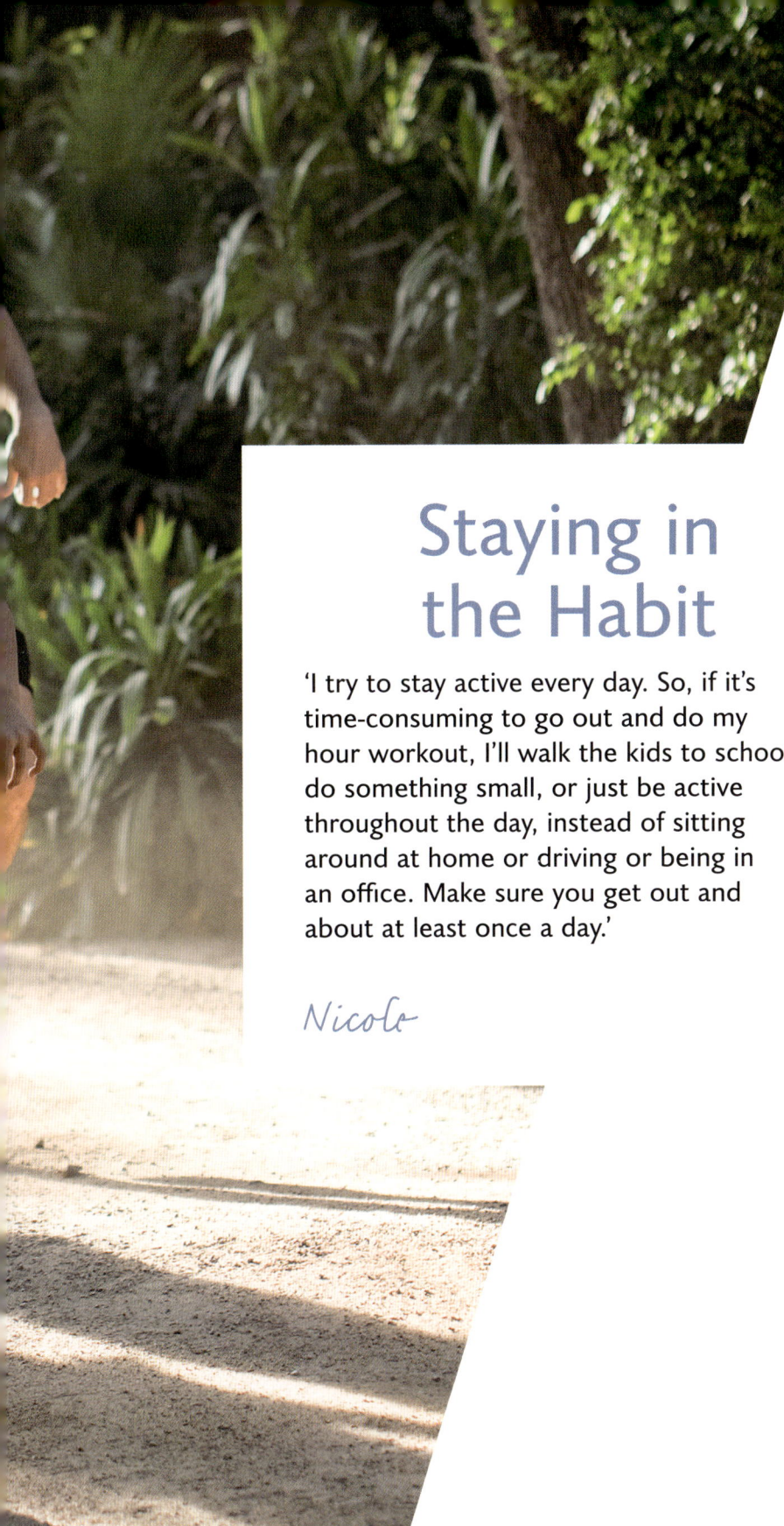

Staying in the Habit

'I try to stay active every day. So, if it's time-consuming to go out and do my hour workout, I'll walk the kids to school, do something small, or just be active throughout the day, instead of sitting around at home or driving or being in an office. Make sure you get out and about at least once a day.'

Nicole

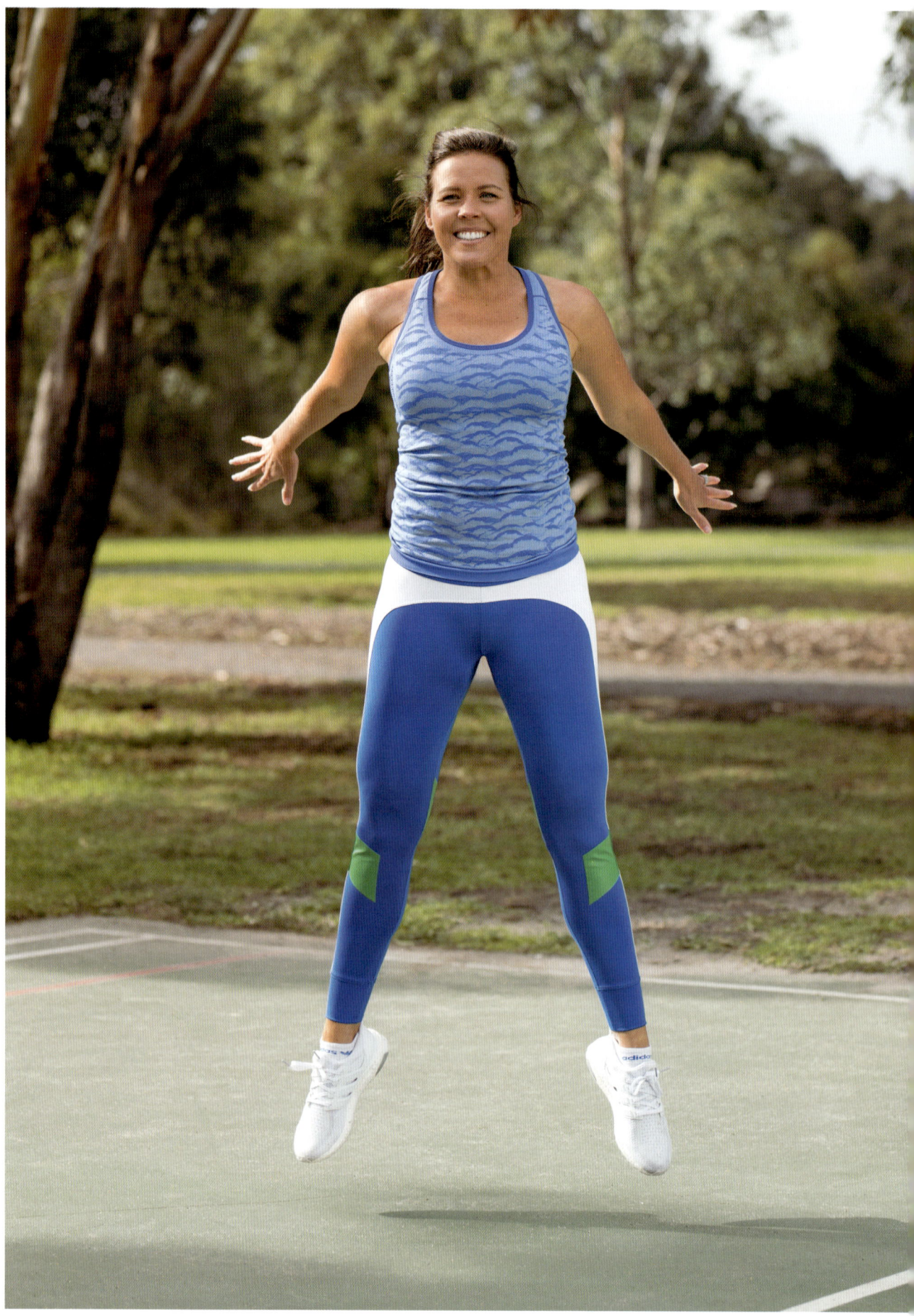

BLOCK 6: VICTORIA

'Nicole, the kids and myself have become very settled here and love calling it our home. As a family, we take every opportunity to get outside into a park, take our dog Buddy for a walk or go for a bike ride. We move outside as much as possible and share a bunch of great times as a family.'

Billy

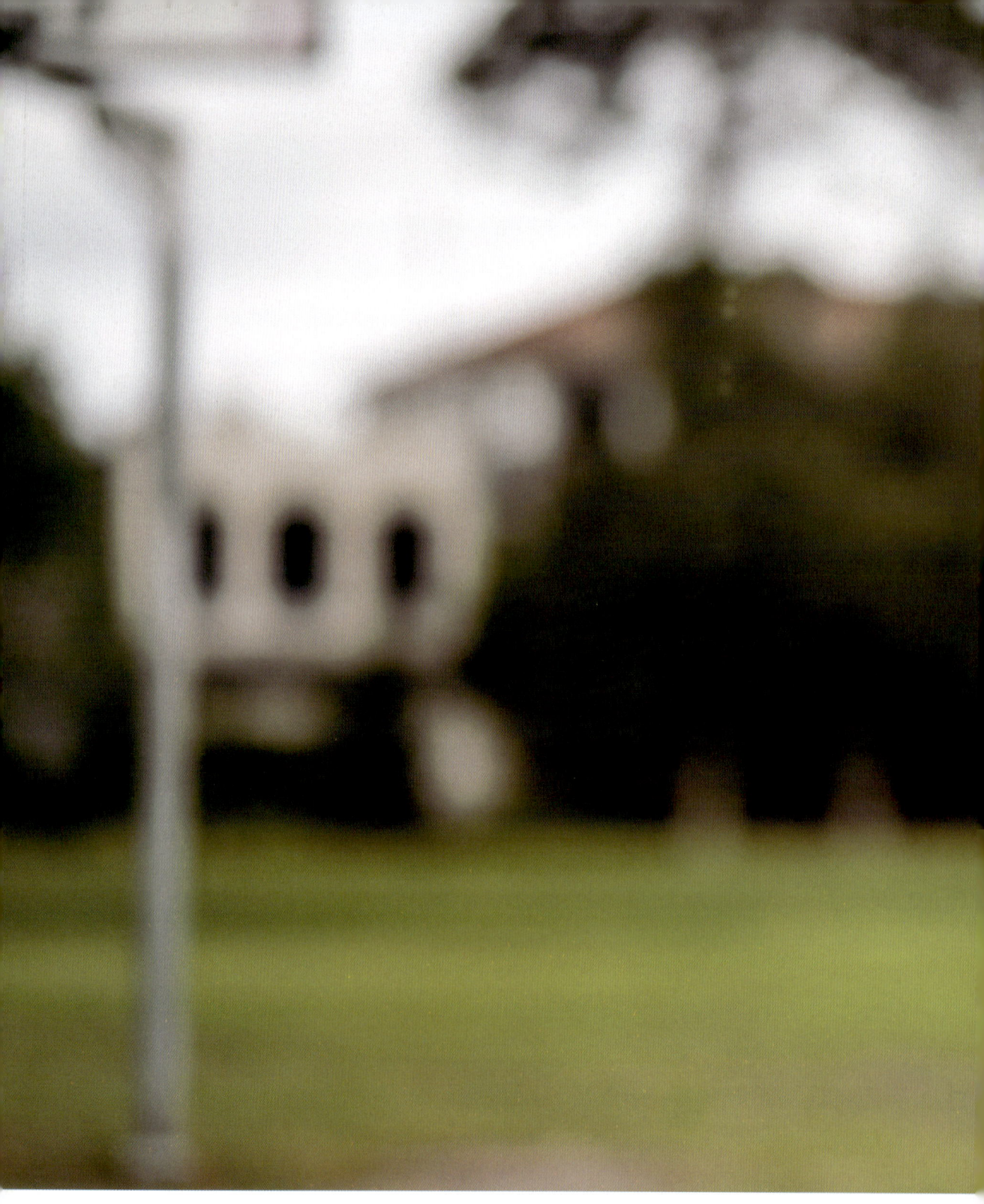

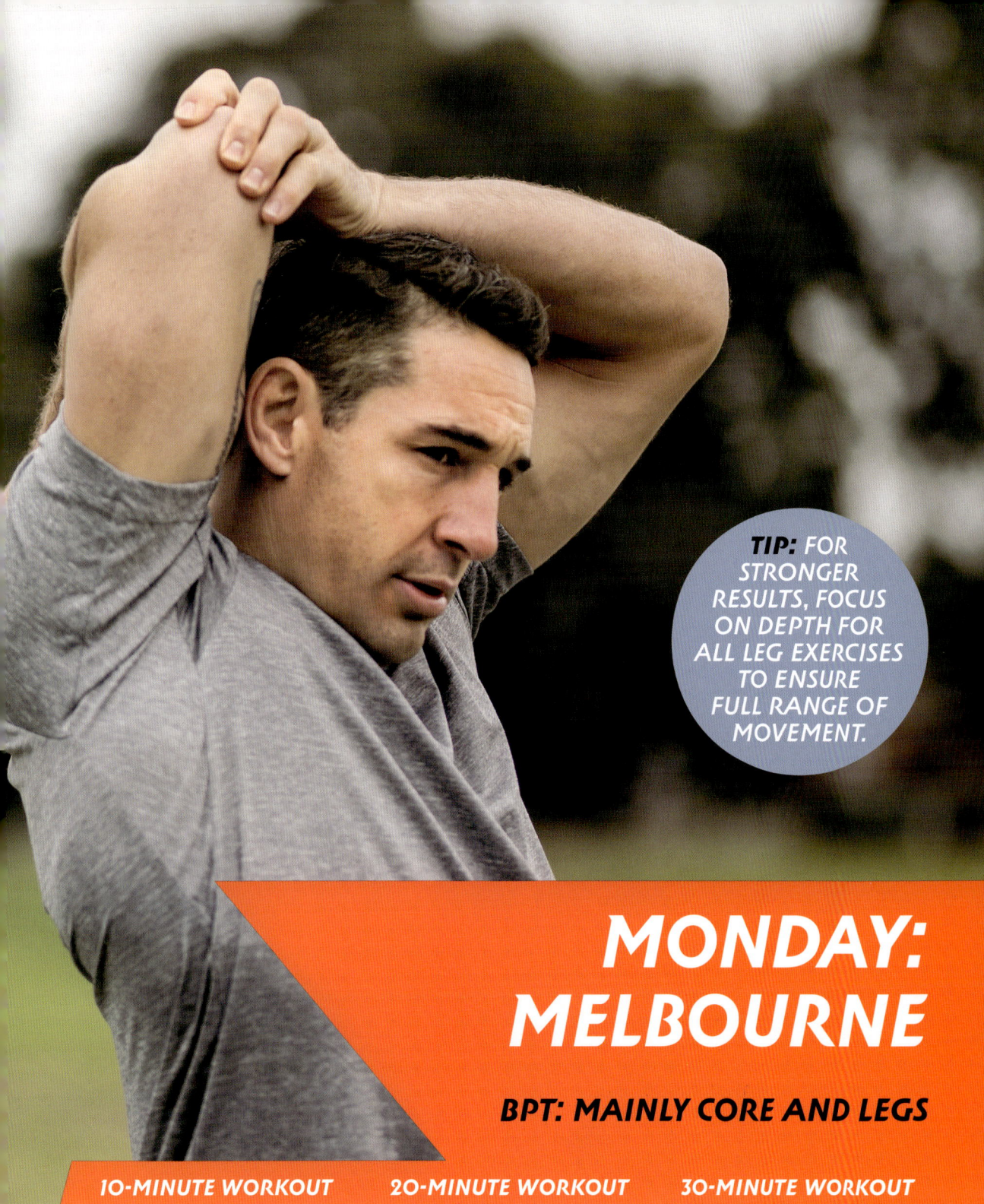

TIP: FOR STRONGER RESULTS, FOCUS ON DEPTH FOR ALL LEG EXERCISES TO ENSURE FULL RANGE OF MOVEMENT.

MONDAY: MELBOURNE

BPT: MAINLY CORE AND LEGS

10-MINUTE WORKOUT

20 seconds movement /
10 seconds rest
2 sets of each exercise
(one lap)

20-MINUTE WORKOUT

20 seconds movement /
10 seconds rest
2 sets of each exercise
(two laps)

30-MINUTE WORKOUT

20 seconds movement /
10 seconds rest
2 sets of each exercise
(three laps)

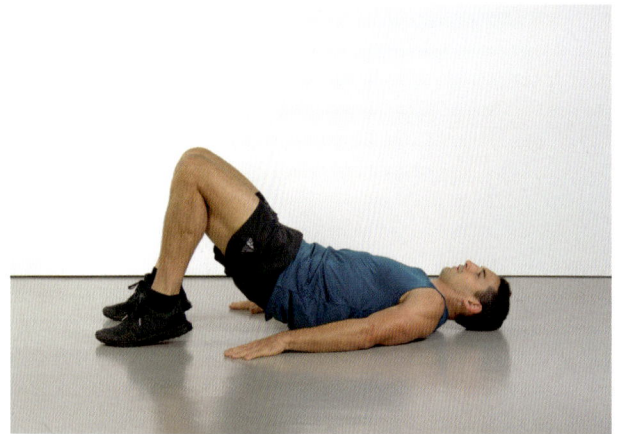

1. **Double-leg glute bridge**
   Lie on your back with your hands on your hips or with your arms straight or beside your body on the ground and your palms facing down. Bring your heels as close as you can to your butt, raising your hips and pressing down on the balls of your feet. Squeeze your butt cheeks (glutes) before lowering yourself down. Don't allow yourself to collapse – stay tight through your core and make sure your butt doesn't hit the ground.

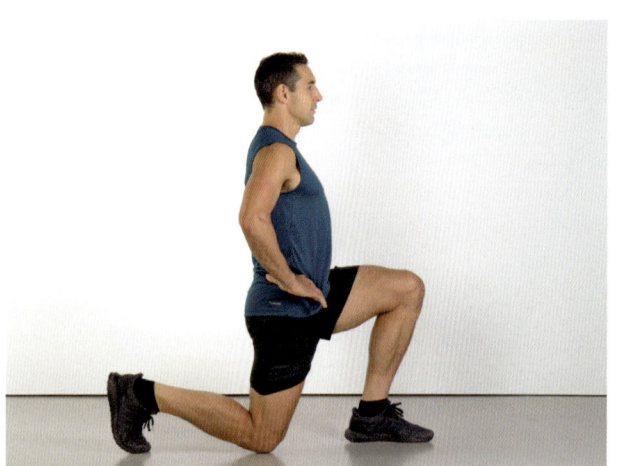

2. **Reverse lunges**
   Stand with your feet shoulder-width apart and your hands on your hips. Step one leg back and then lower it until it is 90 degrees to the ground. Step forward to the starting position. Repeat on the other side to complete the movement.

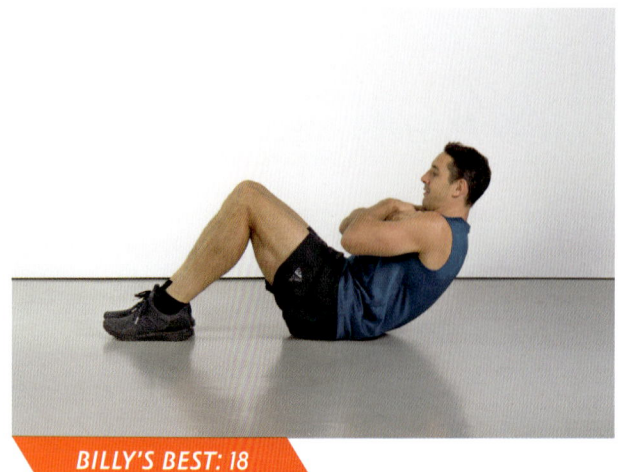

3. **Sit-ups**
   Lie on your back, bend your legs and place your feet firmly on the ground to stabilise your lower body. Cross your arms over your chest, then curl your upper body all the way up to touch your knees. Slowly lower yourself down to return to the starting point.

BILLY'S BEST: 18

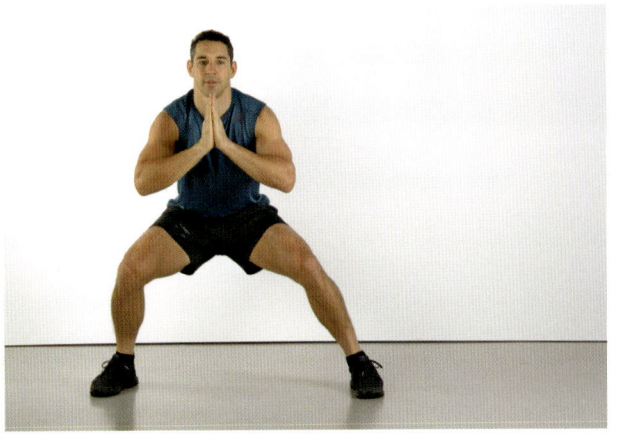

4 Crab walks

Stand with your feet shoulder-width apart and bend at the hips to come down into a squatting position. With your hands in front of your chest and staying low, step two to your left and then two to your right. Try to stay low throughout the time allocated.

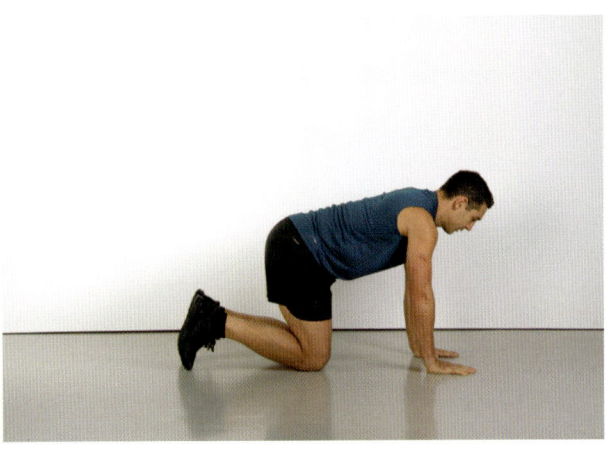

5 Contralateral limb raises

Place your hands, knees and toes firmly on the ground. From here, raise one arm and the opposite leg. Kick the leg out straight, squeezing your core, and then return to the starting position. Repeat on the other side.

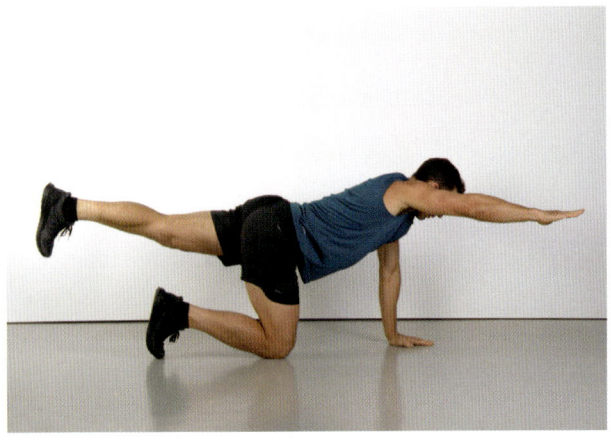

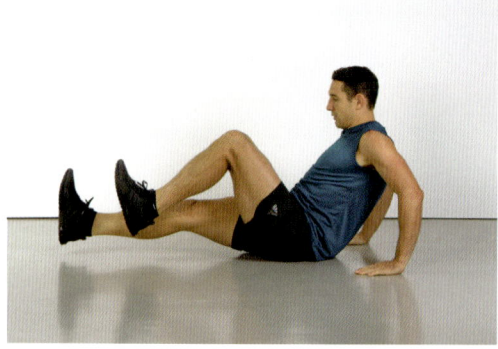

6 Bicycle crunches

Start by sitting on the ground with your hands on the floor by your side and your legs extended in front of you. From here, lean back, engaging your core so your feet are off the ground. Now bring one knee towards your chest, keeping the other leg straight. Return your knee to the earlier position and swap to bring your other knee towards your chest.

Advanced: Take your hands off the ground and bring the opposite elbow to your knee.

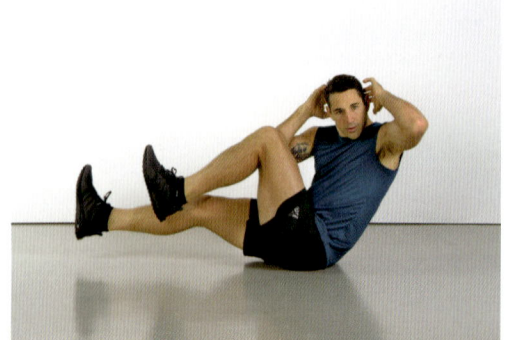

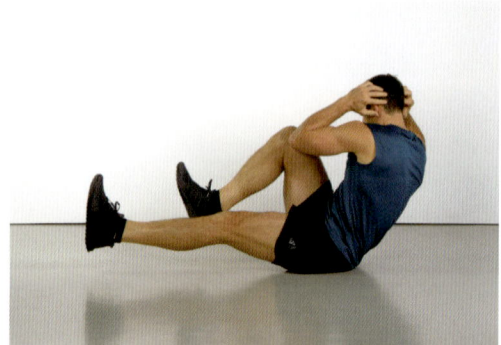

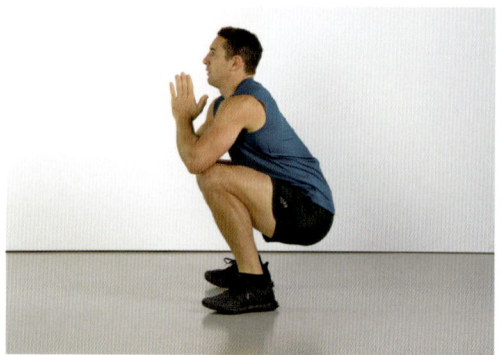

7 Squats

Stand with your feet just past shoulder-width apart and your feet slightly pointed outwards so your knees track with your feet. Bending at the hips, stick your butt out and bend your knees until they are at a 90-degree angle. Return to starting position.

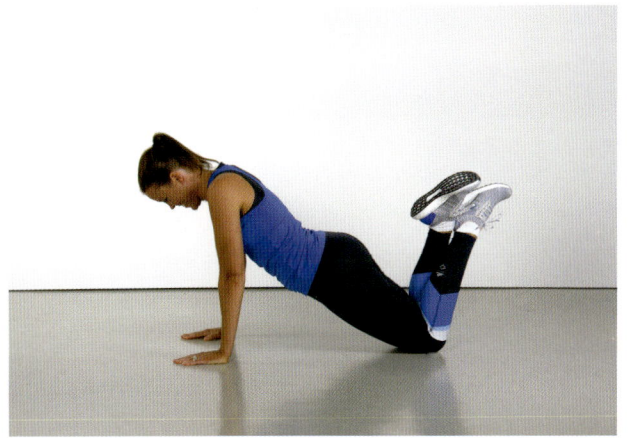

8 Push-ups

8.1 Get into high plank position with your hands shoulder-width apart, your shoulders over your wrists and your feet elevated on your toes. This is the starting position. Now lower yourself down to transfer all your weight into your shoulders and back. Press back up to the starting position.

8.2 Alternatively, place one ankle over the other while your knees are on the floor in the starting position. Now lift yourself up so your shoulders are over your wrists. Lower yourself down to the ground and then press back up to the starting position.

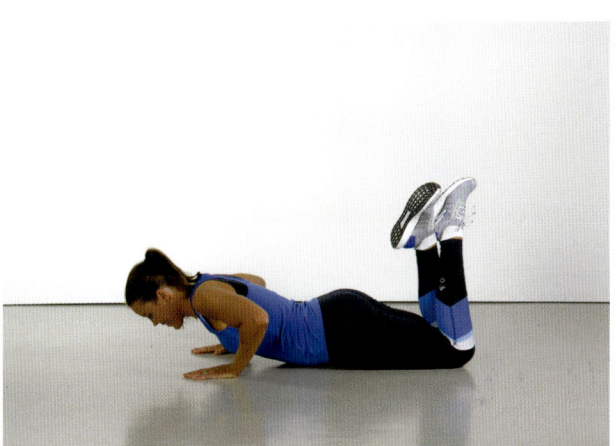

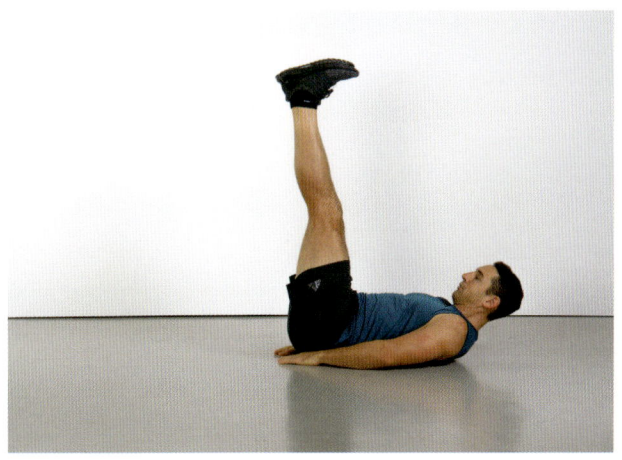

9 Double-leg raises

Lie on your back and tuck both your thumbs under your lower lumbar. Raise your legs and then lower them, keeping your heels off the ground.

Advanced: Do the exercise with your arms crossed over your chest.

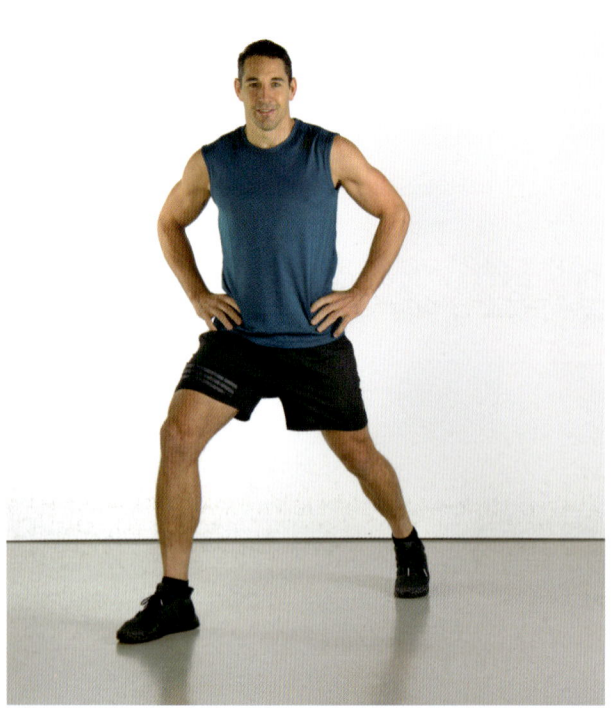

10 Lateral lunges

Stand with your feet shoulder-width apart and your hands on your hips or by your side. Take a half-step to one side and then bend at the knee and lunge, sticking your butt out and keeping your chest up and your core tight. Lunge back to the starting position. Repeat on the other side.

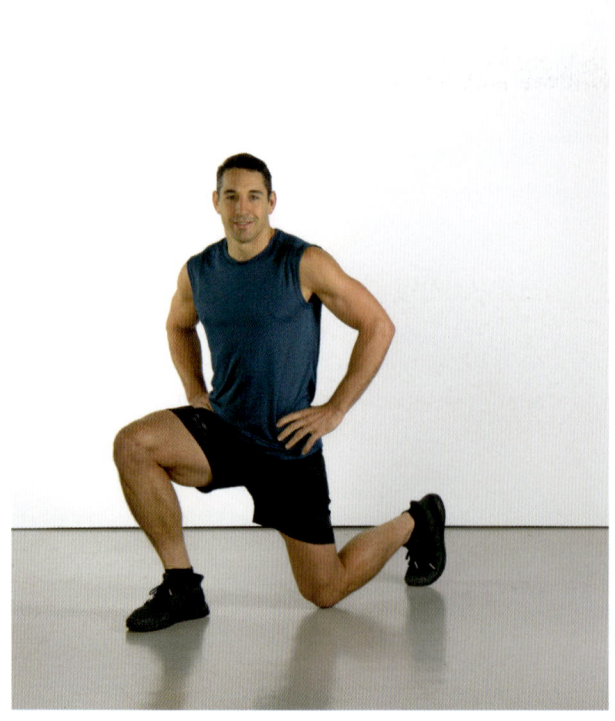

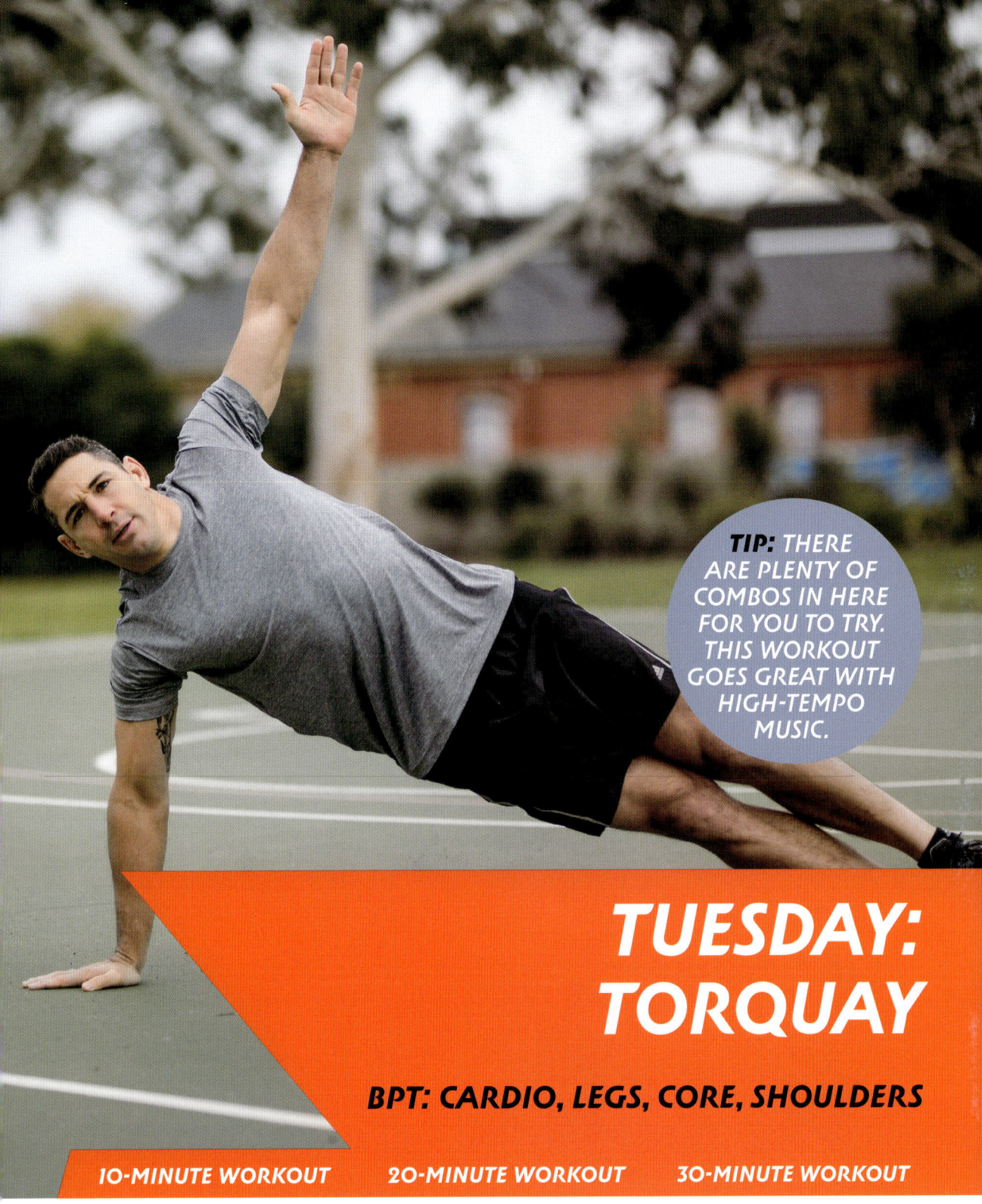

TIP: THERE ARE PLENTY OF COMBOS IN HERE FOR YOU TO TRY. THIS WORKOUT GOES GREAT WITH HIGH-TEMPO MUSIC.

TUESDAY: TORQUAY

BPT: CARDIO, LEGS, CORE, SHOULDERS

10-MINUTE WORKOUT	20-MINUTE WORKOUT	30-MINUTE WORKOUT
20 seconds movement / 10 seconds rest 2 sets of each exercise (one lap)	20 seconds movement / 10 seconds rest 2 sets of each exercise (two laps)	20 seconds movement / 10 seconds rest 2 sets of each exercise (three laps)

BLOCK 6: VICTORIA

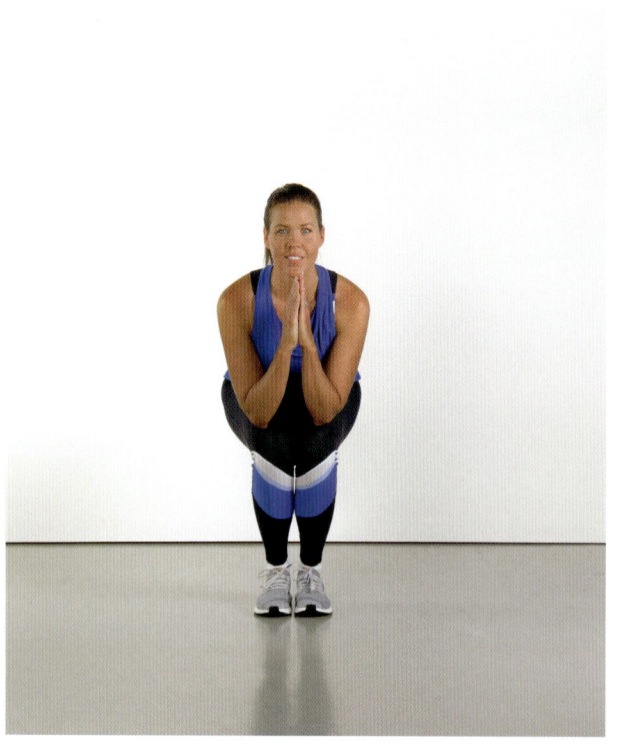

1 **Feet-together pulse squats**
Stand with your feet together and your hands on your hips or in a comfortable position. Bend your hips and come down as deep as you can into a squat position. From here, move up and down slightly to make pulse movements.

2 **Plyometric split lunges**

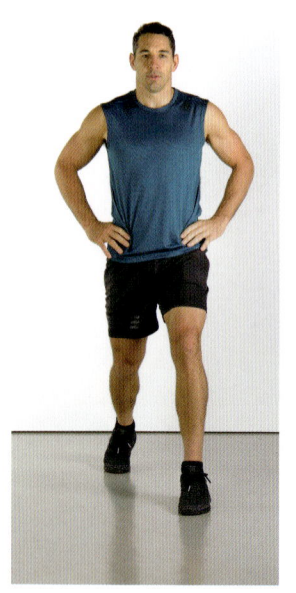 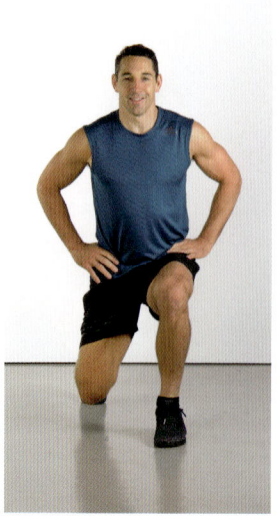

2.1 Start with your feet shoulder-width apart and your hands on your hips. Split your legs before dropping your back knee down in line with the heel of your leading foot – both legs should be at a 90-degree angle – then push up and repeat on the other side.

2.2 Alternatively, stand with your feet shoulder-width apart and your hands on your hips. Step one leg back and then lower it until it is 90 degrees to the ground. Step forward to the starting position. Repeat on the other side to complete the movement.

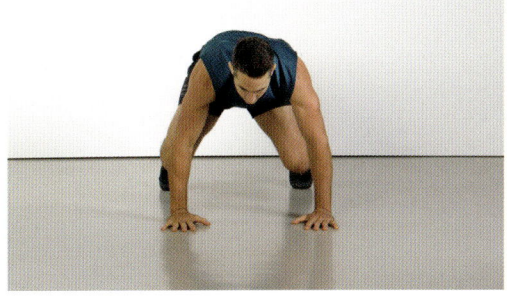

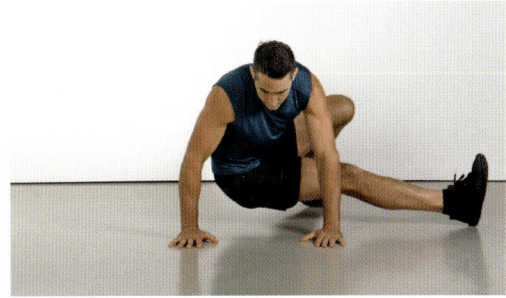

3 **Lateral shoot-throughs**
Start in high plank position with your hands firmly on the ground and your shoulders above your wrists. Bend your knees at a 90-degree angle and have your toes firmly on the ground and your knees off the ground. This is the starting position. Now turn your left foot so it is flat on the ground. Kick your right foot in front of your left foot and out to the side, so your right leg is now straight and your left foot is firmly on the ground. Now pull your right leg back to the starting position. Repeat on the other side.

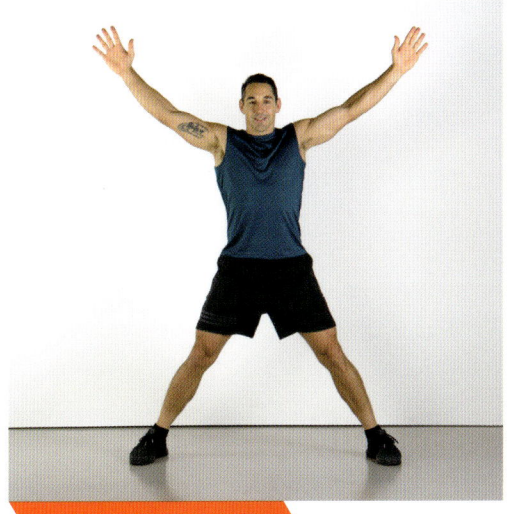

4 **Star tucks**
Stand with your feet shoulder-width apart. Jump your feet out wide with your arms straight above your head. Now jump your feet back together and squat into a ball as low as you can go before exploding back up to the starting position.

BILLY'S BEST: 18

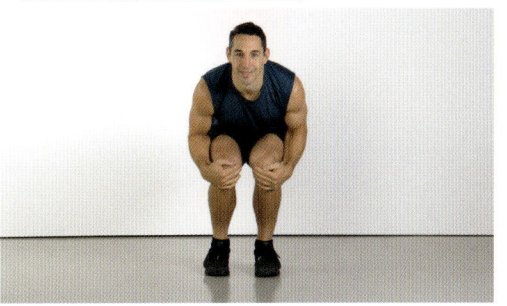

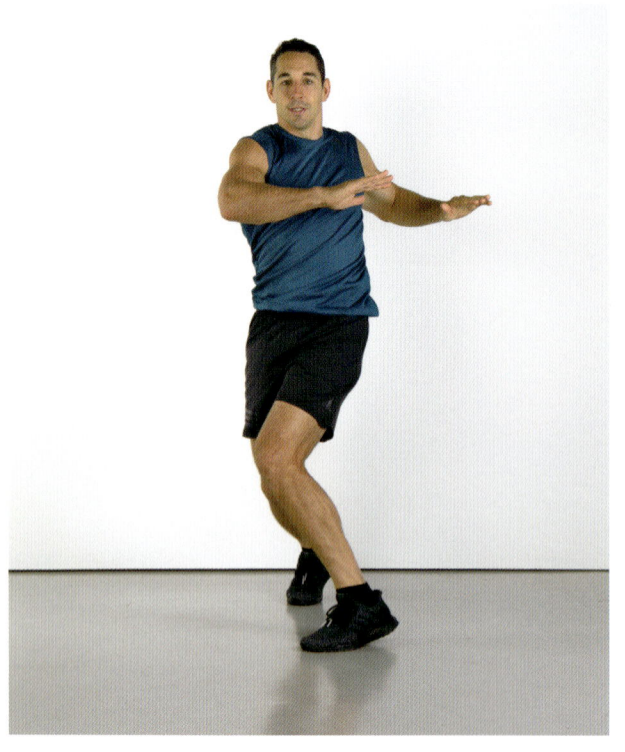

5 2 x torsion twists, 1 x deep squat

For the torsion twists, stand with your feet shoulder-width apart and your arms out nice and wide at shoulder height. Slightly jump to your right, twisting your left hip to your right side and keeping your chest forward. Now come back to the starting position. Repeat on the other side.

For the deep squat, stand with your feet shoulder-width apart, slightly tracked out. Holding your hands together, bend forward at your hips and lower your body down, keeping your feet flat on the ground and going as low as you can before pressing back up through your heels to the starting position.

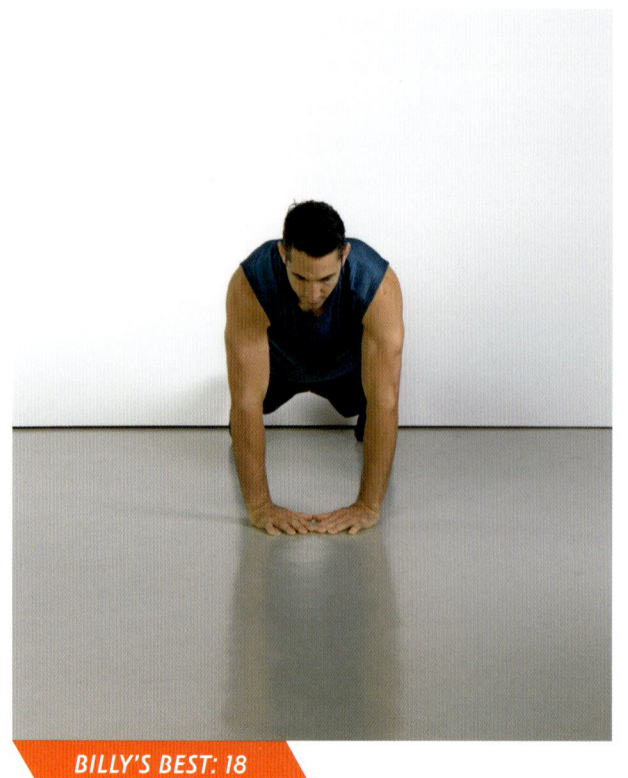

6 Diamond push-ups

Kneel on the ground with your ankles crossed, and set your hands so your thumbs and index fingers are touching in line with your chin. From here, lower your body towards the ground and then press back up to the starting position. You should feel this movement in your triceps.

Advanced: Do the exercise in high plank position with your knees off the ground.

BILLY'S BEST: 18

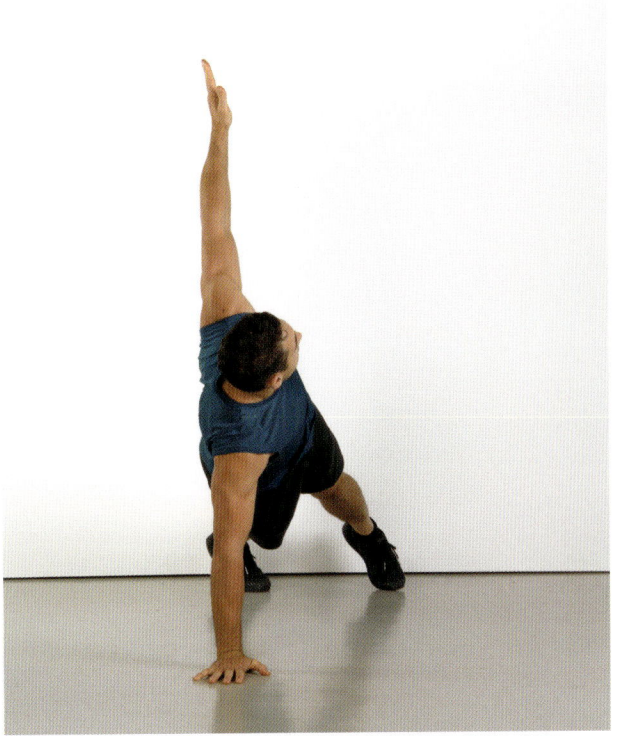

7 **Single-arm plank rotations**
Start in the side plank position. From here, reach up to the sky and bring your arm down and under your opposite armpit before returning to the side plank position. Repeat on the other side.

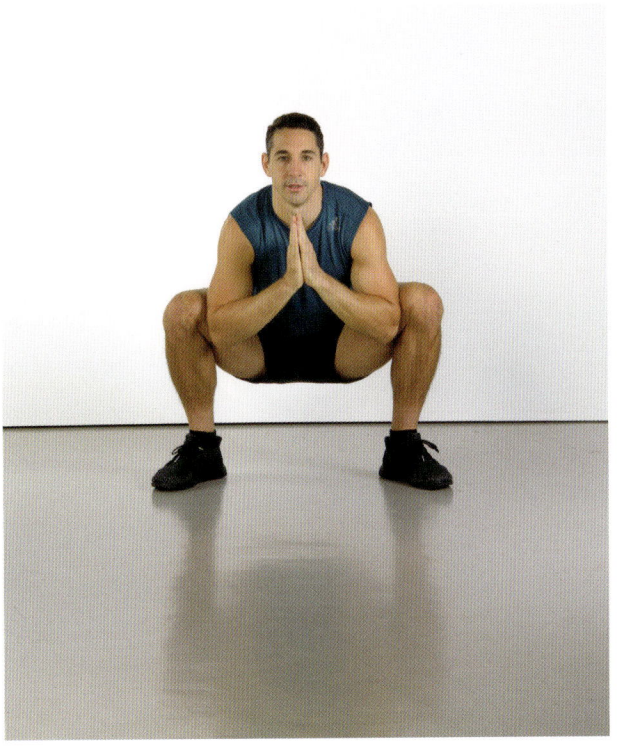

8 **Frog squats**
Stand with your feet shoulder-width apart and your feet slightly tracked out. Bend down to full squat position with your elbows tucked inside your legs. This is the starting position. From here, raise your hips and then lower them back to the starting position.

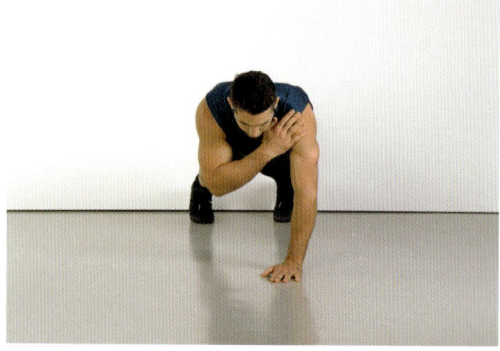

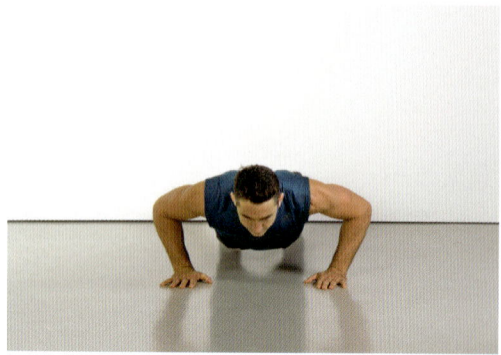

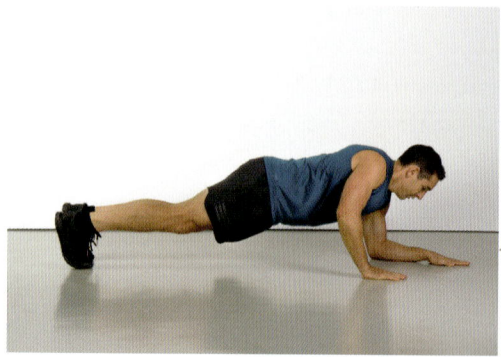

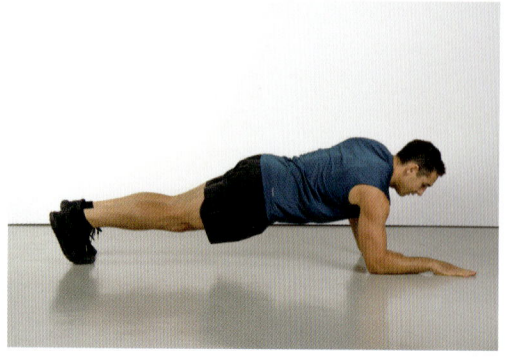

9   **2 x shoulder taps, 1 x push-up**
For the shoulder taps, start in high plank position. Engaging your core, transfer your weight into your right arm, and with your left hand touch your right shoulder. Return to the starting position and repeat on the left side.

9.1 Remain in the starting position. Now lower yourself down to transfer all your weight into your shoulders and back. Press back up to the starting position.

9.2 Alternatively, kneel down and place one ankle over the other while your knees are on the floor in the starting position. Lift yourself up so your shoulders are over your wrists. Lower yourself down to the ground and then press back up to the starting position.

10 **Moving plank**
Lie with your forearms on the ground, your knees off the ground and your feet together. From here, with your toes touching the ground, lean slightly forward to engage your core, lifting yourself up into the high plank position. Keep alternating between the high and low plank positions. (Note: Your back should not be sagging or bent.)

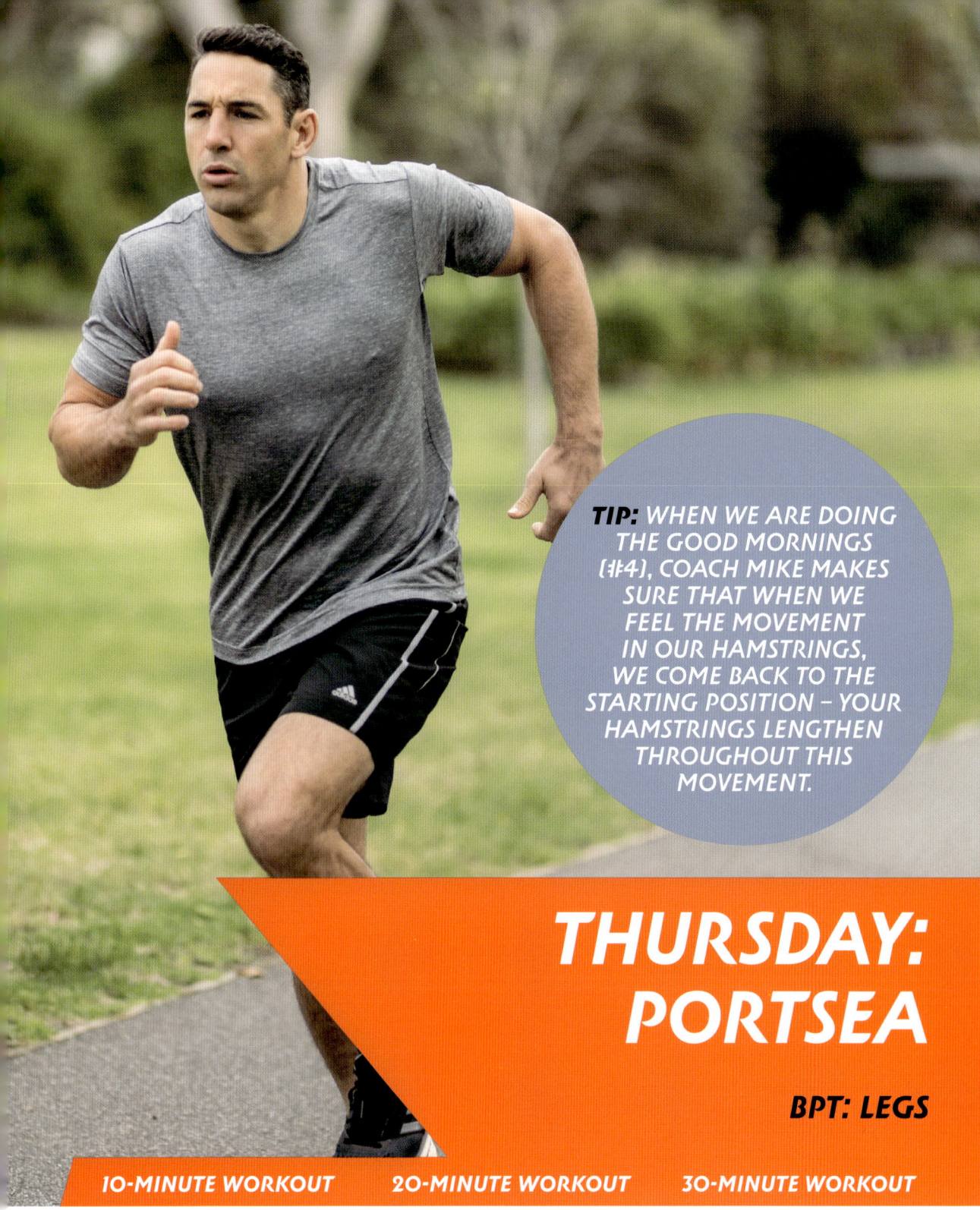

TIP: WHEN WE ARE DOING THE GOOD MORNINGS (#4), COACH MIKE MAKES SURE THAT WHEN WE FEEL THE MOVEMENT IN OUR HAMSTRINGS, WE COME BACK TO THE STARTING POSITION – YOUR HAMSTRINGS LENGTHEN THROUGHOUT THIS MOVEMENT.

THURSDAY: PORTSEA

BPT: LEGS

10-MINUTE WORKOUT	20-MINUTE WORKOUT	30-MINUTE WORKOUT
20 seconds movement / 10 seconds rest 2 sets of each exercise (one lap)	20 seconds movement / 10 seconds rest 2 sets of each exercise (two laps)	20 seconds movement / 10 seconds rest 2 sets of each exercise (three laps)

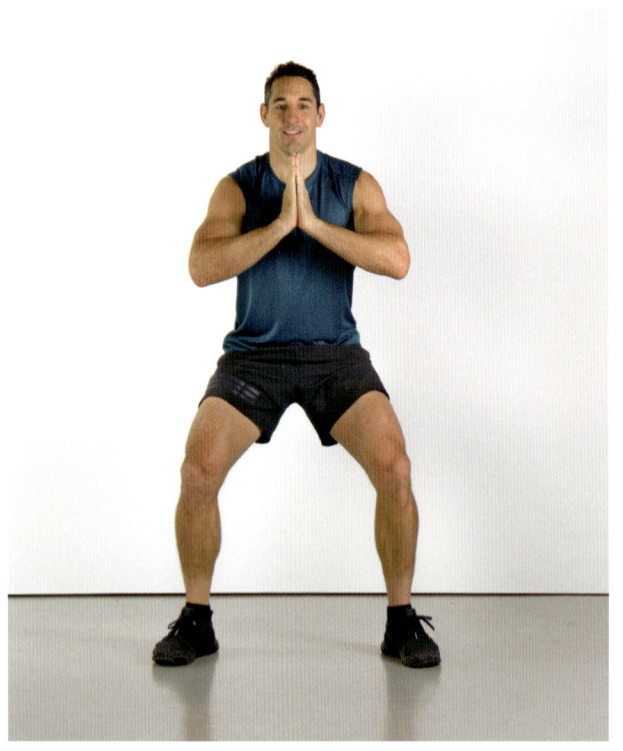

1 **Pulse squats**
Stand with your feet just past shoulder-width apart and slightly tracked out. Squat with your hips back and your legs at a 90-degree angle, then pulse up and down.

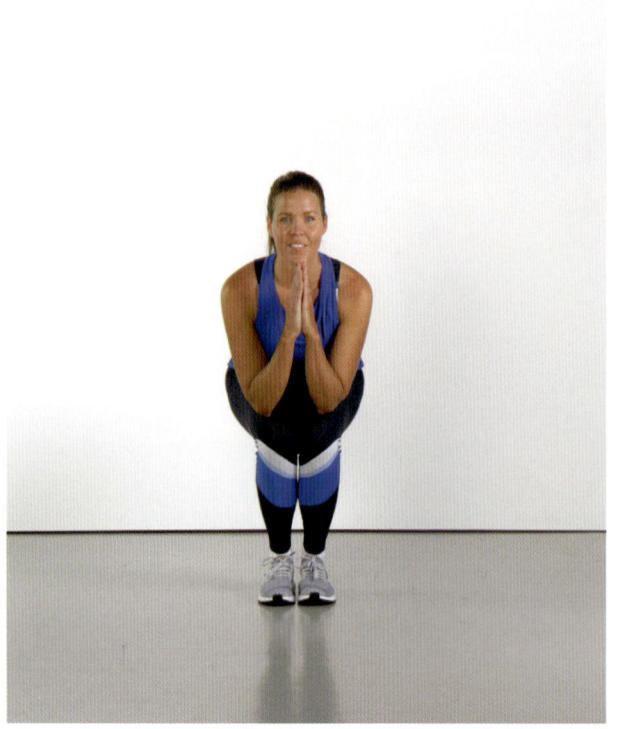

2 **2 x close-feet squats, 2 x squats**
Standing near a wall with your feet together, hands on hips. Bend at the hips and stick your butt out to the wall, lowering yourself down as deep as you can go with all your weight in the back of your heels. From here, drive through your heels back up to the starting position.

For the squats, stand with your feet just past shoulder-width apart and your feet slightly pointed outwards so your knees track with your feet. Bending at the hips, stick your butt out and bend your knees until they are at a 90-degree angle. Return to starting position.

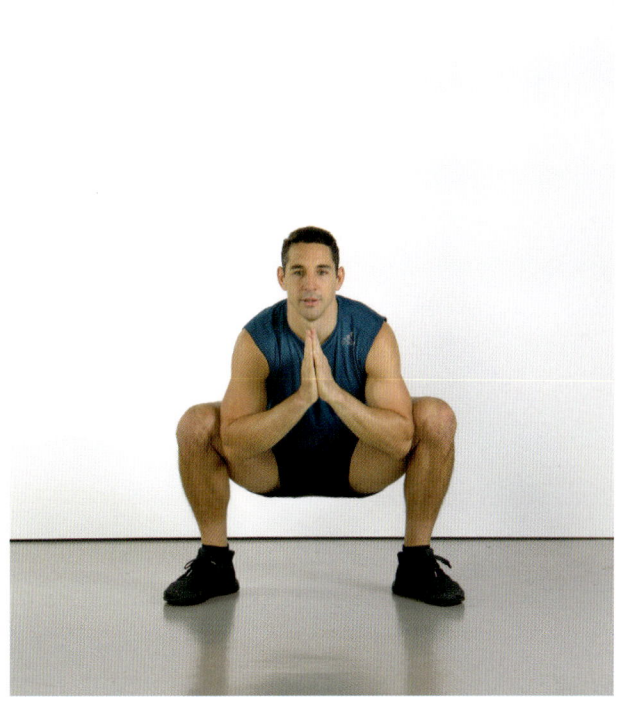

3 Frog squats

Stand with your feet shoulder-width apart and your feet slightly tracked out. Bend down to full squat position with your elbows tucked inside your legs. This is the starting position. From here, raise your hips and then lower them back to the starting position.

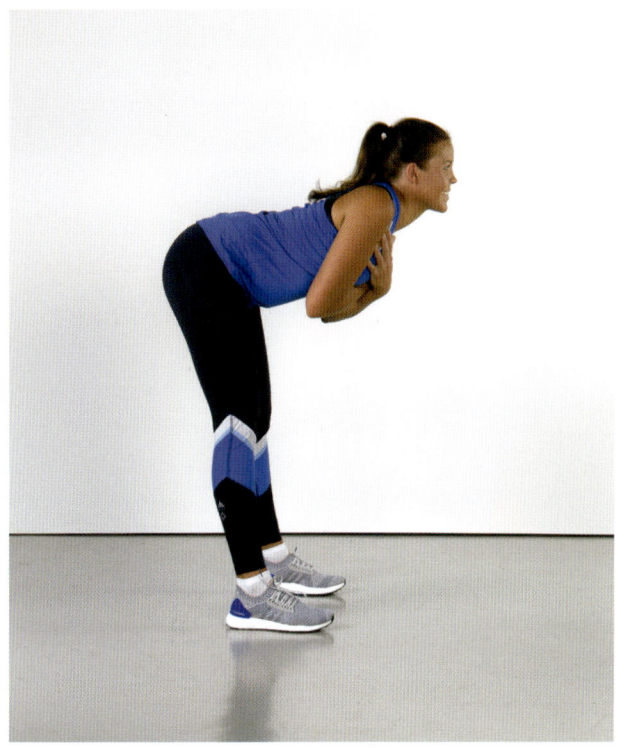

4 Good mornings

Stand with your feet wider than shoulder-width apart, your knees slightly bent and your arms crossed over your chest. Sticking your butt out, lean forward, keeping your knees slightly bent. Return to the starting position.

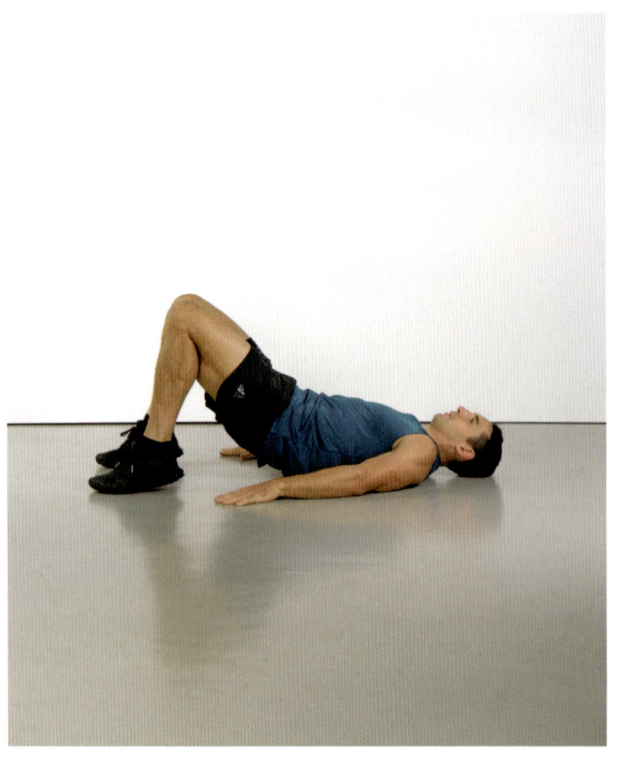

5 Double-leg glute bridge

Lie on your back with your hands on your hips or with your arms straight or beside your body on the ground and your palms facing down. Bring your heels as close as you can to your butt, raising your hips and pressing down on the balls of your feet. Squeeze your butt cheeks (glutes) before lowering yourself down. Don't allow yourself to collapse – stay tight through your core and make sure your butt doesn't hit the ground.

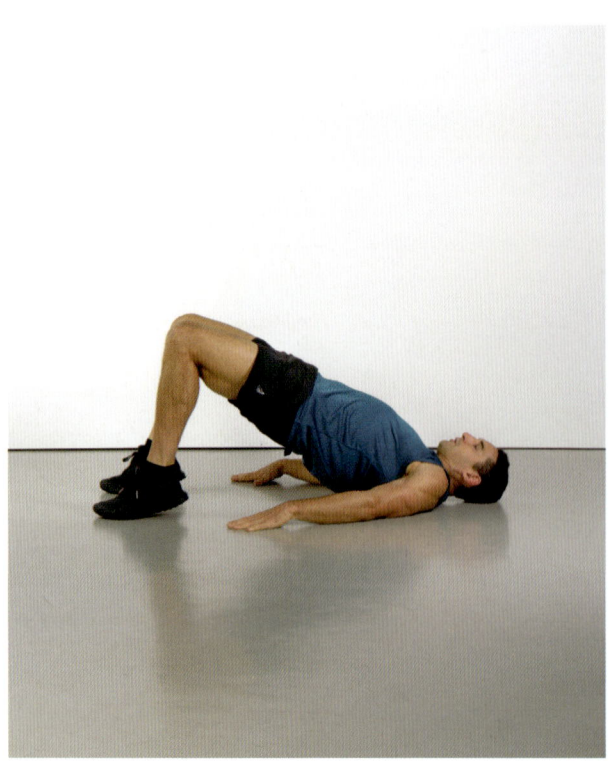

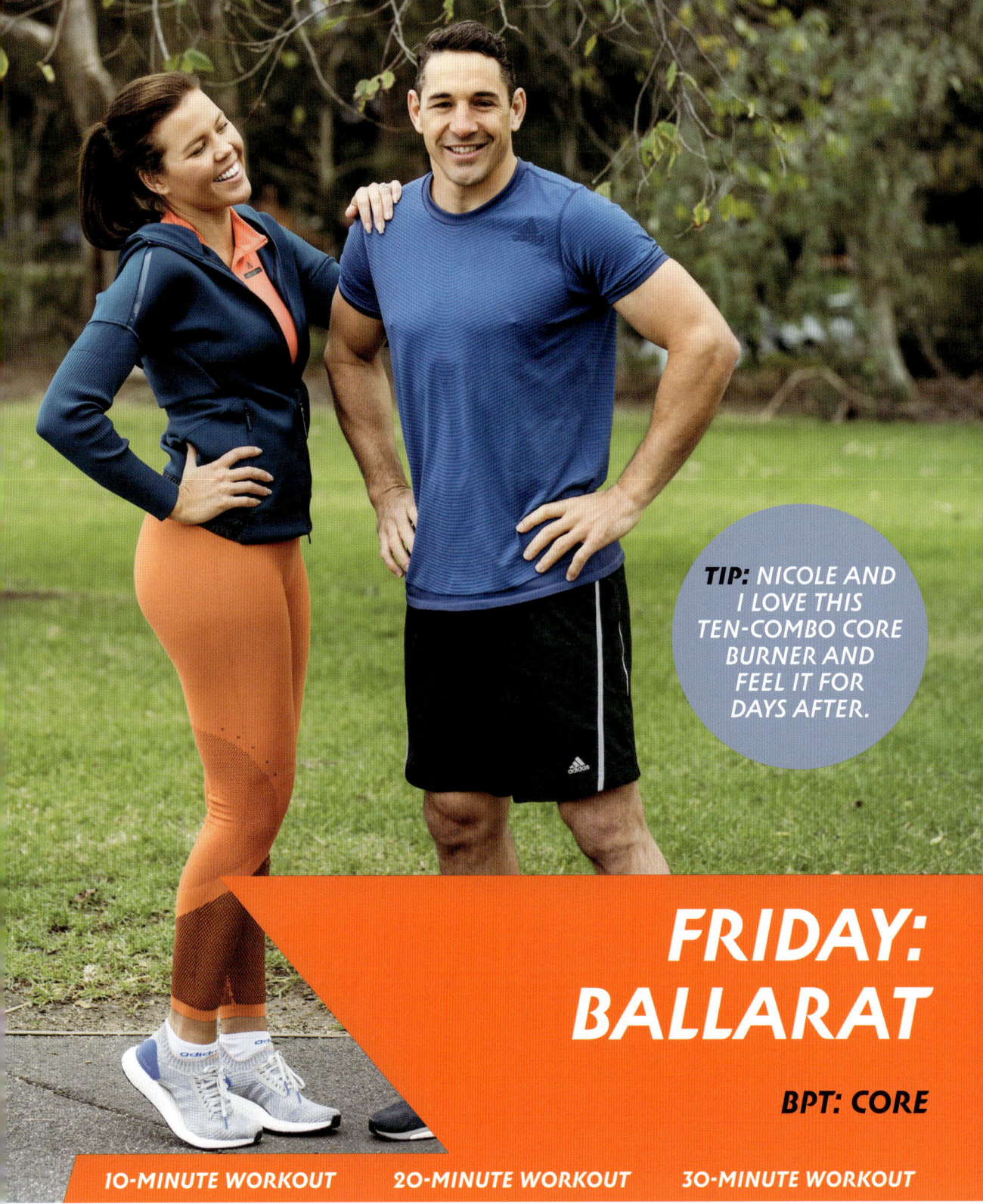

TIP: NICOLE AND I LOVE THIS TEN-COMBO CORE BURNER AND FEEL IT FOR DAYS AFTER.

FRIDAY: BALLARAT

BPT: CORE

10-MINUTE WORKOUT

20 seconds movement /
10 seconds rest
2 sets of each exercise
(one lap)

20-MINUTE WORKOUT

20 seconds movement /
10 seconds rest
2 sets of each exercise
(two laps)

30-MINUTE WORKOUT

20 seconds movement /
10 seconds rest
2 sets of each exercise
(three laps)

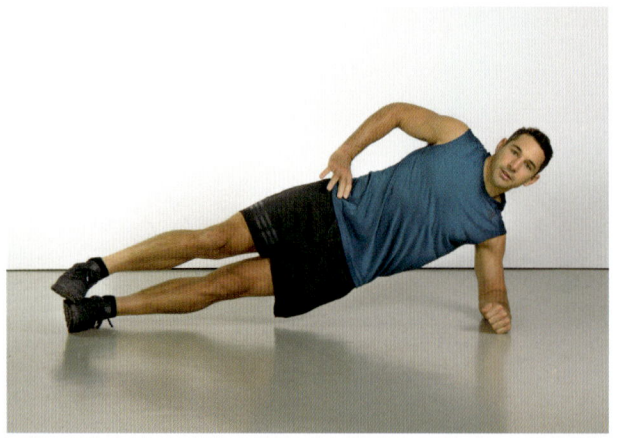

1 **Side plank**

Lie on your side with your feet together. With your lower forearm firmly on the ground, raise your hips up and place your other hand firmly on your waist. From here, press down into your shoulders and raise your hips, squeezing your core. Hold.

Advanced: Have your other hand raised straight up in the air instead of on your waist throughout the entire movement.

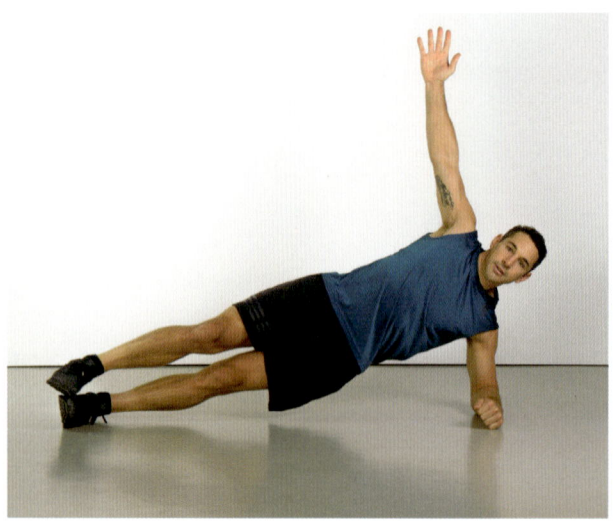

2 **Side plank – alternate side**

Lie on your side with your feet together. Raise your upper arm so it is at a 90-degree angle parallel to your shoulder. Keep your opposite arm firmly on the ground in line with your opposite wrist. From here, press down into your shoulders and raise your hips, squeezing your core. Hold.

Advanced: Have your other hand raised straight up in the air instead of on your waist throughout the entire movement.

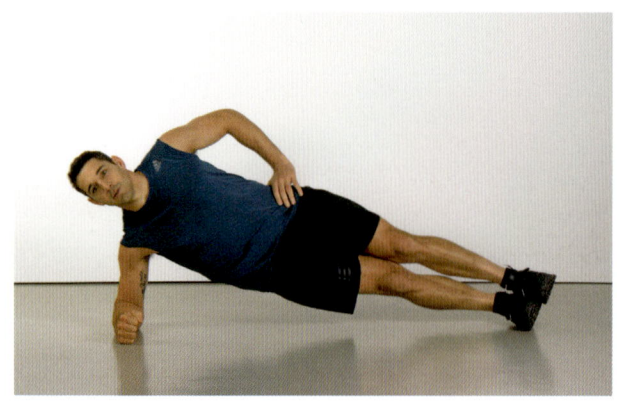

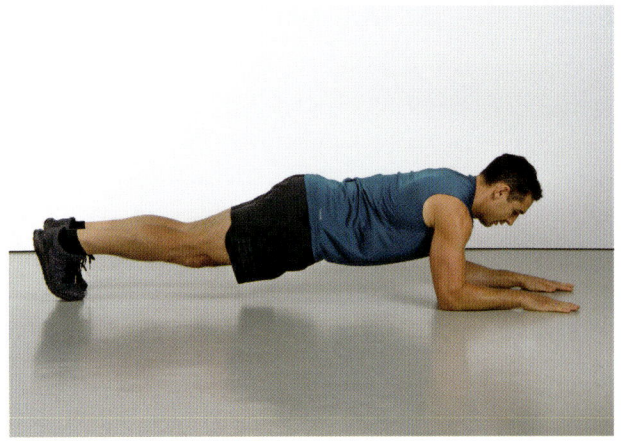

3 Plank

Place your forearms on the ground and lift your knees off the ground with your feet together and your toes touching the ground. From here, lean slightly forward to engage your core. Hold the position for the duration of time. (Note: Your back should not be sagging or bent.)

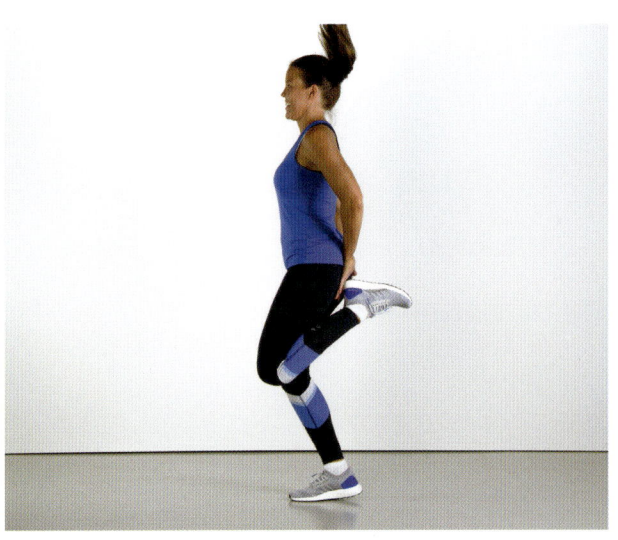

4 Butt kicks

Stand with your feet shoulder-width apart and your hands flat behind your back with your palms facing outwards. Bring one heel up to touch your butt, then do the same with the other heel. Try to keep your feet nice and soft and land back on the ball of your foot each time.

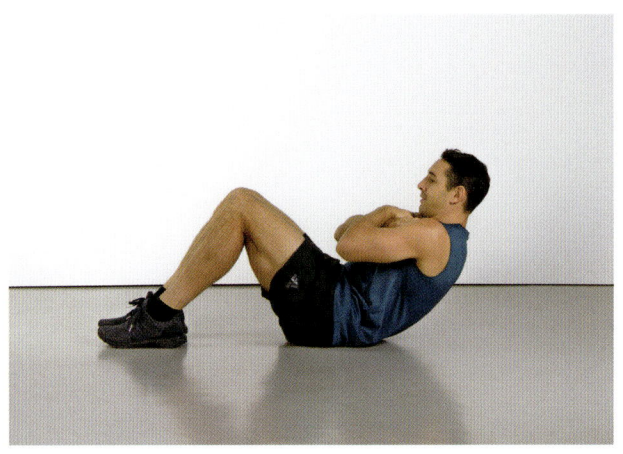

5 Sit-ups

Lie on your back, bend your legs and place your feet firmly on the ground to stabilise your lower body. Cross your arms over your chest, then curl your upper body all the way up to touch your knees. Slowly lower yourself down to return to the starting point.

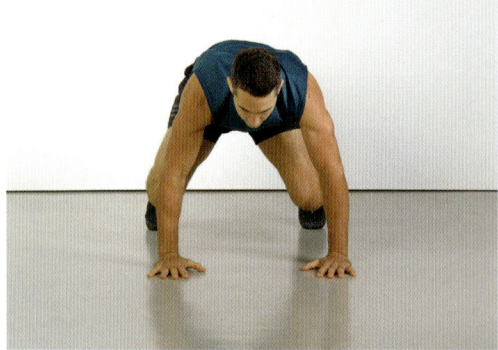

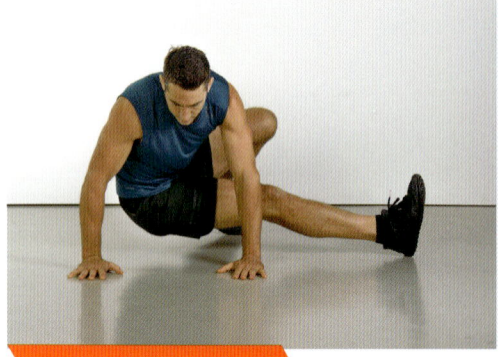

BILLY'S BEST: 16

6 Lateral shoot-throughs

Start in high plank position with your hands firmly on the ground and your shoulders above your wrists. Bend your knees at a 90-degree angle and have your toes firmly on the ground and your knees off the ground. This is the starting position. Now turn your left foot so it is flat on the ground. Kick your right foot in front of your left foot and out to the side, so your right leg is now straight and your left foot is firmly on the ground. Now pull your right leg back to the starting position. Repeat on the other side.

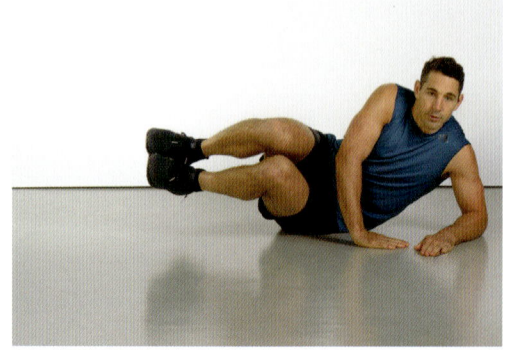

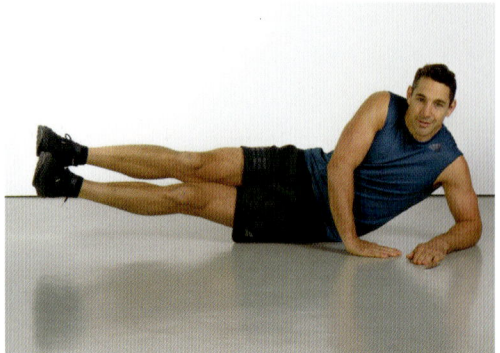

7 Oblique kick-outs

Sit on the ground with your knees together and slightly bent, and your hands touching the ground. Bring your knees diagonally across your chest, then straighten your legs out. Repeat on the other side.

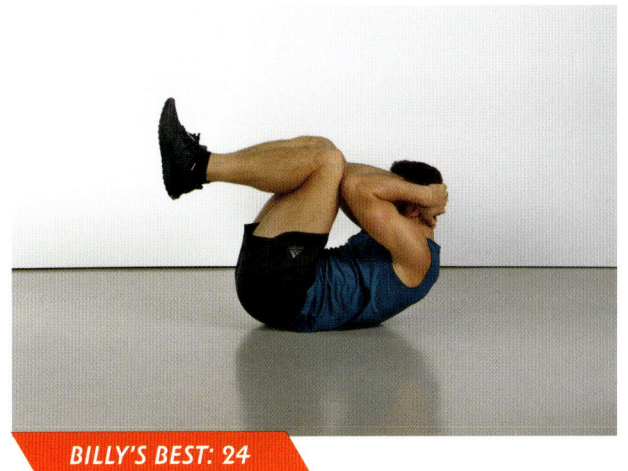

BILLY'S BEST: 24

8 Crunches

Lie on your back with your legs off the ground, with knees bent at a 90-degree angle to your body. With your hands crossed behind your head, bring your elbows in next to your ears. Bring your elbows up to your knees and then return to the starting position.

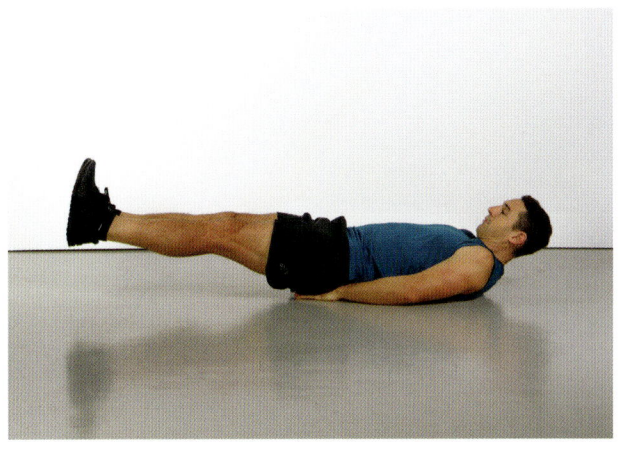

9 Double-leg raises

Lie on your back and tuck both your thumbs under your lower lumbar (base of your back). Raise your legs then lower them, keeping your heels off the ground.

Advanced: Do the exercise with your arms crossed over your chest.

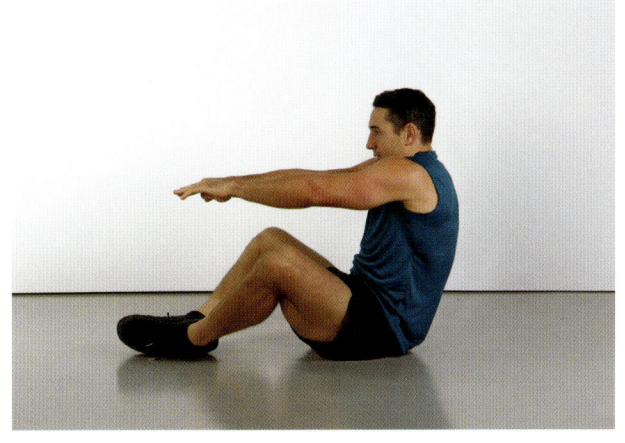

10 Butterfly sit-ups

Sit on the ground with your feet together and as close as possible to your butt, with your knees out wide. From here, lean back until you are lying flat on the ground. Lift your head and then your body back up to the starting position.

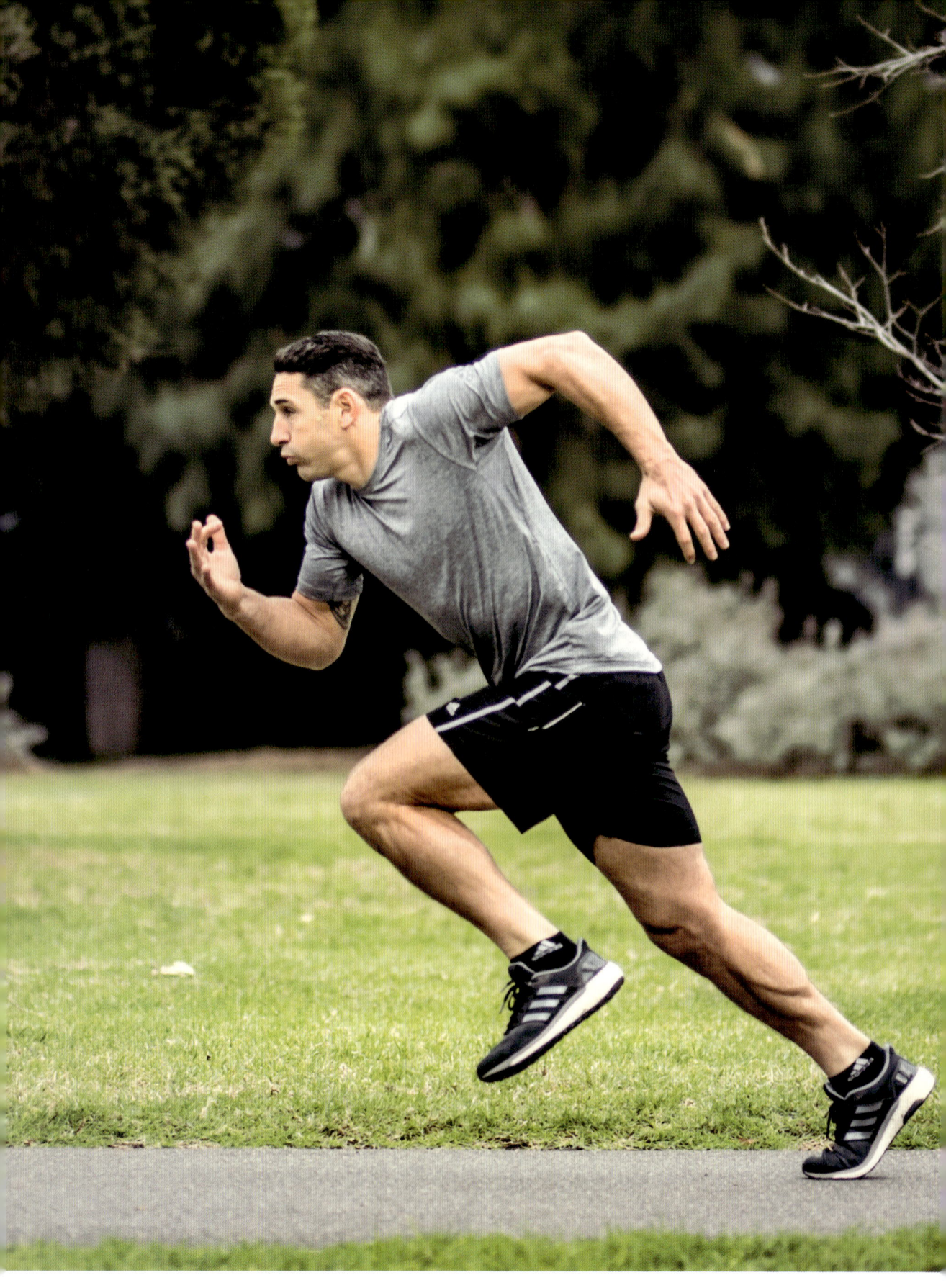

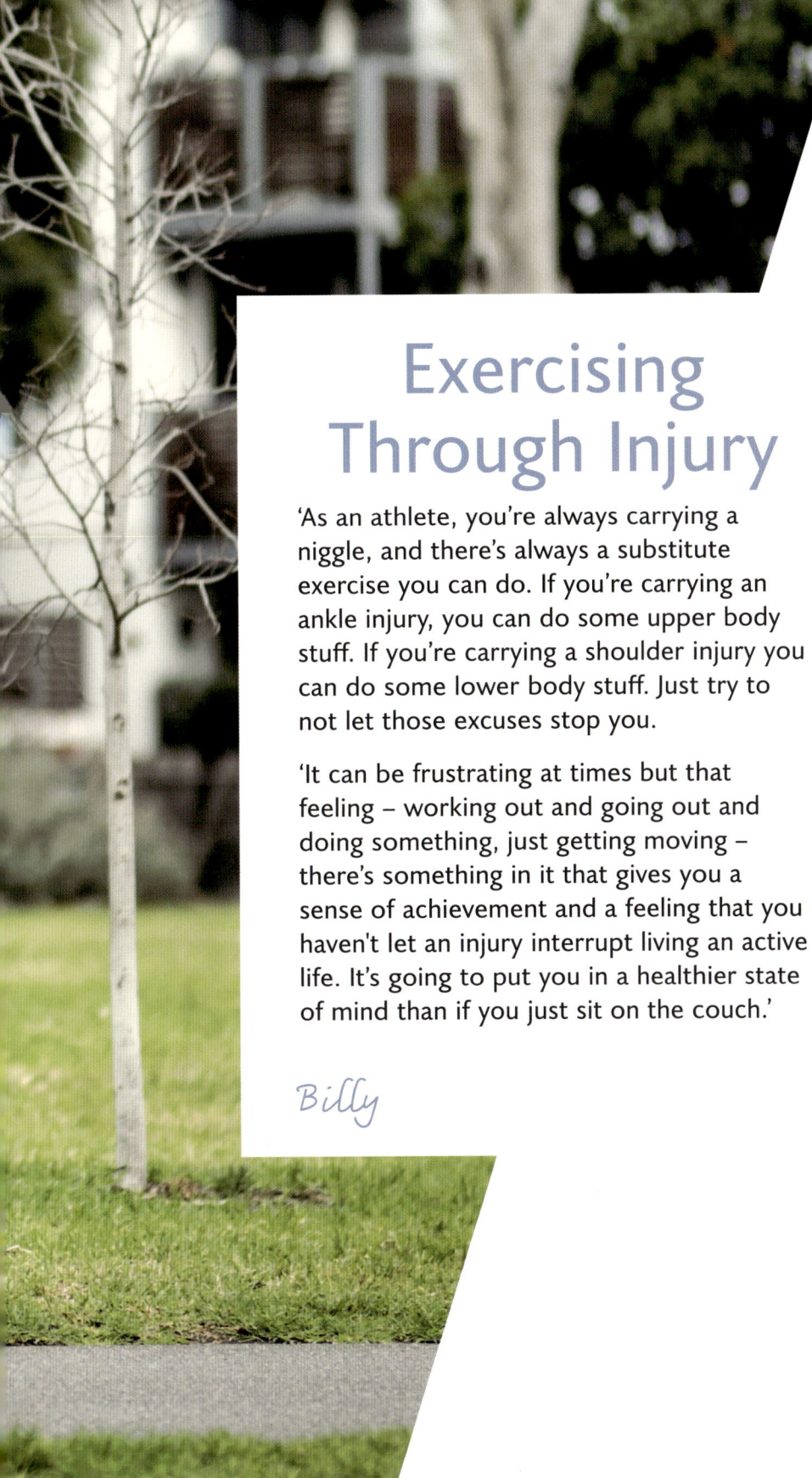

Exercising Through Injury

'As an athlete, you're always carrying a niggle, and there's always a substitute exercise you can do. If you're carrying an ankle injury, you can do some upper body stuff. If you're carrying a shoulder injury you can do some lower body stuff. Just try to not let those excuses stop you.

'It can be frustrating at times but that feeling – working out and going out and doing something, just getting moving – there's something in it that gives you a sense of achievement and a feeling that you haven't let an injury interrupt living an active life. It's going to put you in a healthier state of mind than if you just sit on the couch.'

Billy

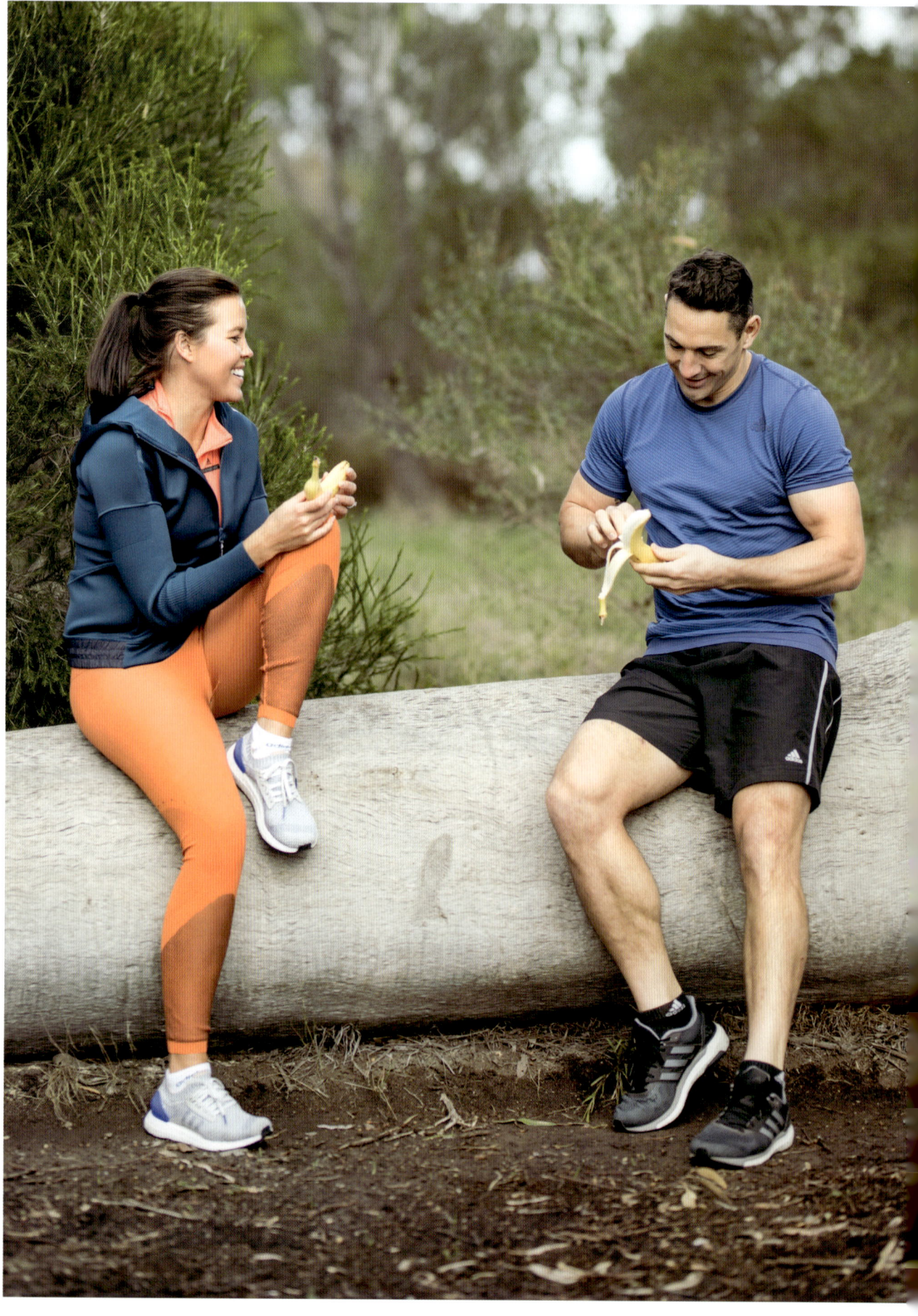

BLOCK 7: TASMANIA

'Peaceful and serene. Tasmania is a wonderful state for getting outside and perhaps on the bike. It's a great place to tour around. There are plenty of good spots to enjoy the natural beauty of Australia and get a workout in.'

Billy

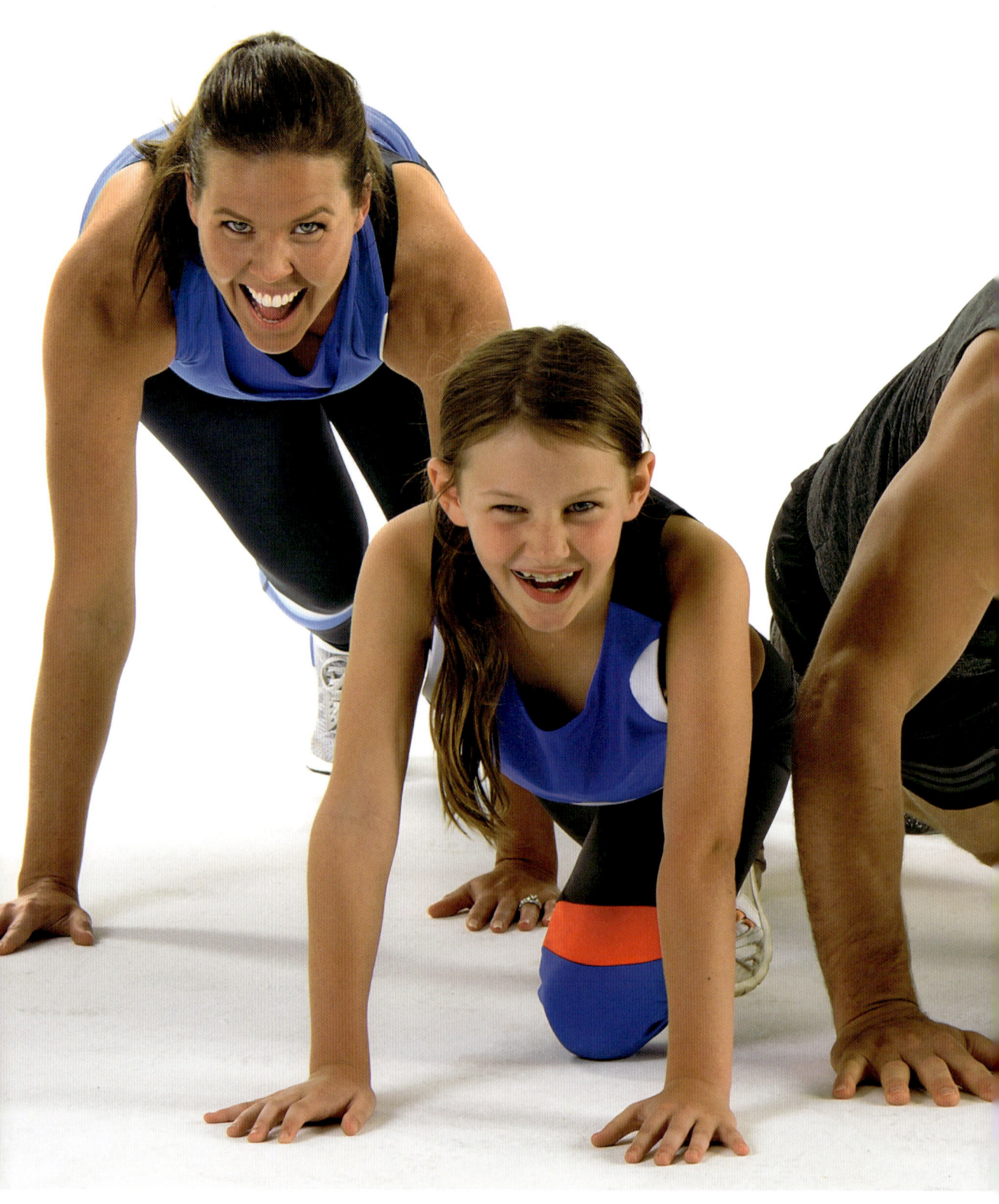

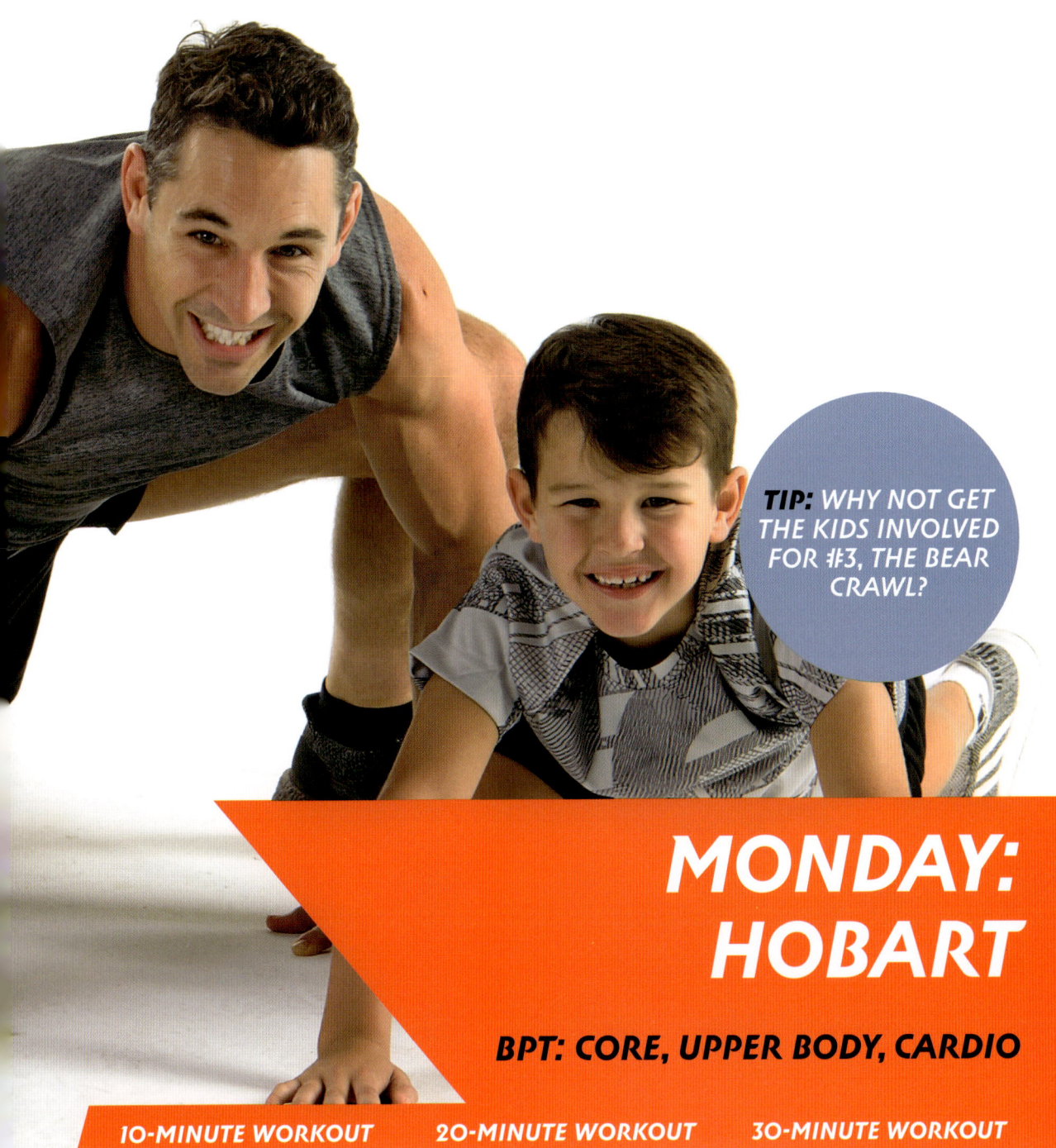

TIP: WHY NOT GET THE KIDS INVOLVED FOR #3, THE BEAR CRAWL?

MONDAY: HOBART

BPT: CORE, UPPER BODY, CARDIO

10-MINUTE WORKOUT

20 seconds movement /
10 seconds rest
2 sets of each exercise
(one lap)

20-MINUTE WORKOUT

20 seconds movement /
10 seconds rest
2 sets of each exercise
(two laps)

30-MINUTE WORKOUT

20 seconds movement /
10 seconds rest
2 sets of each exercise
(three laps)

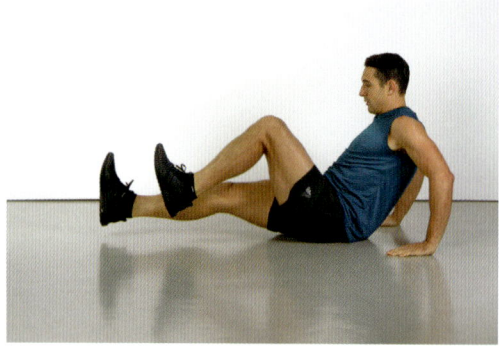

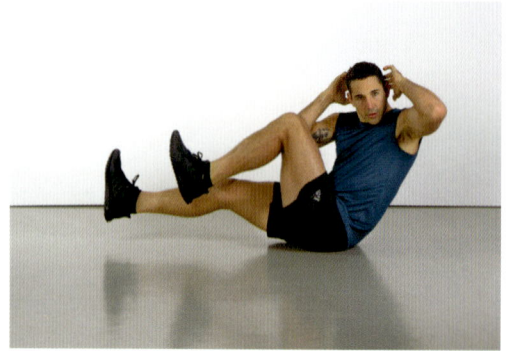

1. **Bicycle crunches**

   Start by sitting on the ground with your hands on the floor by your side and your legs extended in front of you. From here, lean back, engaging your core so your feet are off the ground. Now bring one knee towards your chest, keeping the other leg straight. Return your knee to the earlier position and swap to bring your other knee towards your chest.

   Advanced: Take your hands off the ground and bring the opposite elbow to your knee.

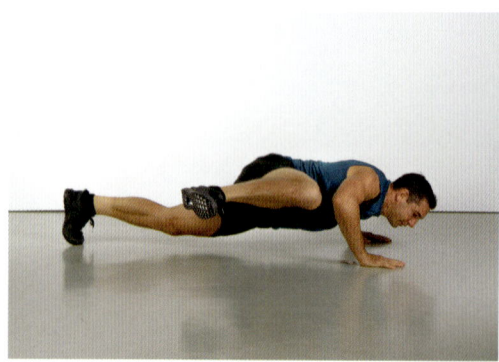

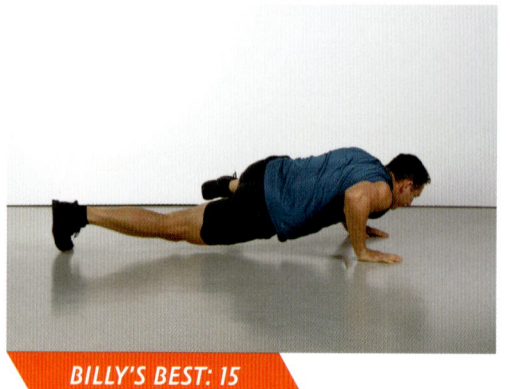

2. **Elbow to knee push-ups**

   Lie in high plank position with your hands shoulder-width apart, your shoulders over your wrists and your feet elevated on your toes. This is the starting position. Now lower yourself down to transfer all your weight into your shoulders and back. Press back up to the starting position. From here, bring your right knee towards your chest and your right elbow towards your knee. Return to the starting position. Repeat on the other side.

BILLY'S BEST: 15

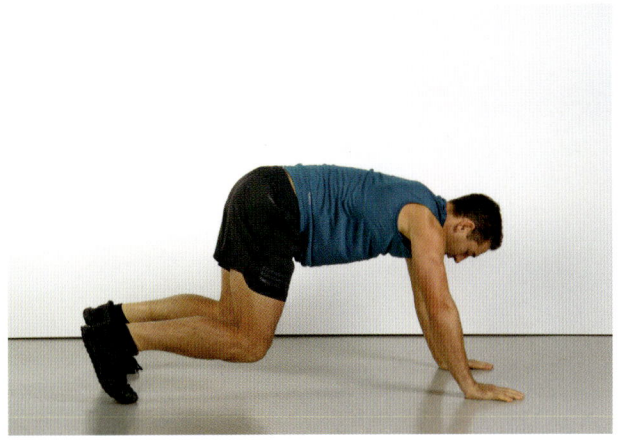

3 Bear crawl

Start in the push-up position with your knees bent at a 90-degree angle and positioned directly under your hips. Engage your core and do not raise or round your back. This is your starting position. Walk your right hand and your left foot forward, and then your left hand and your right foot forward. Continue until you reach 5 metres. Now, keeping your hips down and your core engaged, reverse the movement by walking your left arm and your right foot back, and then your right arm and your left leg back. Continue until you have returned to your starting position.

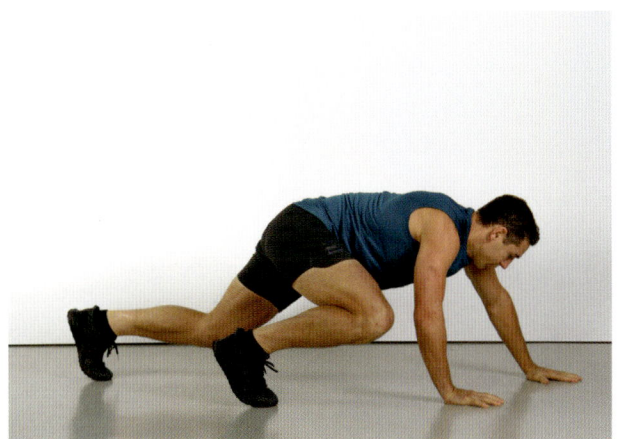

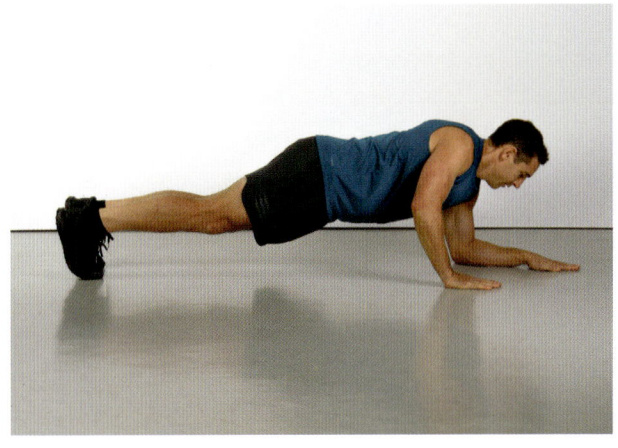

4 Moving plank

Lie with your forearms on the ground, your knees off the ground and your feet together. From here, with your toes touching the ground, lean slightly forward to engage your core, lifting yourself up into the high plank position. Keep alternating between the high and low plank positions. (Note: Your back should not be sagging or bent.)

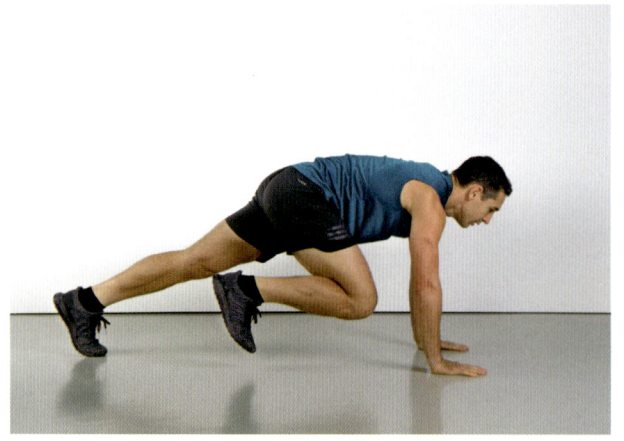

5 Mountain climbers

Start in a high plank position, with your shoulders over your wrists, your feet together and your core engaged. From here, bring one knee up towards your chest and then return it to the starting position. Repeat on the other side.

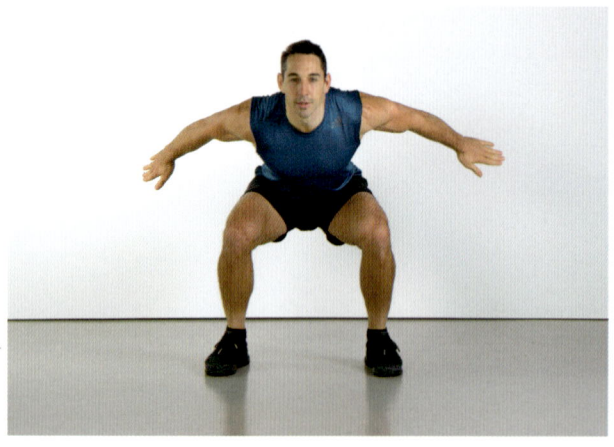

6 Squat jumps

Stand with your feet just past shoulder-width apart and slightly pointed outwards so your knees track with your feet. Bend at the hips, stick your butt out and bend your knees until they are at a 90-degree angle. This is the starting position. With your hands clasped together, drive through your legs and explode up so your feet are off the ground. As you land, lower your body back to the starting position.

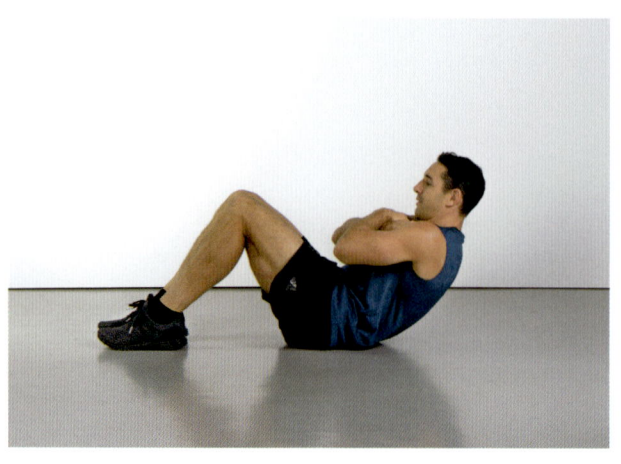

7 Sit-ups

Lie on your back, bend your legs and place your feet firmly on the ground to stabilise your lower body. Cross your arms over your chest, then curl your upper body all the way up to touch your knees. Slowly lower yourself down to return to the starting point.

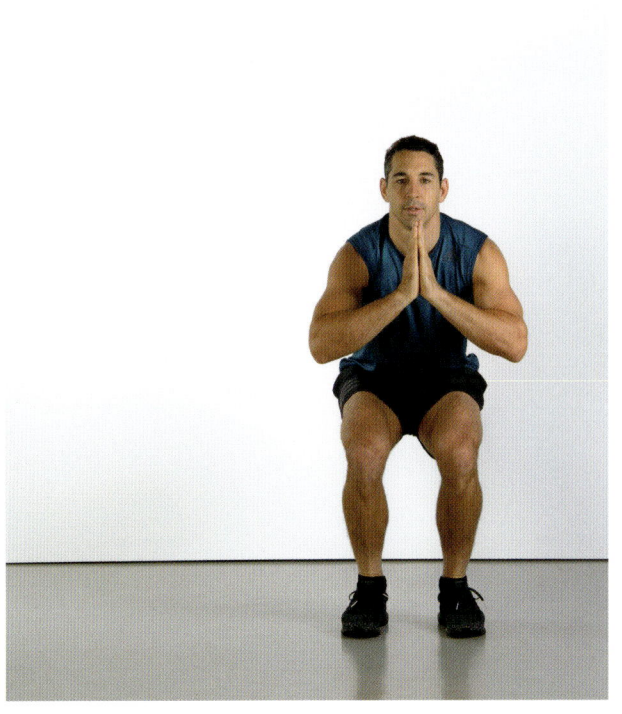

8 Crab walks

Stand with your feet shoulder-width apart and bend at the hips to come down into a squatting position. With your hands in front of your chest and staying low, step two to your left and then two to your right. Try to stay low throughout the time allocated.

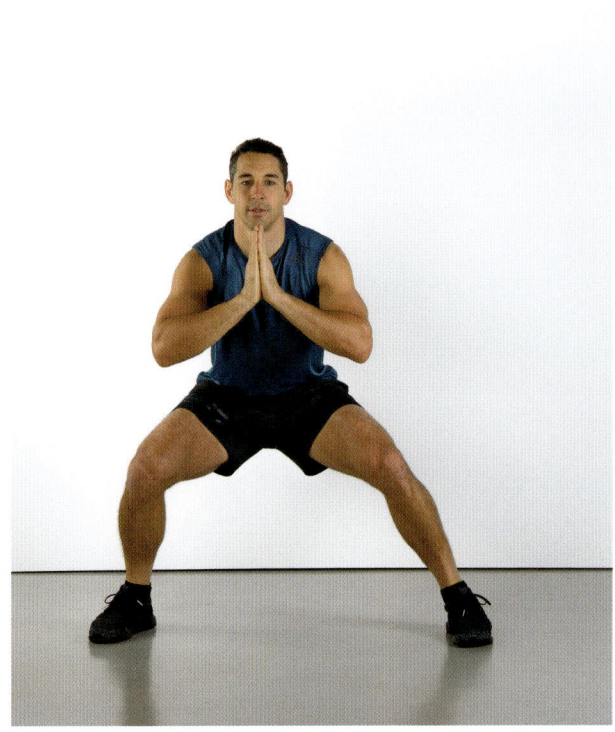

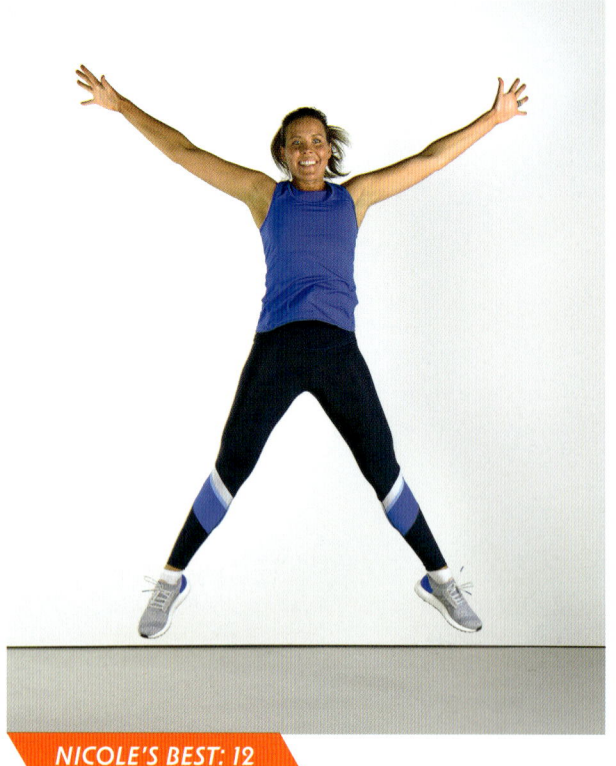

NICOLE'S BEST: 12

9 Star jumps

Begin in a relaxed stance with your arms close to your body. Jump your feet out wide past shoulder-width and raise both your arms above your head, then land back in the starting position.

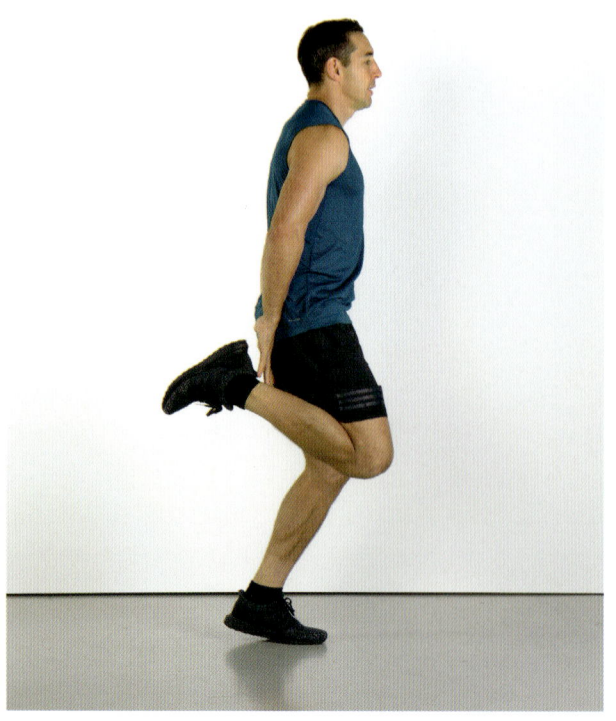

10 Butt kicks

Stand with your feet shoulder-width apart and your hands flat behind your back with your palms facing outwards. Bring one heel up to touch your butt, then do the same with the other heel. Try to keep your feet nice and soft and land back on the ball of your foot each time.

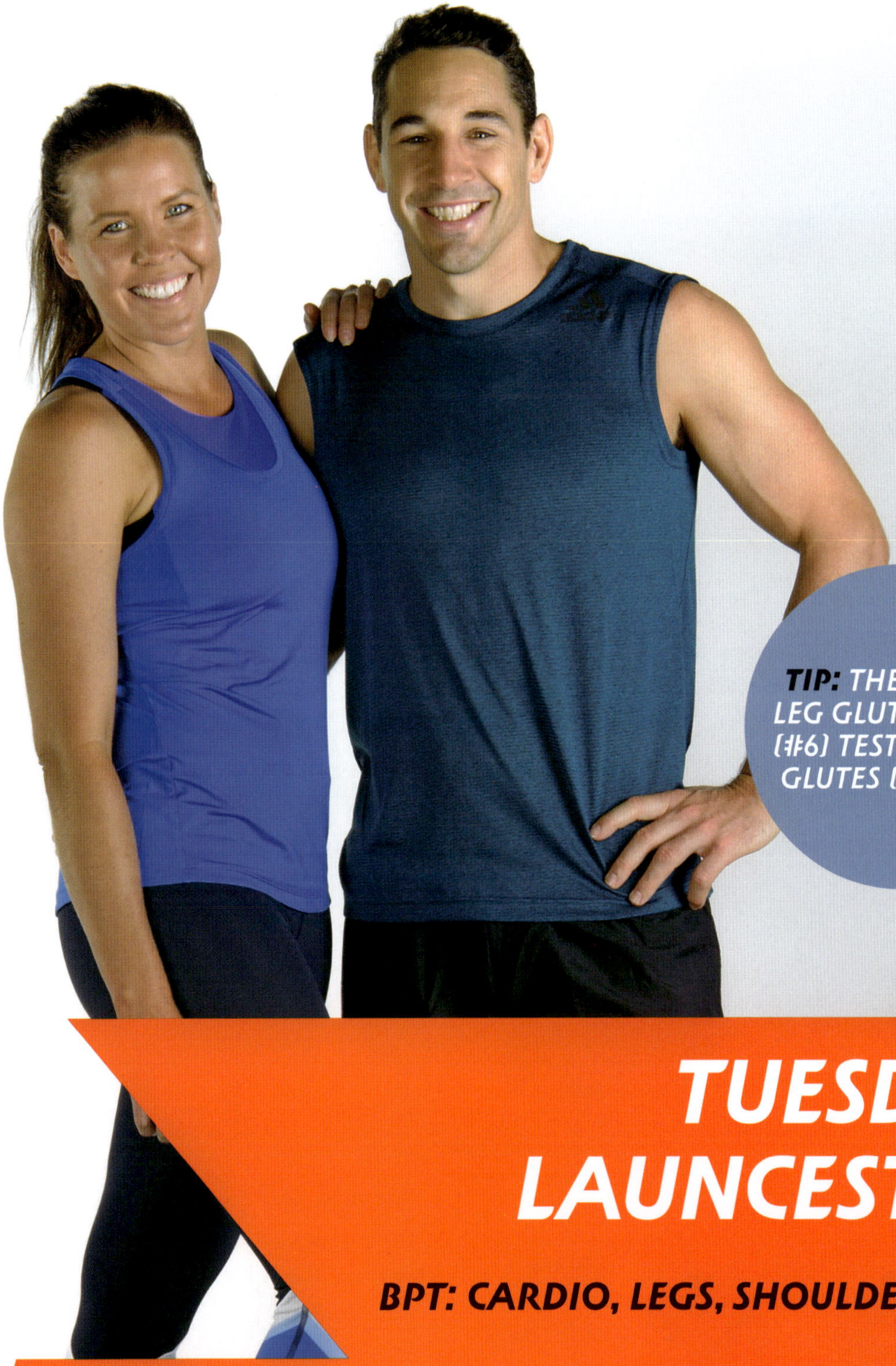

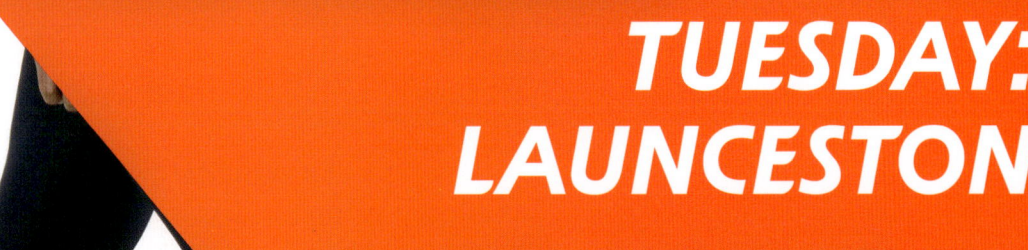

TIP: *THE SINGLE-LEG GLUTE BRIDGE (#6) TESTS OUT MY GLUTES (OUCHIE).*

TUESDAY: LAUNCESTON

BPT: CARDIO, LEGS, SHOULDERS, CORE

10-MINUTE WORKOUT

20 seconds movement /
10 seconds rest
2 sets of each exercise
(one lap)

20-MINUTE WORKOUT

20 seconds movement /
10 seconds rest
2 sets of each exercise
(two laps)

30-MINUTE WORKOUT

20 seconds movement /
10 seconds rest
2 sets of each exercise
(three laps)

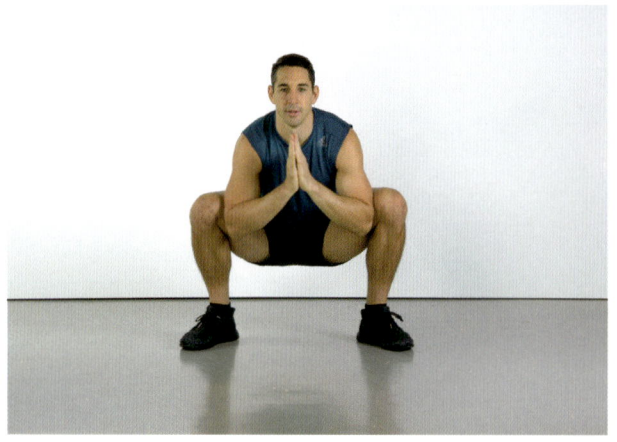

1. **Frog squats**
   Stand with your feet shoulder-width apart and your feet slightly tracked out. Bend down to full squat position with your elbows tucked inside your legs. This is the starting position. From here, raise your hips and then lower them back to the starting position.

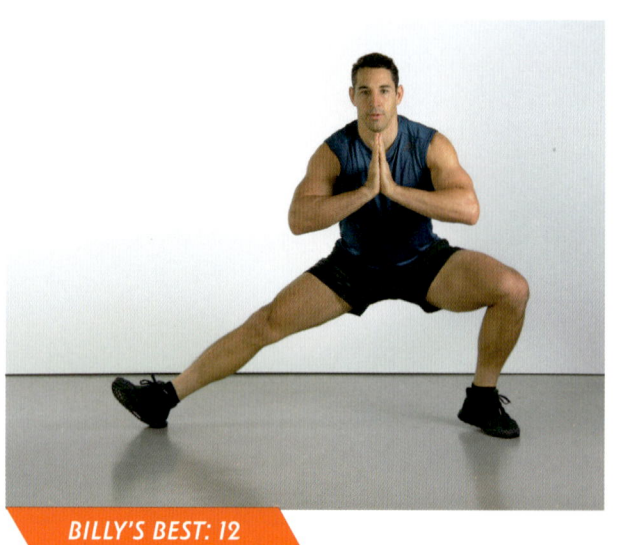

2. **Cossack squats (side lunges)**
   Stand with your feet wide apart and your toes pointing out to the side. From here, squat to one side as low as you can – your opposite heel should be on the ground. Stand back up to the starting position and repeat on the other side.

BILLY'S BEST: 12

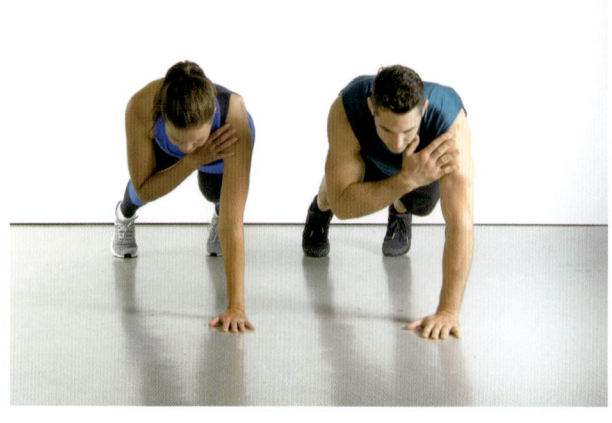

3. **2 x shoulder taps, 1 x push-up**
   For the shoulder taps, start in high plank position. Engaging your core, transfer your weight into your right arm, and with your left hand touch your right shoulder. Return to the starting position and repeat on the left side.

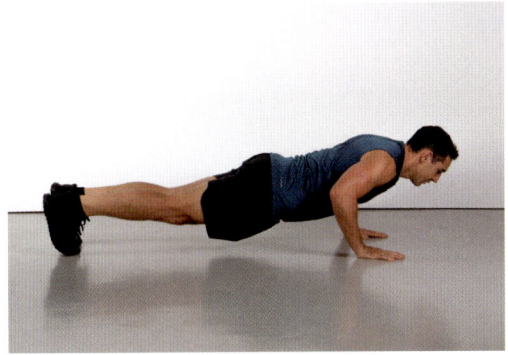

3.1 Remaining in the starting position with your hands shoulder-width apart, lift yourself up so your shoulders are over your wrists and your feet are elevated on your toes. This is the starting position. Now lower yourself down to transfer all your weight into your shoulders and back. Press back up to the starting position.

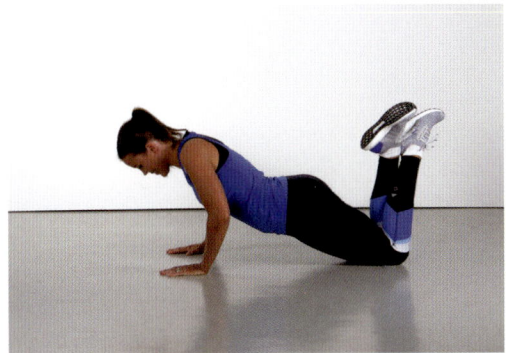

3.2 Alternatively, kneel down and place one ankle over the other while your your knees are on the floor in the starting position. Now lift yourself up so your shoulders are over your wrists. Lower yourself down to the ground and then press back up to the starting position.

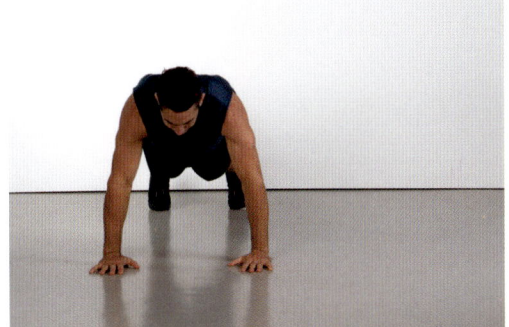

4   **Plank lateral moves**

Starting in plank position, lift and move the same arm and same leg out to one side. Now in wide stance, both arms and feet are in a wide position. Bring the opposite arm and leg back together to the starting position, alternating each side.

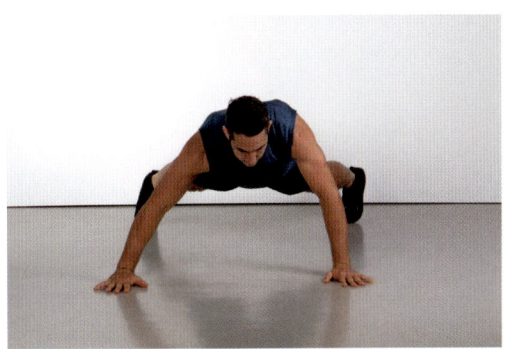

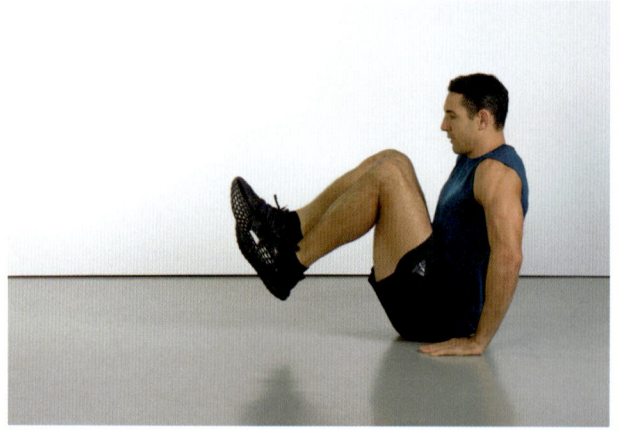

5 **Crossed-leg knee to chest**
Sit on the ground with your legs out straight and your ankles crossed. Put your hands just behind your butt and lean back. This is the starting position. Lift your legs off the ground and slowly bring your knees to your chest. From here, straighten your legs back out to the starting position. Continue throughout the allotted time without letting your heels touch the ground.

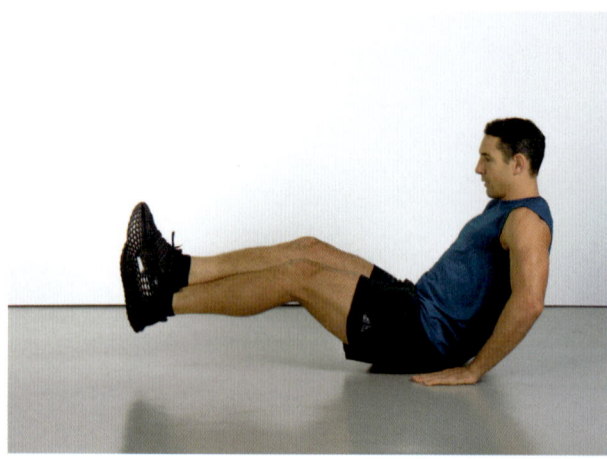

6 **Glute bridge**
Lie on your back with your arms by your sides and one leg out straight. Bend the opposite leg and bring the heel as close as you can to your butt. Now raise your hips, keeping the straight leg off the ground and squeezing your butt, before lowering yourself back to the starting position. Swap sides and repeat.

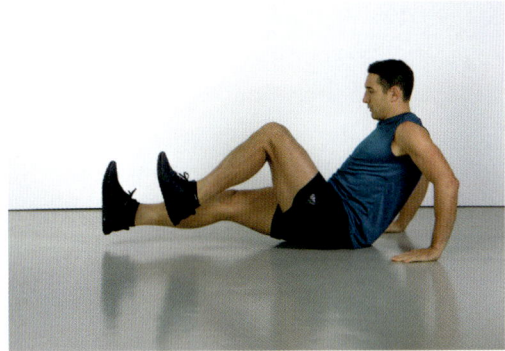

7 Bicycle crunches

Start by sitting on the ground with your hands on the floor by your side and your legs extended in front of you. From here, lean back, engaging your core so your feet are off the ground. Now bring one knee towards your chest, keeping the other leg straight. Return your knee to the earlier position and swap to bring your other knee towards your chest.

Advanced: Take your hands off the ground and bring the opposite elbow to your knee.

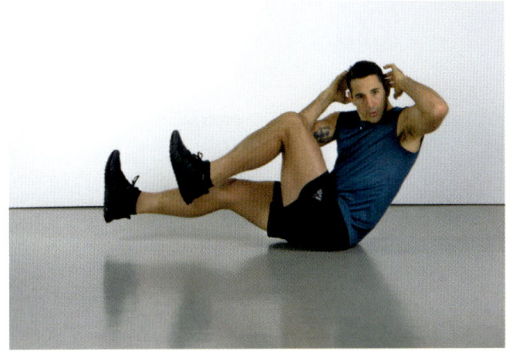

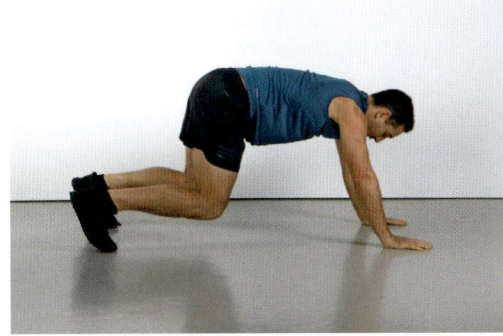

8 Bear crawl

Start in the push-up position with your knees bent at a 90-degree angle and positioned directly under your hips. Engage your core and do not raise or round your back. This is your starting position. Walk your right hand and your left foot forward, and then your left hand and your right foot forward. Continue until you reach 5 metres. Now, keeping your hips down and your core engaged, reverse the movement by walking your left arm and your right foot back, and then your right arm and your left leg back. Continue until you have returned to your starting position.

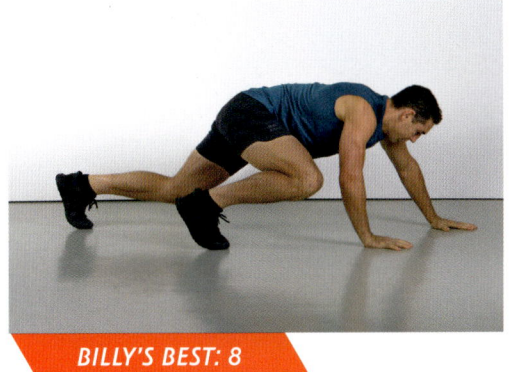

BILLY'S BEST: 8

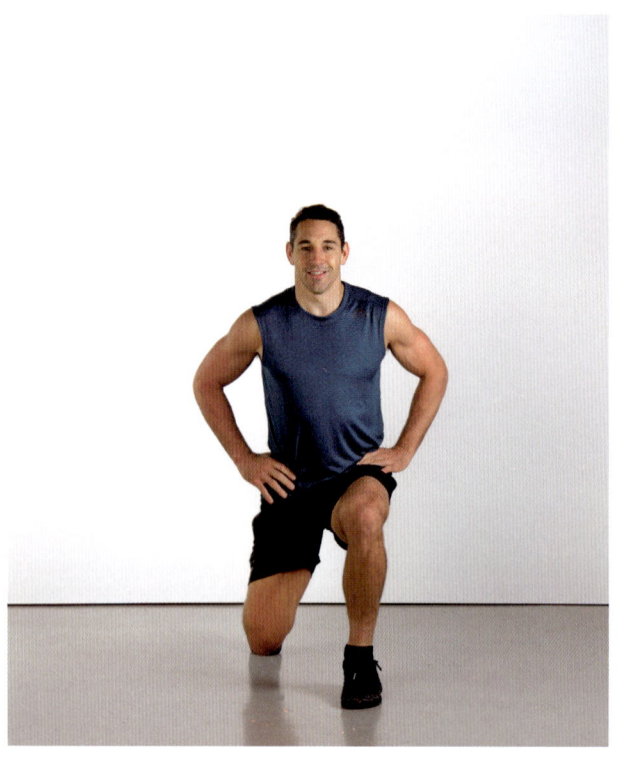

9 **Plyometric split lunges**

9.1 Start with your feet shoulder-width apart and your hands on your hips. Split your legs before dropping your back knee down in line with the heel of your leading foot – both legs should be at a 90-degree angle – then push up and repeat on the other side.

9.2 Alternatively, stand with your feet shoulder-width apart and your hands on your hips. Step one leg back and then lower it until it is 90 degrees to the ground. Step forward to the starting position. Repeat on the other side to complete the movement.

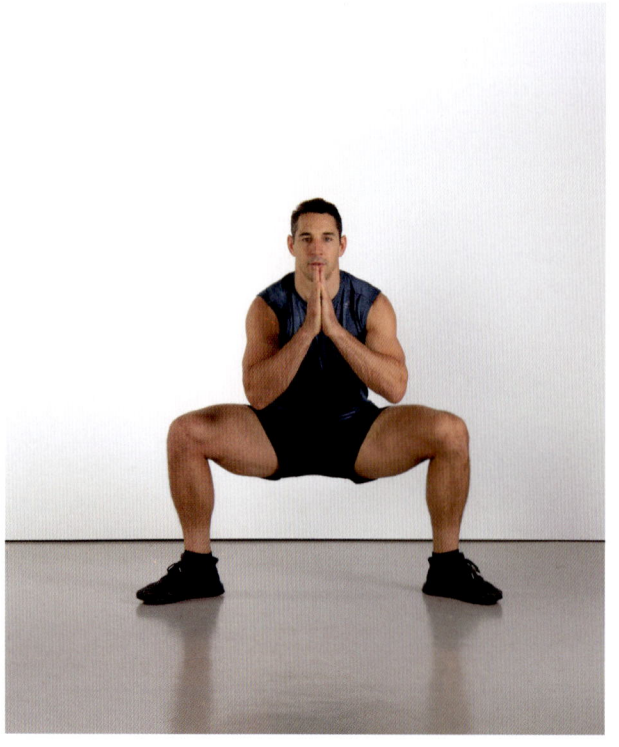

10 **Sumo squats**

Stand with your feet wide apart and slightly tracked out, and your hands on your hips. Bend at the hips and lower your butt towards the ground, bending your knees and keeping your shoulders back and your chest tight. Lower yourself down as far as is comfortable. Return to starting position.

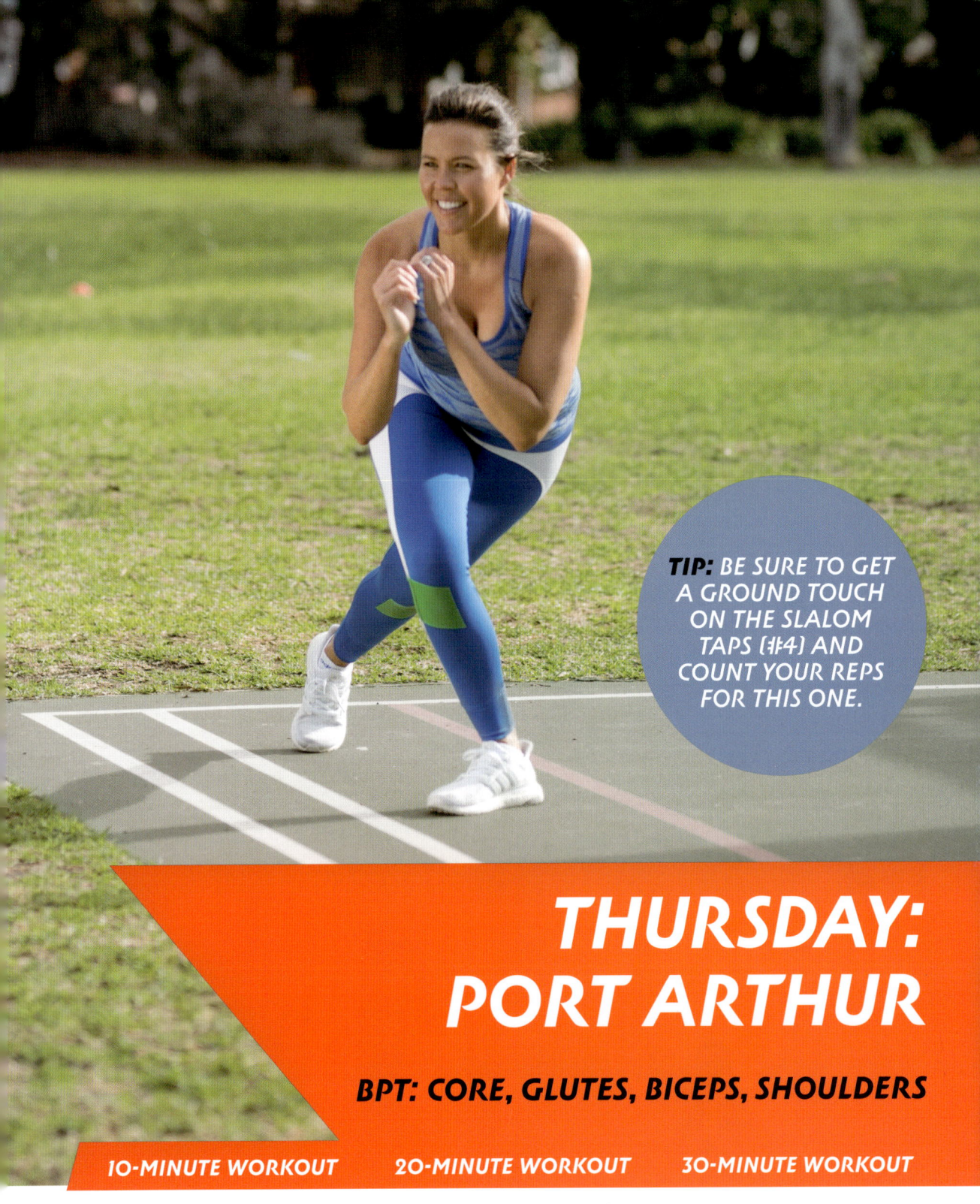

TIP: BE SURE TO GET A GROUND TOUCH ON THE SLALOM TAPS (#4) AND COUNT YOUR REPS FOR THIS ONE.

THURSDAY: PORT ARTHUR

BPT: CORE, GLUTES, BICEPS, SHOULDERS

10-MINUTE WORKOUT

20 seconds on / 10 seconds off
2 sets per exercise
1 lap of circuit

20-MINUTE WORKOUT

40 seconds on / 20 seconds off
1 set per exercise
1 lap of circuit

30-MINUTE WORKOUT

50 seconds on / 10 seconds off
1 set per exercise
1 lap of circuit

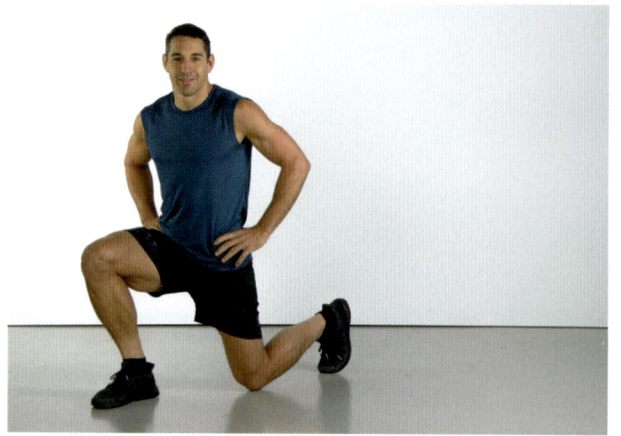

1. **Lateral lunges**

   Stand with your feet shoulder-width apart and your hands on your hips or by your side. Take a half-step to one side and then bend at the knee and lunge, sticking your butt out and keeping your chest up and your core tight. Lunge back to the starting position. Repeat on the other side.

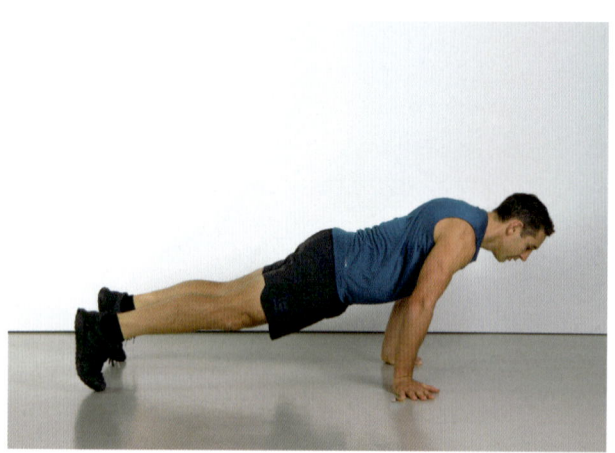

2. **Planche push-ups**

   Start in an assisted or full push-up position with your hands slightly tracked out. Lean forward so that your arms are straight and you are comfortable. From here, lower yourself until your chest is just off the ground, and then press back up. You should feel this movement in your shoulders and biceps.

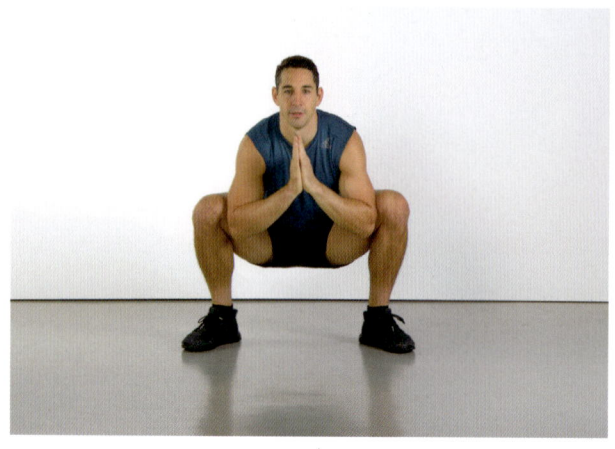

3. **Frog squats**

   Stand with your feet shoulder-width apart and your feet slightly tracked out. Bend down to full squat position with your elbows tucked inside your legs. This is the starting position. From here, raise your hips and then lower them back to the starting position.

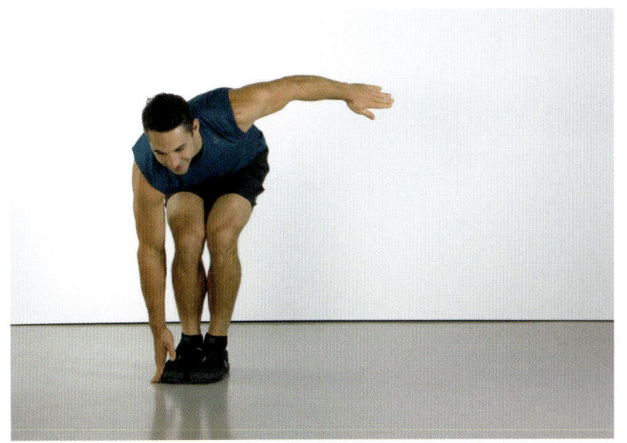

4 Slalom taps

Start with your feet together, then jump to the left to land on both feet, touching your left hand down next to your left foot. Then jump to the right with both feet, touching your right hand to your right foot.

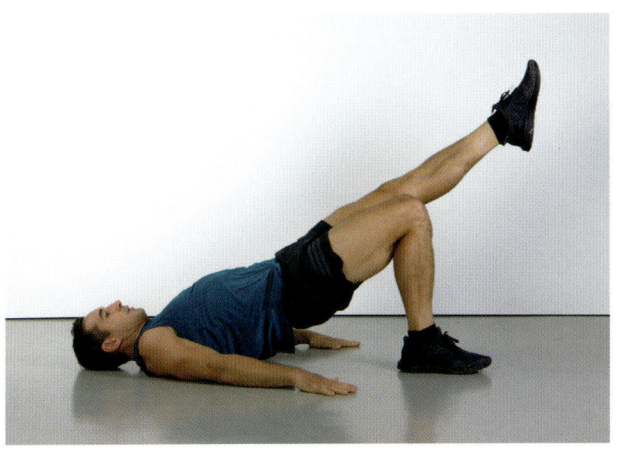

5 Glute bridge

Lie on your back with your arms by your sides and one leg out straight. Bend the opposite leg and bring the heel as close as you can to your butt. Now raise your hips, keeping the straight leg off the ground and squeezing your butt, before lowering yourself back to the starting position.

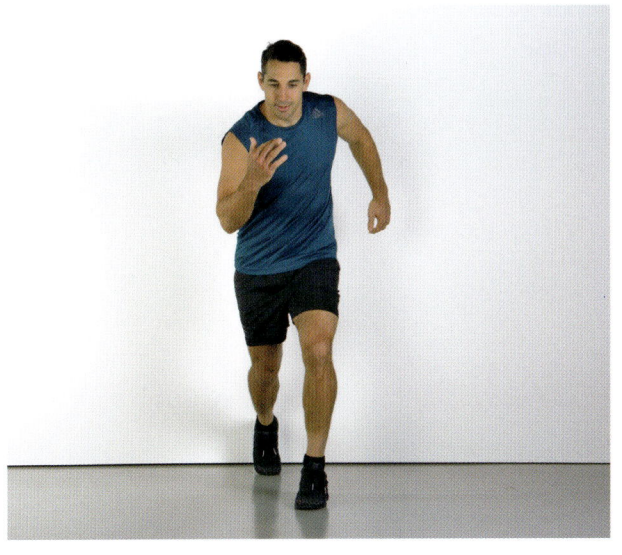

6 Shuttle run

Picking a distance that suits your environment, run up and back for the duration of time.

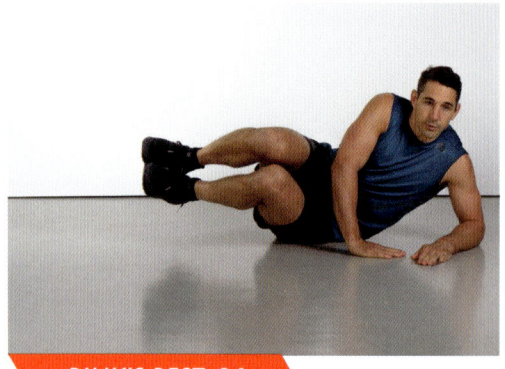

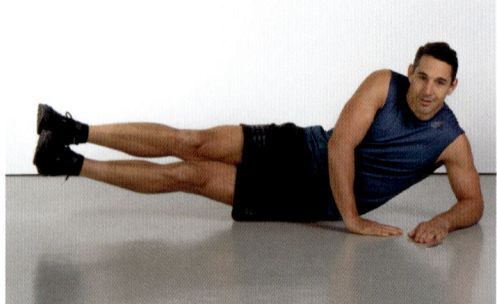

BILLY'S BEST: 24

7 **Oblique kick-outs**

Sit on the ground with your knees together and slightly bent, and your hands touching the ground. Bring your knees diagonally across your chest, then straighten your legs out. Repeat on the other side.

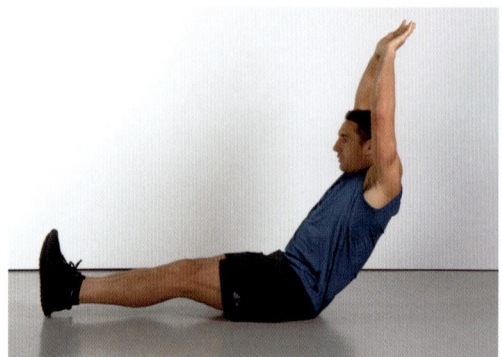

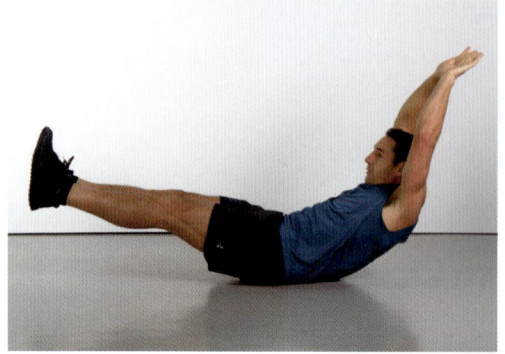

8 **Body rocks**

Sit on the ground with your legs extended in front and lean back, raising your hands above your head, contracting your core and lifting your legs off the ground. From here, rock back and forth with your heels off the ground and, if you like, your knees slightly bent.

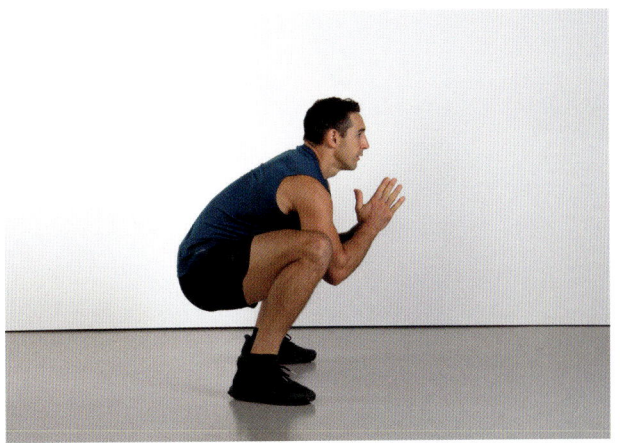

9 **Sprawls**

Stand with your feet just shoulder-width apart. Squat until both your hands and both your feet are firmly on the ground. From this position, transfer your weight into your shoulders and shoot your feet back so that your legs are out wide, then jump your feet back up and stand up into the starting position.

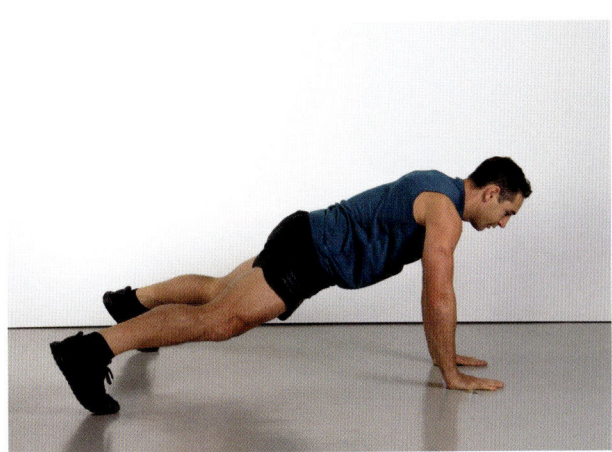

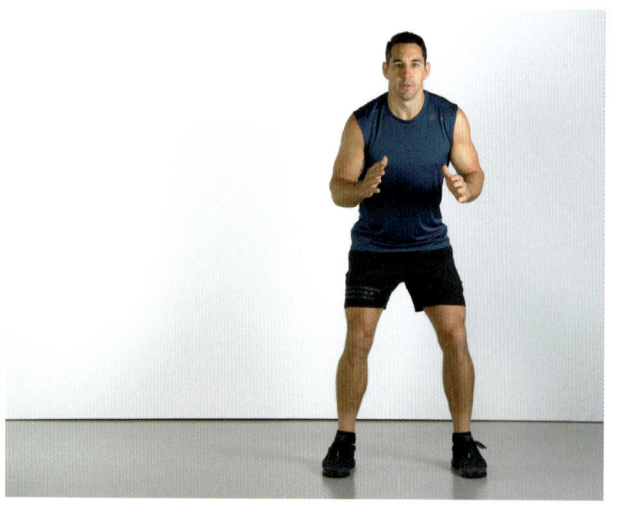

10 Ice skaters

Start with your feet shoulder-width apart. Step half a foot to your left, swing your right leg behind your left leg, and with your right hand touch your left toe. From here, step to your right, swing your left leg behind your right leg, and with your left hand touch your right toe.

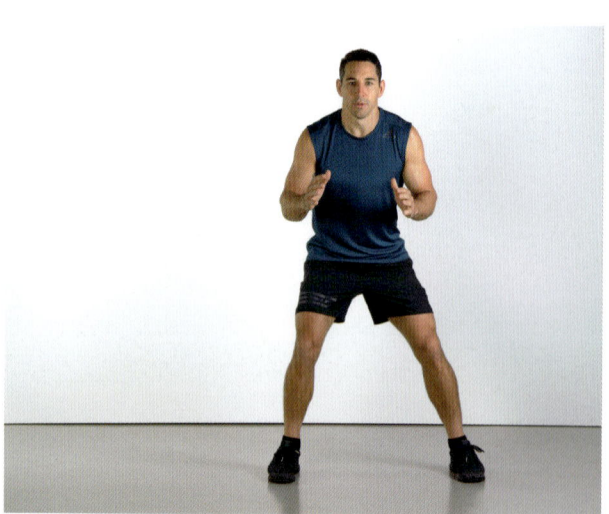

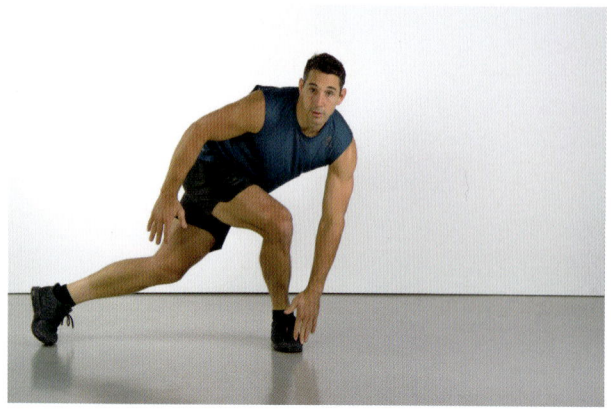

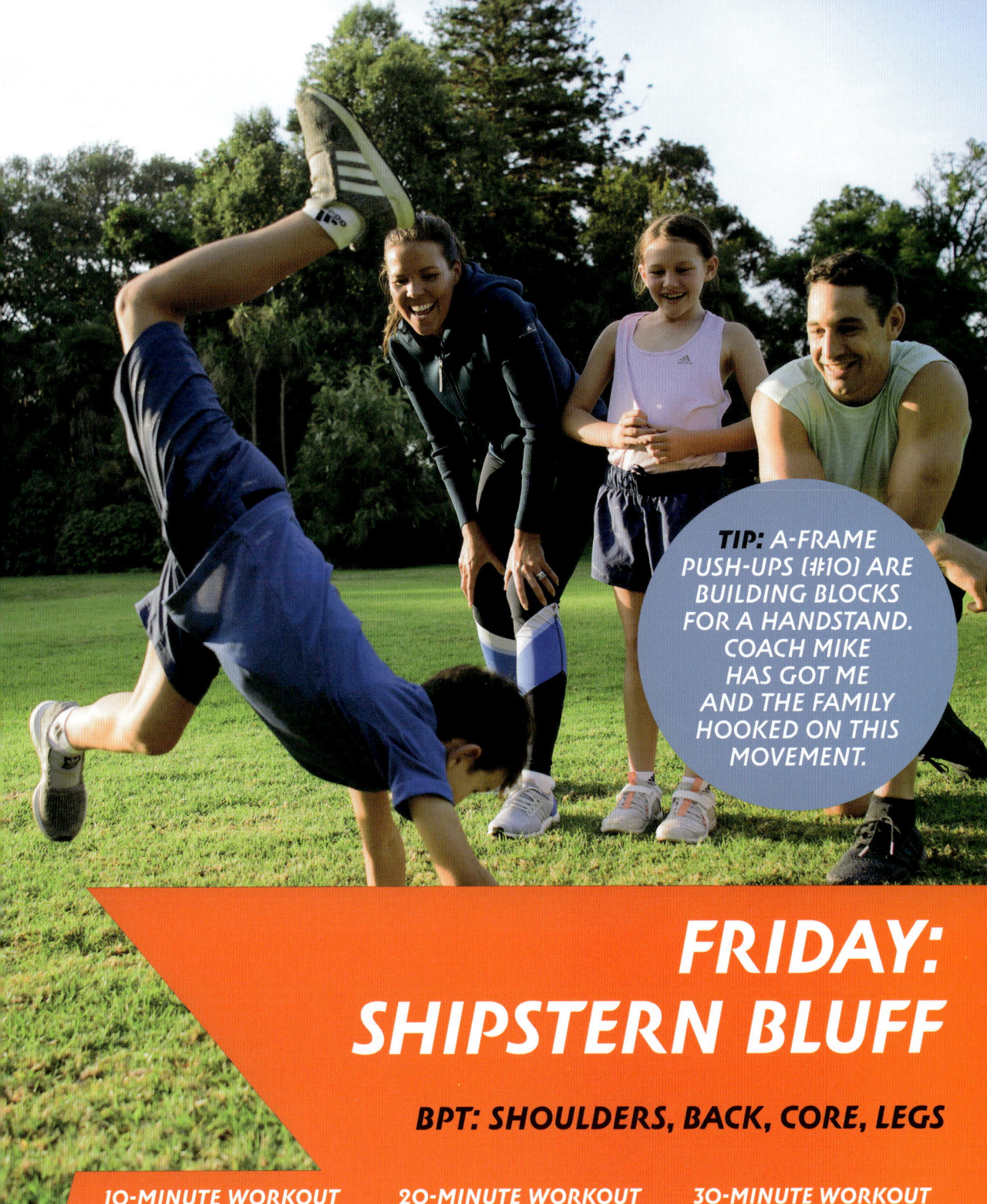

TIP: A-FRAME PUSH-UPS (#10) ARE BUILDING BLOCKS FOR A HANDSTAND. COACH MIKE HAS GOT ME AND THE FAMILY HOOKED ON THIS MOVEMENT.

FRIDAY: SHIPSTERN BLUFF

BPT: SHOULDERS, BACK, CORE, LEGS

10-MINUTE WORKOUT	20-MINUTE WORKOUT	30-MINUTE WORKOUT
20 seconds movement / 10 seconds rest 2 sets of each exercise (one lap)	20 seconds movement / 10 seconds rest 2 sets of each exercise (two laps)	20 seconds movement / 10 seconds rest 2 sets of each exercise (three laps)

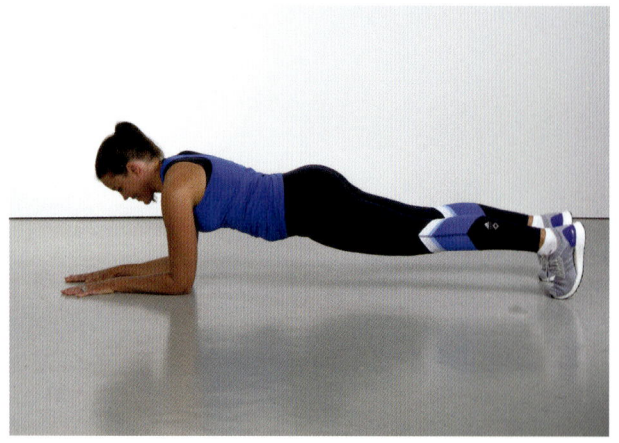

1. **Plank**

   Place your forearms on the ground and lift your knees off the ground with your feet together and your toes touching the ground. From here, lean slightly forward to engage your core. Hold the position for the duration of time. (Note: Your back should not be sagging or bent.)

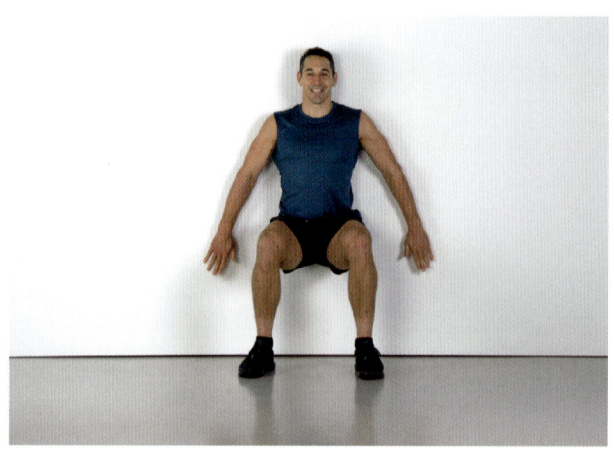

2. **Wall sit**

   Put your back against a wall, feet shoulder-width apart and two steps away from the wall. With your hands firmly against the wall, lower your butt down the wall until your knees are at a 90-degree angle. Hold the position.

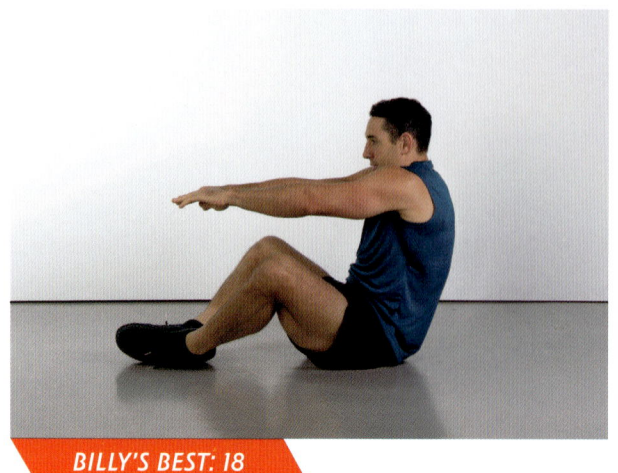

3. **Butterfly sit-ups**

   Sit on the ground with your feet together and as close as possible to your butt, with your knees out wide. From here, lean back until you are lying flat on the ground. Lift your head and then your body back up to the starting position.

BILLY'S BEST: 18

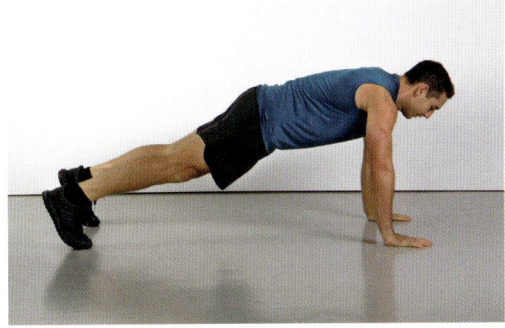

4 Burpees

Stand in a relaxed position with your feet shoulder-width apart. Squat and place your hands firmly on the ground with your feet back. Shoot your legs back so you are in a high plank position, then lower your body so your torso is just touching the ground. Release your hands and then, placing your hands back on the ground, raise your torso and jump your feet back so both hands and both feet are on the ground. Stand back up, then jump up and raise your hands above your head.

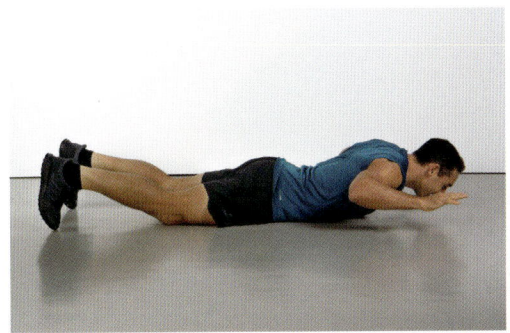

5 Push-ups

5.1 Get into high plank position with your hands shoulder-width apart, your shoulders over your wrists and your feet elevated on your toes. This is the starting position. Now lower yourself down to transfer all your weight into your shoulders and back. Press back up to the starting position.

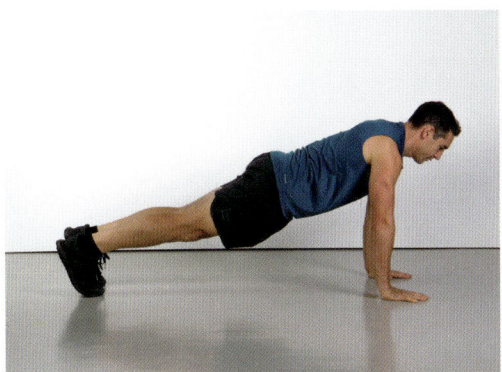

5.2 Alternatively, place one ankle over the other while your knees are on the floor in the starting position. Now lift yourself up so your shoulders are over your wrists. Lower yourself down to the ground and then press back up to the starting position.

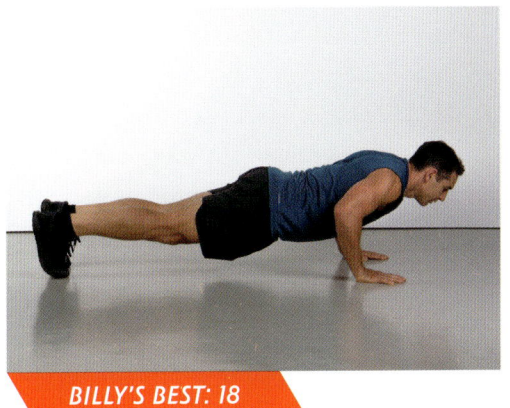

BILLY'S BEST: 18

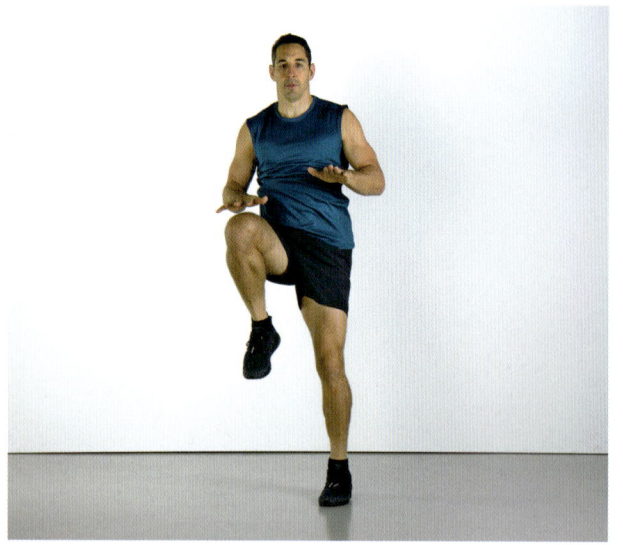

6 **High knees**

Stand with your feet shoulder-width apart. One leg at a time, raise your left knee up as high as you can before alternating to the other leg.

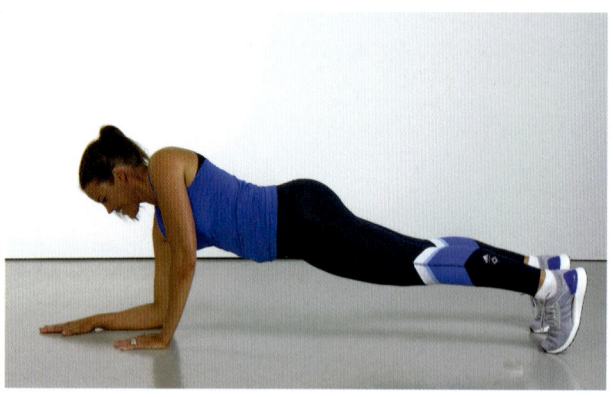

7 **Moving plank**

Lie with your forearms on the ground, your knees off the ground and your feet together. From here, with your toes touching the ground lean slightly forward to engage your core. Shifting your weight to the right, place your right hand firmly on the ground. Shift your weight to the left side and place your left hand on the ground. Finish in the high plank position. (Note: Your back should not be sagging or bent.)

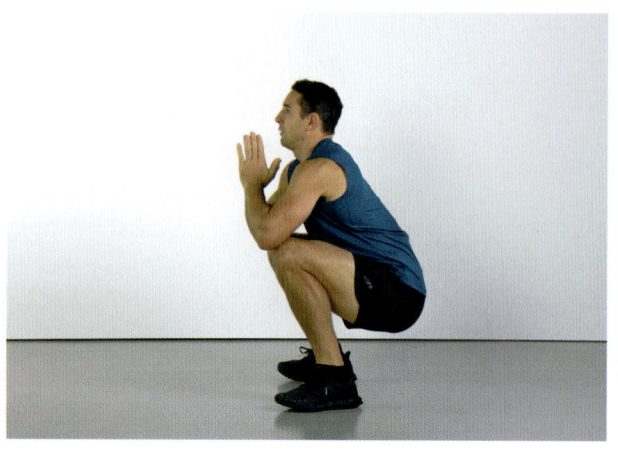

8 **Deep squats**

Stand with your feet shoulder-width apart, slightly tracked out. Holding your hands together, bend forward at your hips and lower your body down, keeping your feet flat on the ground and going as low as you can before pressing back up through your heels to the starting position.

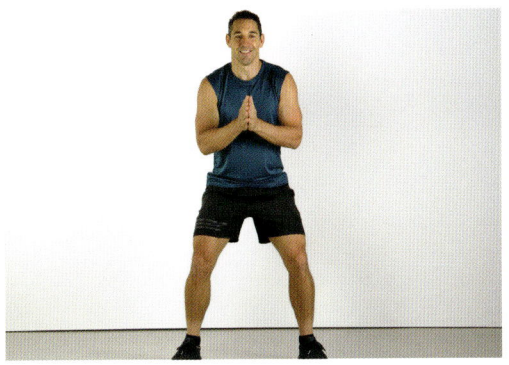

9 Seal jacks

Starting in a relaxed position with your hands touching together in the middle of your chest, jump out so your feet are in a wide stance and your arms split. Bring your feet and hands back together.

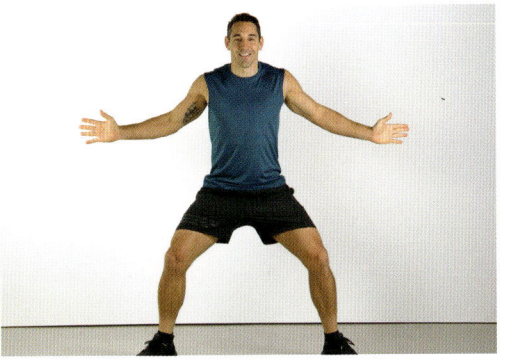

10 A-frame push-ups

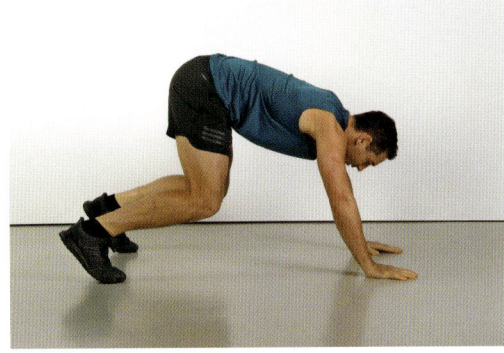

Stand with your feet wide apart and slightly tracked out. With your hands shoulder-width apart, and bending at the hips, lean over to touch the ground with your legs straight or bent and your chin slightly tucked. From this starting position, lower yourself down till the top of your head is just off the ground and you're looking through your legs. Your head should be in line with your hands. From here, press back up to the starting position, transferring all the weight into your palms.

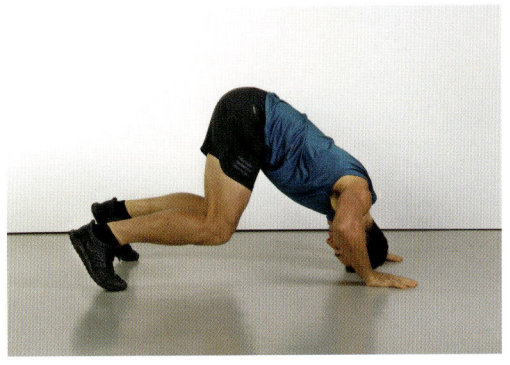

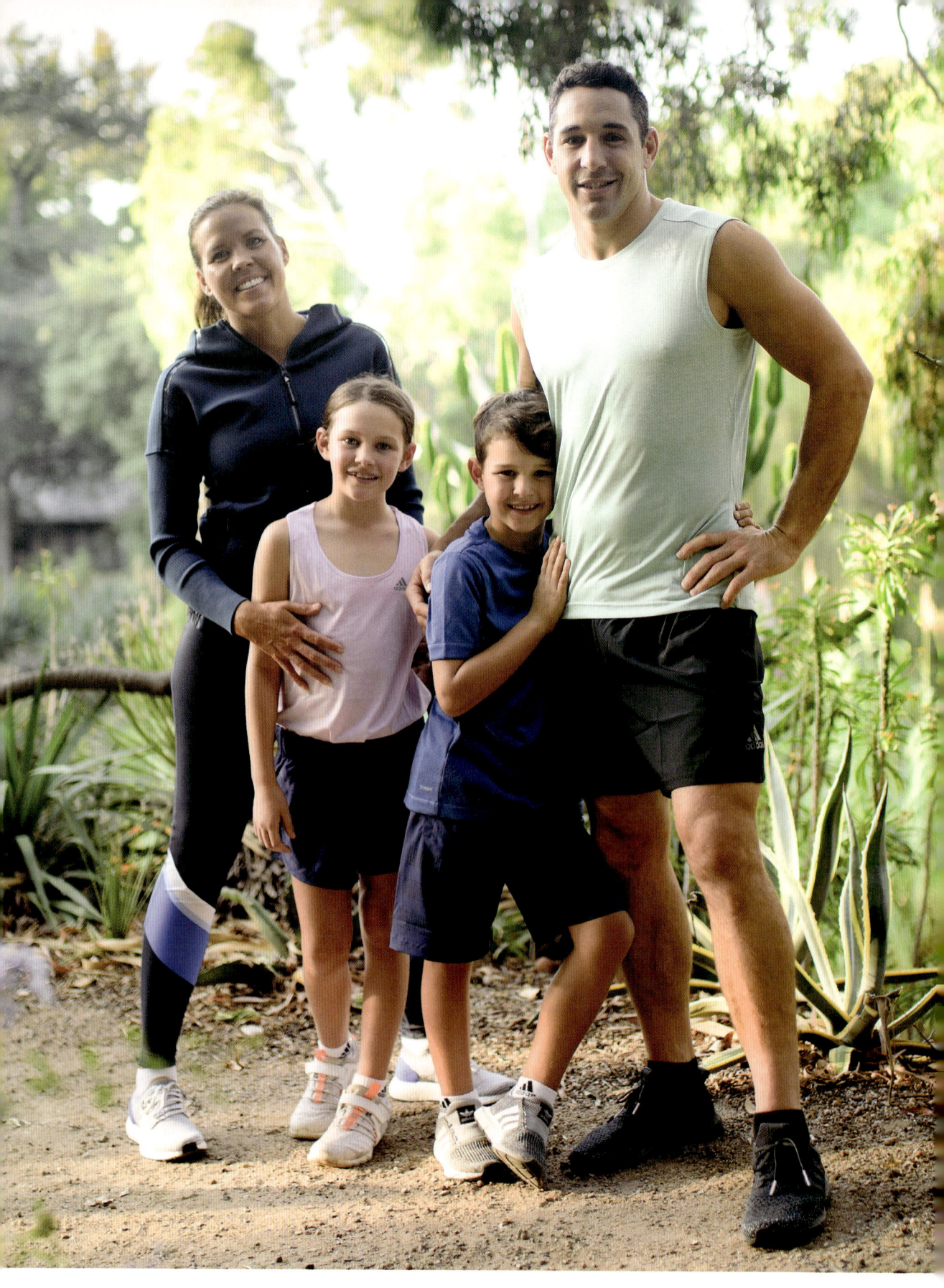

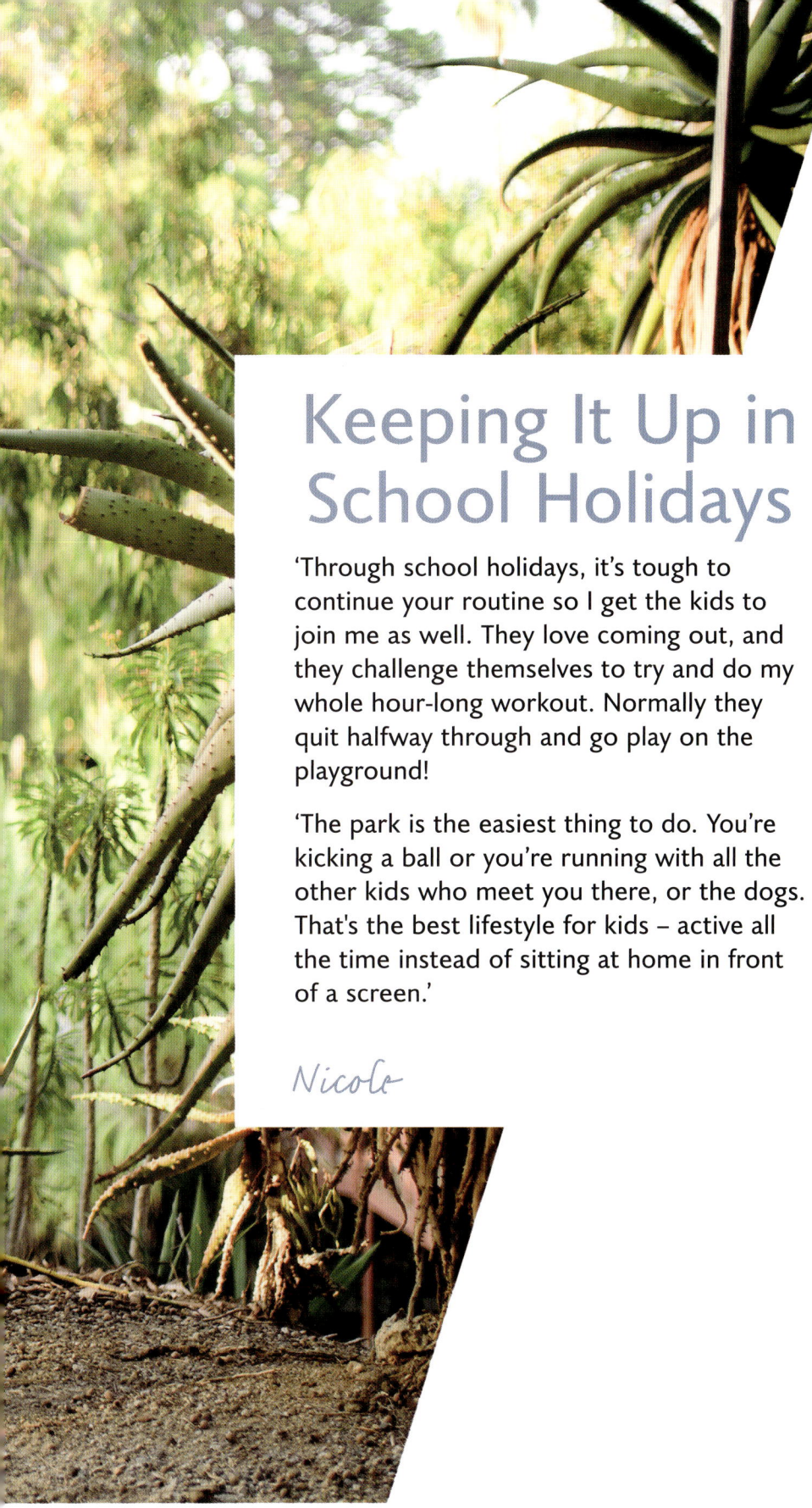

Keeping It Up in School Holidays

'Through school holidays, it's tough to continue your routine so I get the kids to join me as well. They love coming out, and they challenge themselves to try and do my whole hour-long workout. Normally they quit halfway through and go play on the playground!

'The park is the easiest thing to do. You're kicking a ball or you're running with all the other kids who meet you there, or the dogs. That's the best lifestyle for kids – active all the time instead of sitting at home in front of a screen.'

Nicole

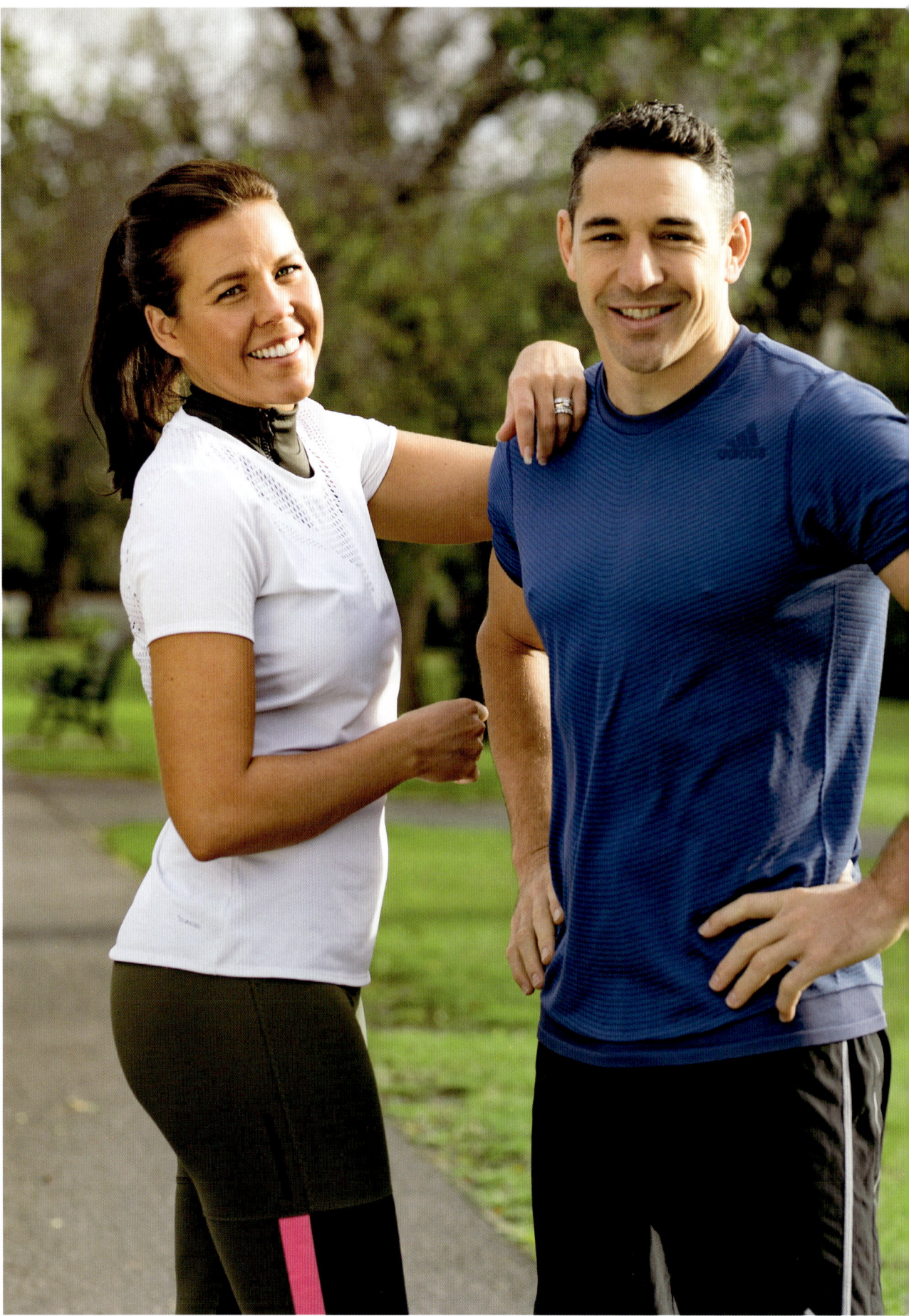

BLOCK 8: NEW ZEALAND

'A stunning location. I've played here a few times over my career. Great people, too! There's a diverse range of scenery, from the cosmopolitan CBDs to the lush landscapes as you travel between the North and South Islands. An excellent place to get moving outside (or even in the snow!).'

Billy

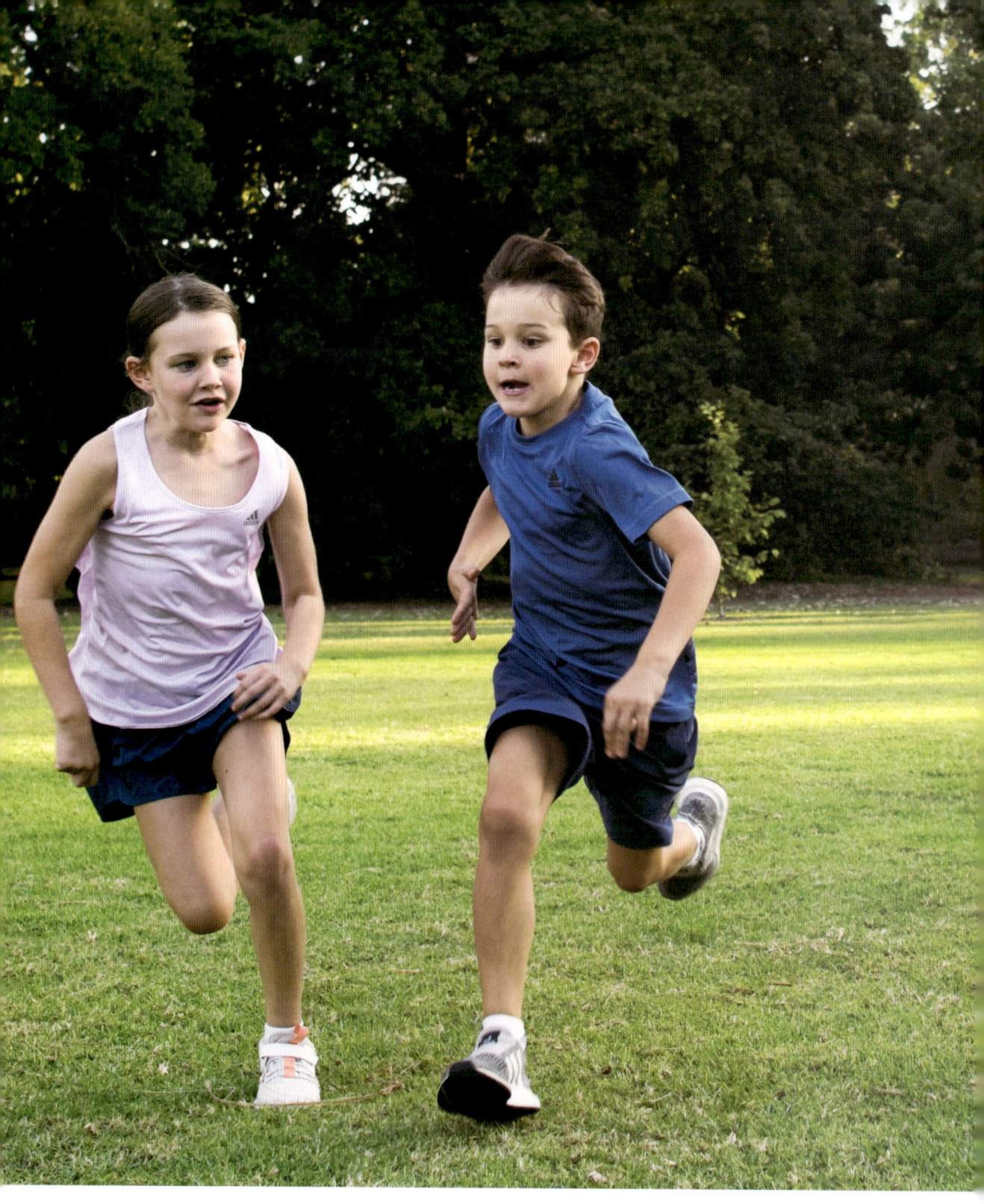

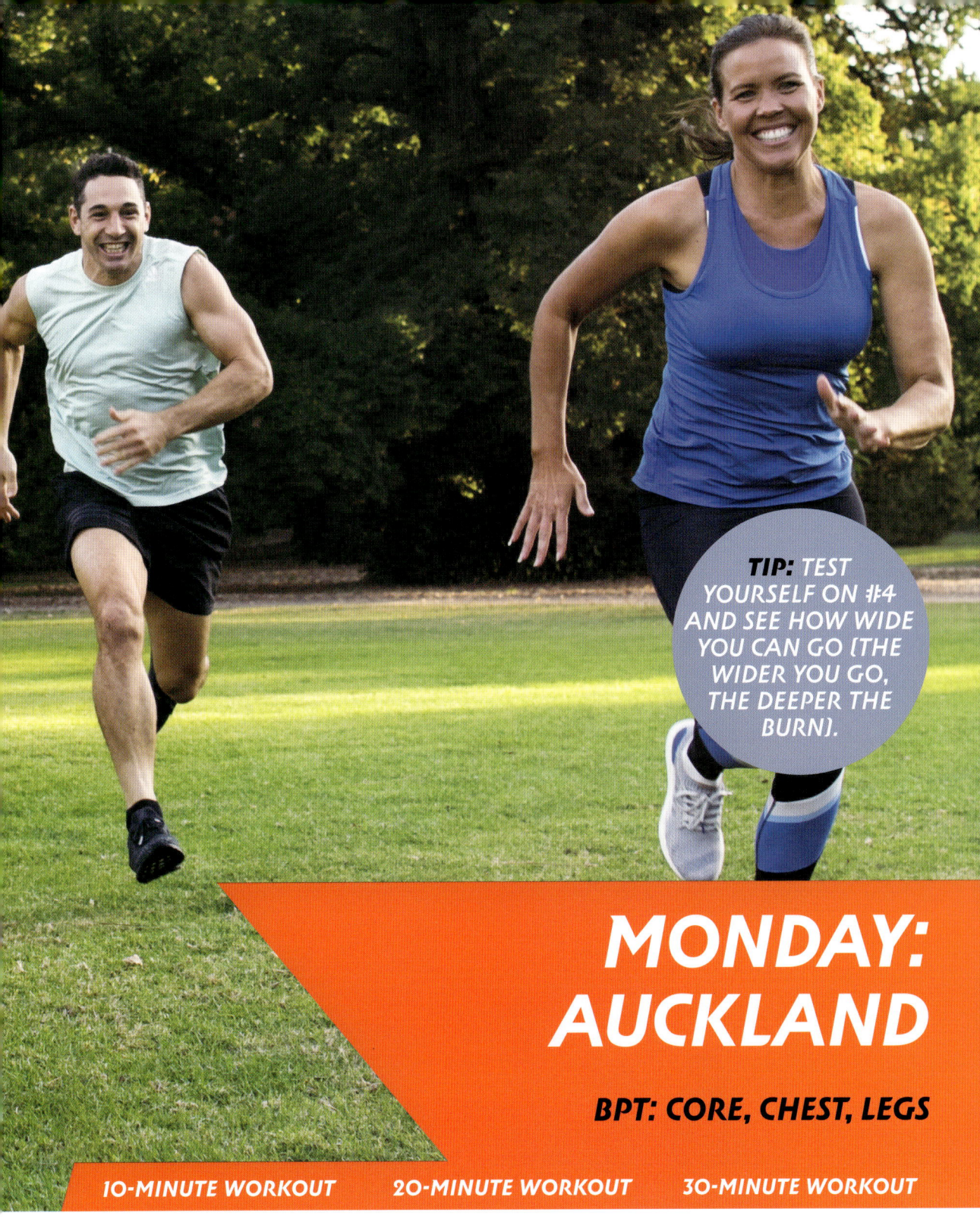

TIP: TEST YOURSELF ON #4 AND SEE HOW WIDE YOU CAN GO (THE WIDER YOU GO, THE DEEPER THE BURN).

MONDAY: AUCKLAND

BPT: CORE, CHEST, LEGS

10-MINUTE WORKOUT

20 seconds movement /
10 seconds rest
2 sets of each exercise
(one lap)

20-MINUTE WORKOUT

20 seconds movement /
10 seconds rest
2 sets of each exercise
(two laps)

30-MINUTE WORKOUT

20 seconds movement /
10 seconds rest
2 sets of each exercise
(three laps)

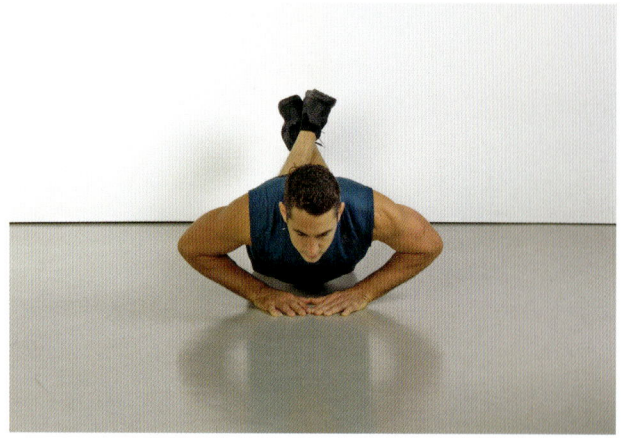

1. **Diamond push-ups**

   Kneel on the ground with your ankles crossed, and set your hands so your thumbs and index fingers are touching in line with your chin. From here, lower your body towards the ground and then press back up to the starting position. You should feel this movement in your triceps.

   Advanced: Do the exercise in high plank position with your knees off the ground.

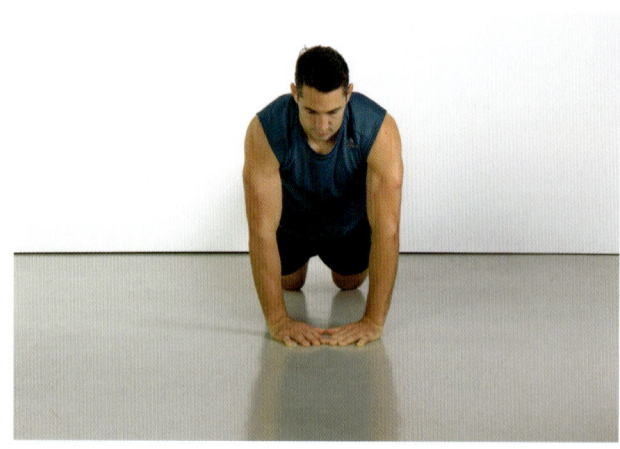

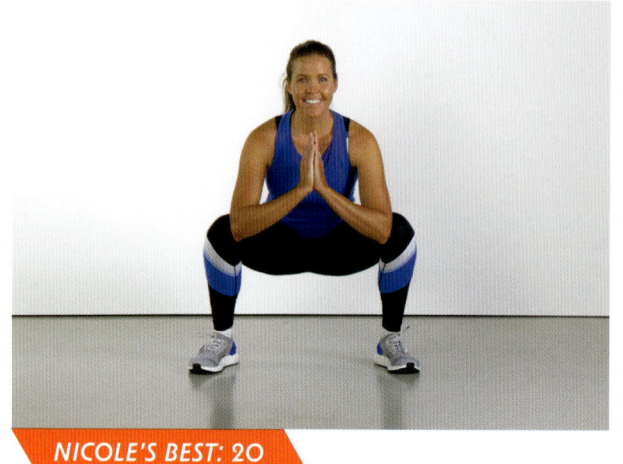

2. **Deep squats**

   Stand with your feet shoulder-width apart, slightly tracked out. Holding your hands together, bend forward at your hips and lower your body down, keeping your feet flat on the ground and going as low as you can before pressing back up through your heels to the starting position.

NICOLE'S BEST: 20

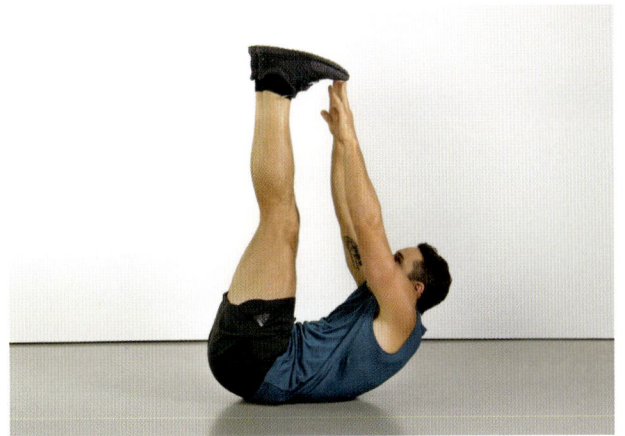

3 Sit-up toe touches

Lie on your back with your legs in the air and your toes flexed. Sitting up, bring both legs up and touch the toes with your hands. Lie back down and repeat.

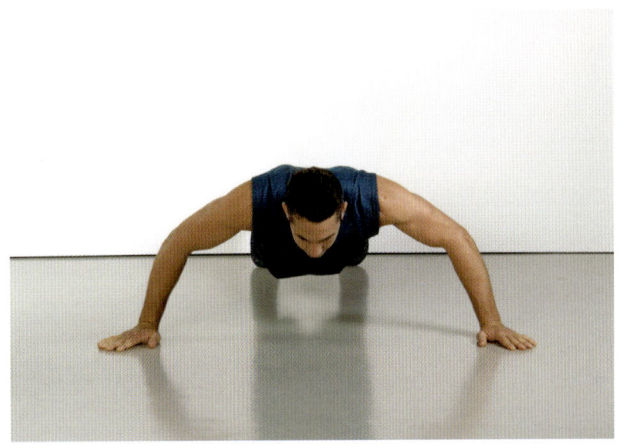

4 Wide push-ups

Get into a high plank position but with your hands slightly wider than shoulder-width, and lift yourself up so your shoulders are over your wrists and your feet are elevated on your toes. Now lower yourself to transfer all your weight into your shoulders and your back. Press back up to the starting position.

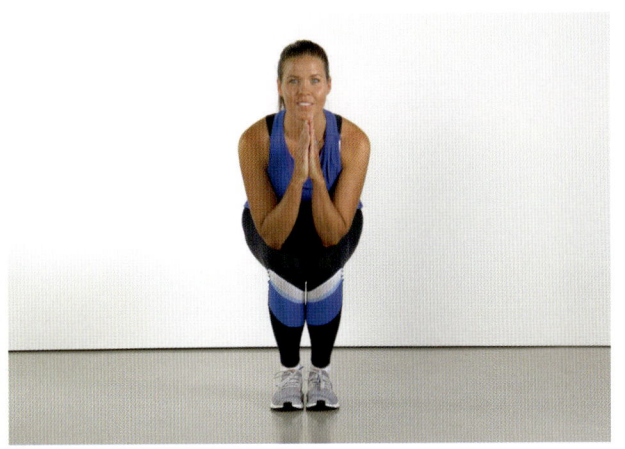

5 Close-feet squats

Stand near a wall with your feet together and your hands on your hips. Bend at the hips, stick your butt out to the wall and lower yourself down as far as you can go with all your weight in the back of your heels. From here, drive through your heels back up to the starting position.

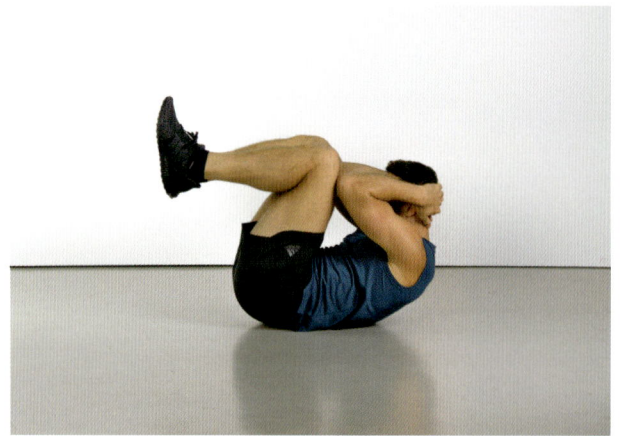

6 Crunches

Lie on your back with your legs off the ground, with knees bent at a 90-degree angle to your body. With your hands crossed behind your head, bring your elbows in next to your ears. Bring your elbows up to your knees and then return to the starting position.

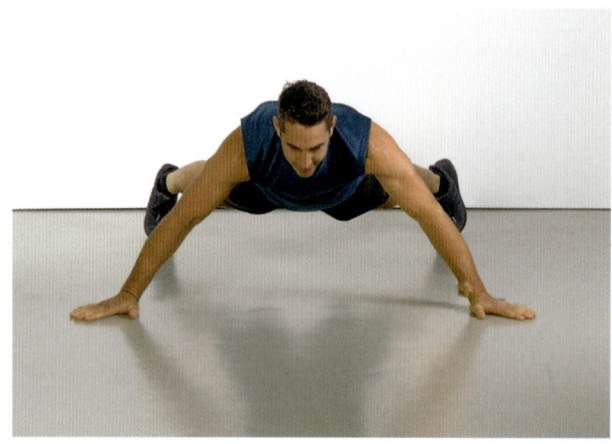

7 Spider-Man holds

Start in a high plank position but with your hands out nice and wide and your legs as wide as your hands. From here, raise your knees and lean forward slightly, engaging your core and squeezing your glutes. You should also feel this movement in your biceps and shoulders.

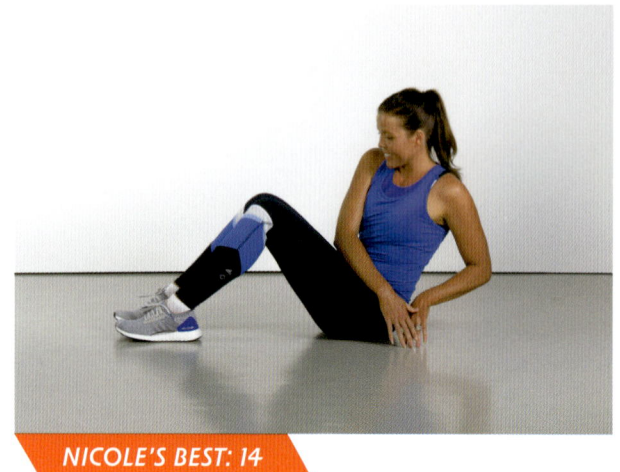

8 Russian twists

Sit on the ground with your knees bent and your feet flat on the ground. Clasping your hands in front of your chest, twist your torso to one side and touch the ground, engaging your core. Then shift your weight and twist your torso to touch the ground on the other side.

NICOLE'S BEST: 14

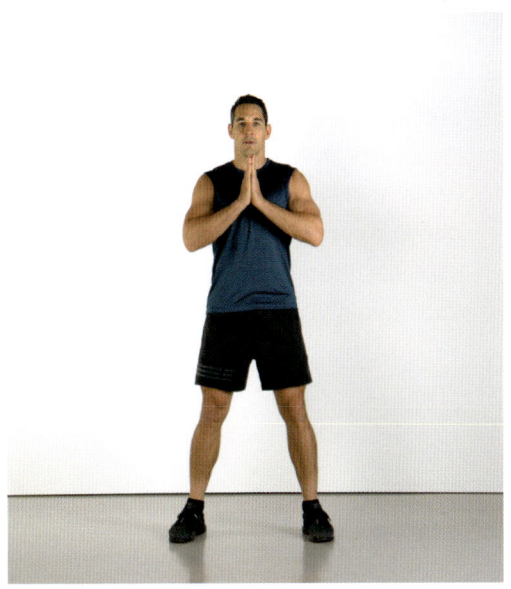

9 **Squat jumps**

Stand with your feet just past shoulder-width apart and slightly pointed outwards so your knees track with your feet. Hinging at the hips, stick your butt out and bend your knees until they are at a 90-degree angle. This is the starting position. With your hands together, drive through your legs and explode up so your feet are off the ground. As you land, lower your body back to the starting position.

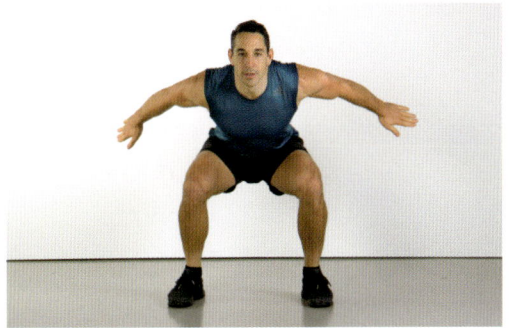

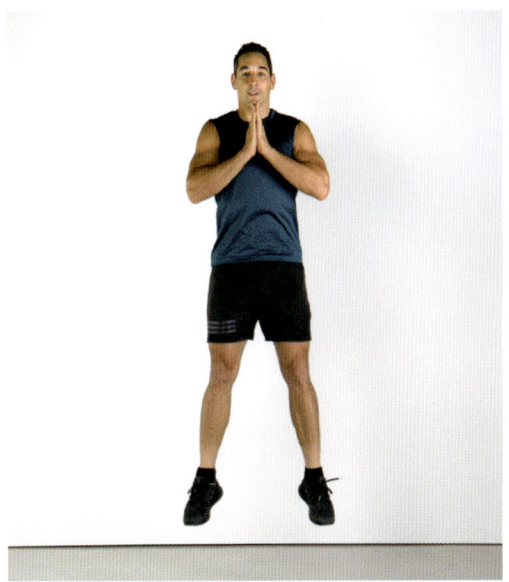

10   Sumo squats

Stand with your feet wide apart and slightly tracked out, and your hands on your hips. Bend at the hips and lower your butt towards the ground, bending your knees and keeping your shoulders back and your chest tight. Lower yourself down as far as is comfortable. Return to starting position.

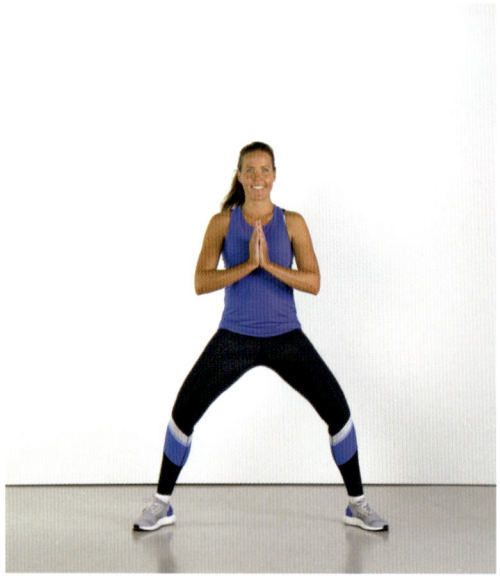

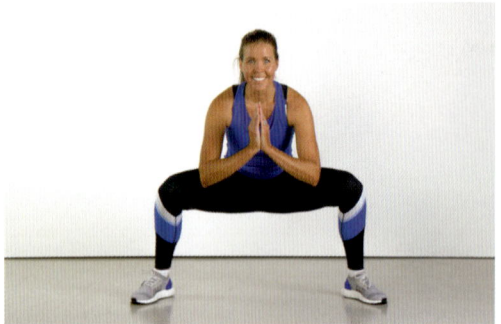

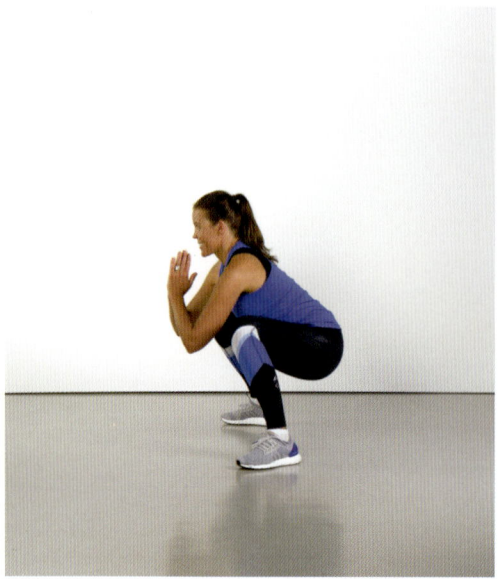

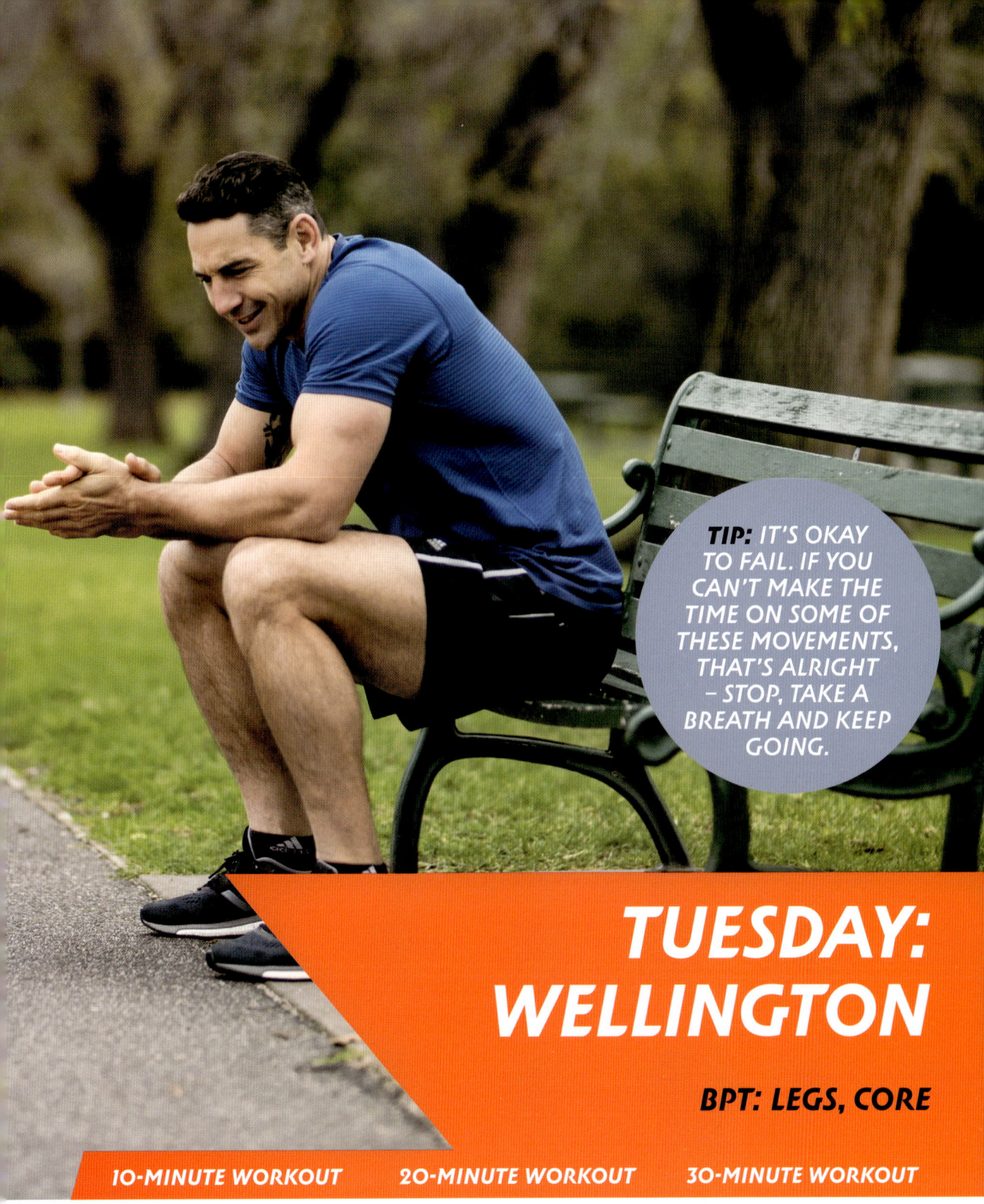

TIP: IT'S OKAY TO FAIL. IF YOU CAN'T MAKE THE TIME ON SOME OF THESE MOVEMENTS, THAT'S ALRIGHT – STOP, TAKE A BREATH AND KEEP GOING.

TUESDAY: WELLINGTON

BPT: LEGS, CORE

10-MINUTE WORKOUT	20-MINUTE WORKOUT	30-MINUTE WORKOUT
20 seconds movement / 10 seconds rest 2 sets of each exercise (one lap)	20 seconds movement / 10 seconds rest 2 sets of each exercise (two laps)	20 seconds movement / 10 seconds rest 2 sets of each exercise (three laps)

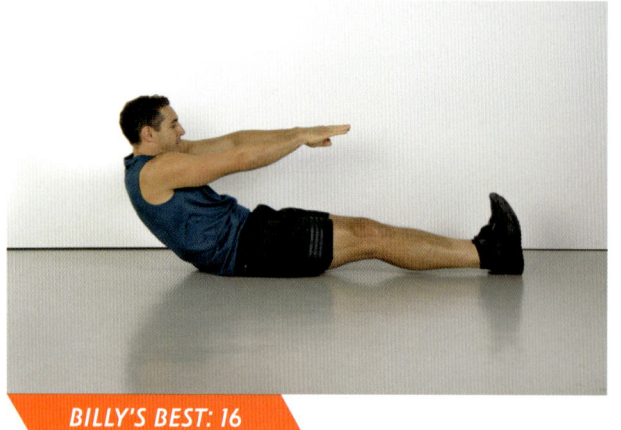

BILLY'S BEST: 16

1 ### Straight-leg sit-ups
Lie flat on the ground with your arms by your sides. Lifting your head up and engaging your core, reach towards your toes, keeping your arms and legs straight. Return to the starting position.

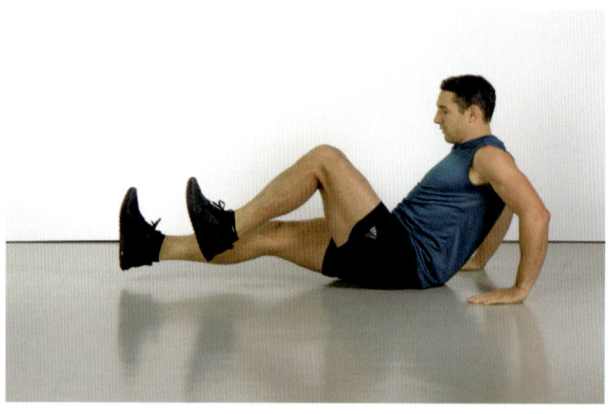

2 ### Bicycle crunches
Start by sitting on the ground with your hands on the floor by your side and your legs extended in front. From here, lean back, engaging your core so your feet are off the ground. Now bring one knee towards your chest, keeping the other leg straight. Return your knee to the earlier position and swap to bring your other knee towards your chest.

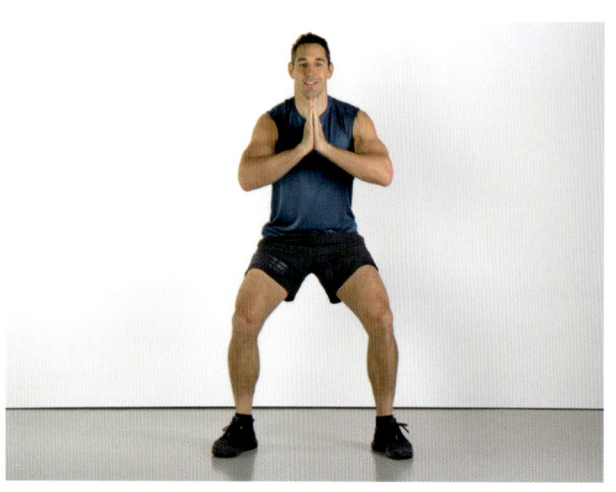

3 ### Pulse squats
Stand with your feet just past shoulder-width apart and slightly tracked out. Squat with your hips back and your legs at a 90-degree angle, then pulse up and down.

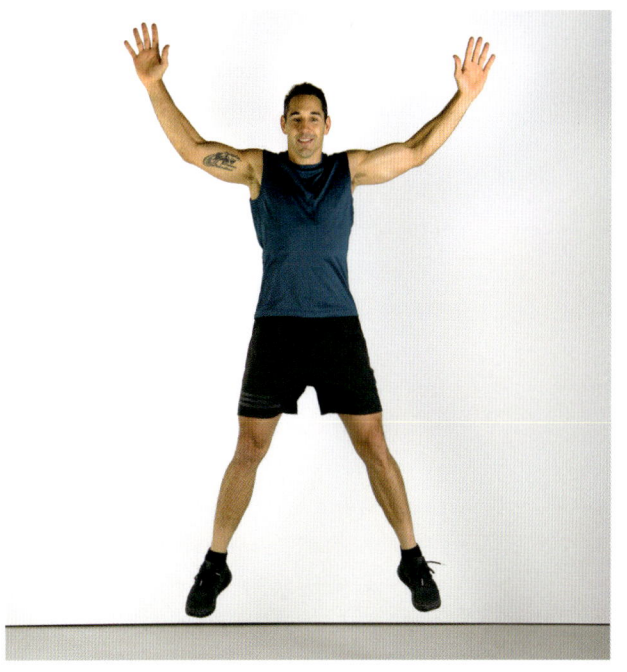

4 Star jumps

Begin in a relaxed stance with your arms close to your body. Jump your feet out wide past shoulder-width and raise both your arms above your head, then land back in the starting position.

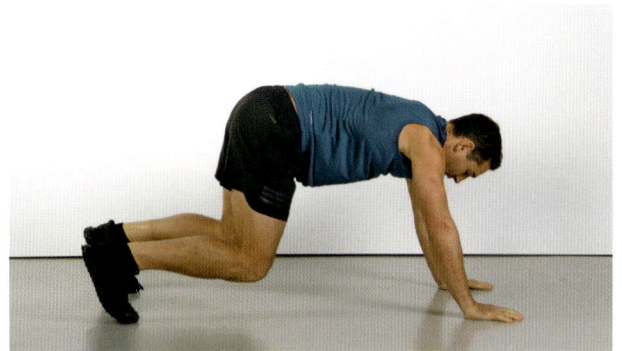

5 Bear crawl

Start in the push-up position with your knees bent at a 90-degree angle and positioned directly under your hips. Engage your core and do not raise or round your back. This is your starting position. Walk your right hand and your left foot forward, and then your left hand and your right foot forward. Continue until you reach 5 metres. Now, keeping your hips down and your core engaged, reverse the movement by walking your left arm and your right foot back, and then your right arm and your left leg back. Continue until you have returned to your starting position.

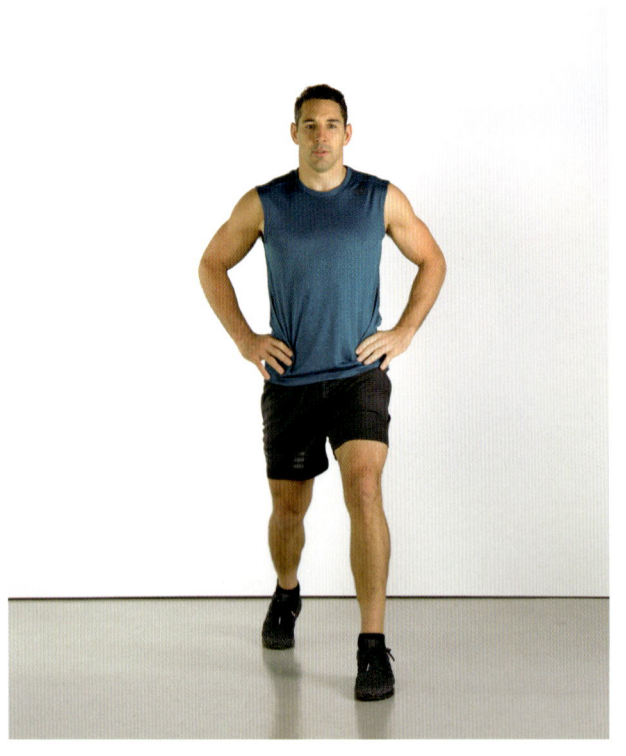

6 Plyometric split lunges

6.1 Start with your feet shoulder-width apart and your hands on your hips. Split your legs before dropping your back knee down in line with the heel of your leading foot – both legs should be at a 90-degree angle – then push up and repeat on the other side.

6.2 Alternatively, stand with your feet shoulder-width apart and your hands on your hips. Step one leg back and then lower it until it is 90 degrees to the ground. Step forward to the starting position. Repeat on the other side to complete the movement.

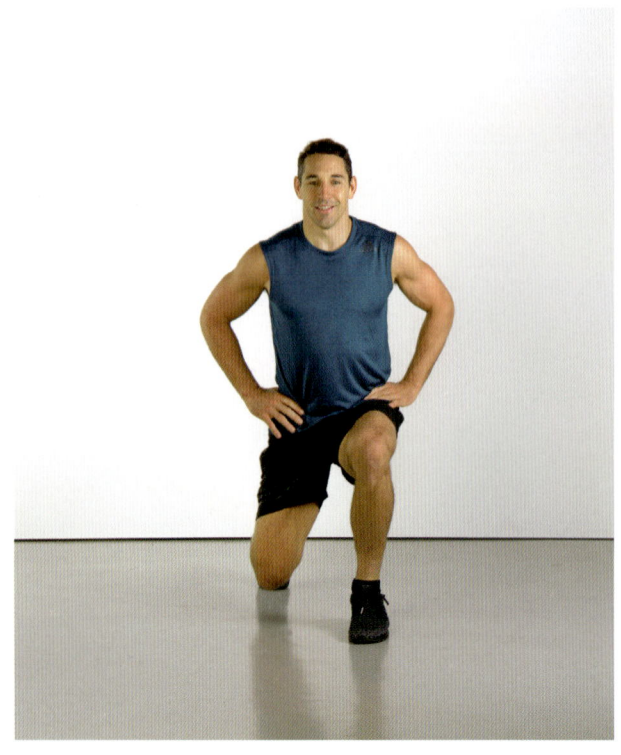

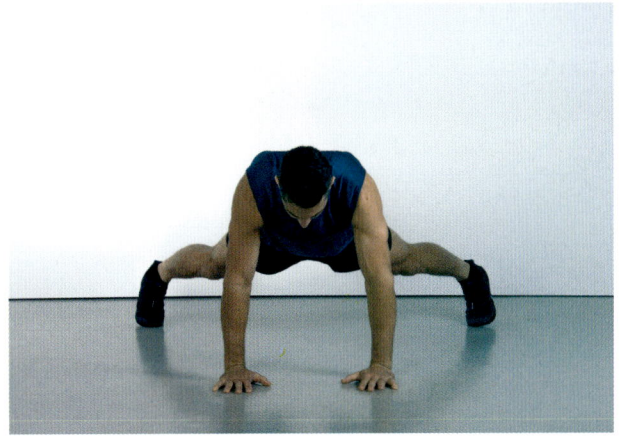

7 Jump sprawls

Stand with your feet just past shoulder-width apart, then jump forward and land softly on both feet before going into a sprawl. Squat until both your hands and both your feet are firmly on the ground. From this position, transfer your weight into your shoulders and shoot your feet back so that your legs are out wide, then jump your feet back up and return to the starting position.

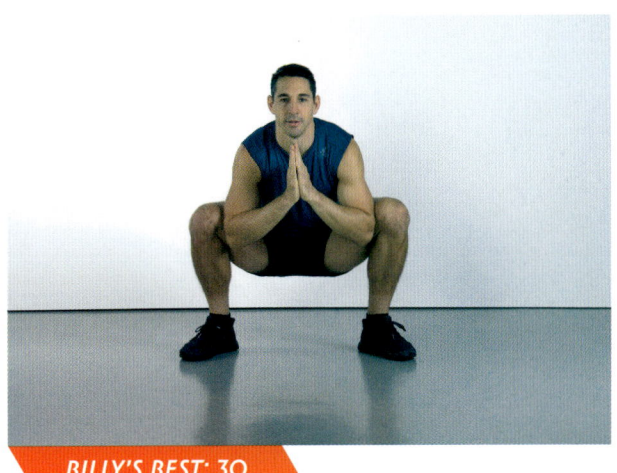

BILLY'S BEST: 30

8 Frog squats

Stand with your feet shoulder-width apart and your feet slightly tracked out. Bend down to full squat position with your elbows tucked inside your legs. This is the starting position. From here, raise your hips and then lower them back to the starting position.

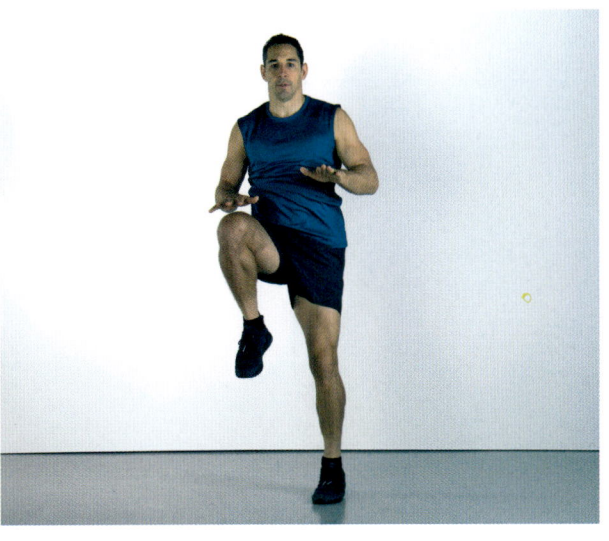

9 High knees

Stand with your feet shoulder-width apart. One leg at a time, raise your left knee up as high as you can before alternating to the other leg.

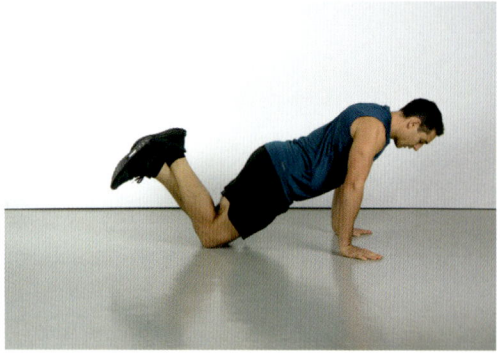

10 Planche push-ups

Start in an assisted (top images) or full push-up position with your hands slightly tracked out. Lean forward so that your arms are straight and you are comfortable. From here, lower yourself until your chest is just off the ground, and then press back up. You should feel this movement in your shoulders and biceps.

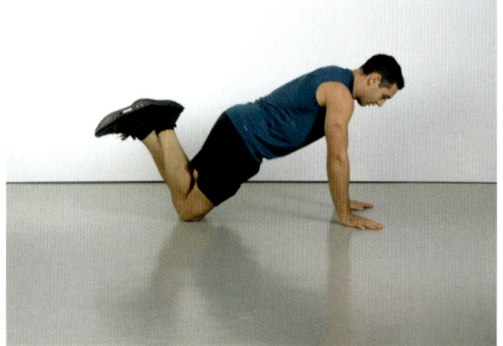

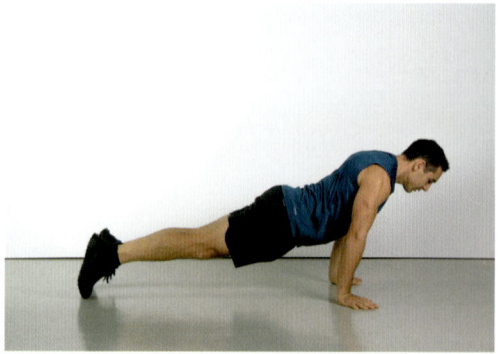

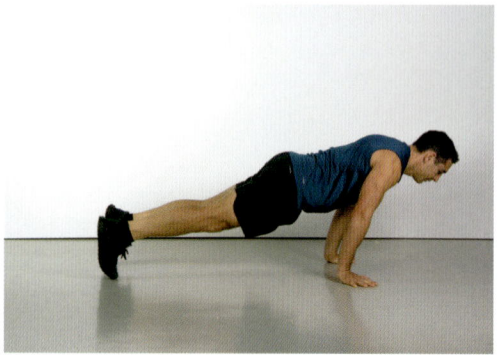

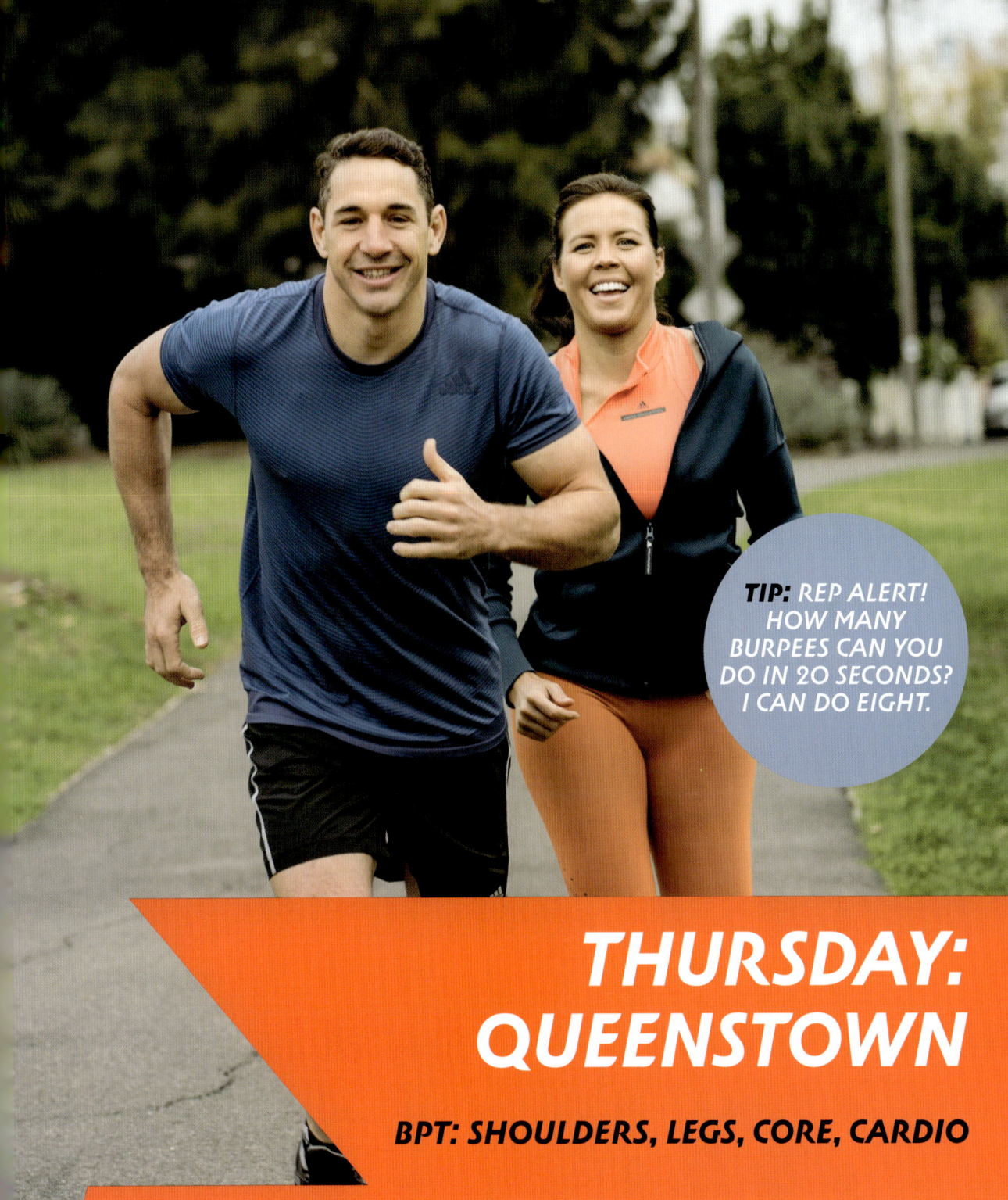

TIP: *REP ALERT! HOW MANY BURPEES CAN YOU DO IN 20 SECONDS? I CAN DO EIGHT.*

THURSDAY: QUEENSTOWN

BPT: SHOULDERS, LEGS, CORE, CARDIO

10-MINUTE WORKOUT

20 seconds movement /
10 seconds rest
2 sets of each exercise
(one lap)

20-MINUTE WORKOUT

20 seconds movement /
10 seconds rest
2 sets of each exercise
(two laps)

30-MINUTE WORKOUT

20 seconds movement /
10 seconds rest
2 sets of each exercise
(three laps)

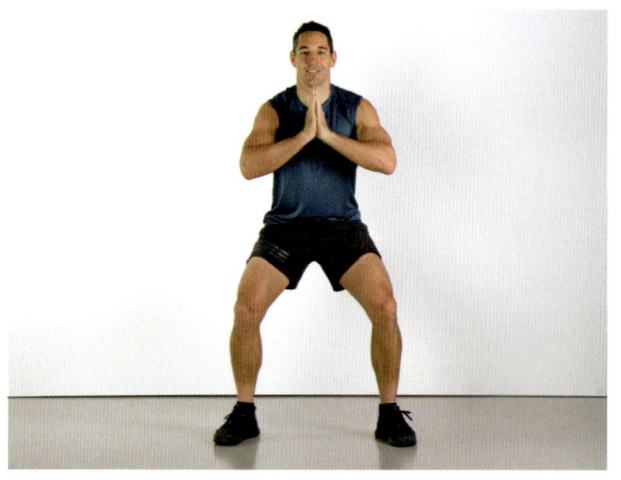

1 Pulse squats
Stand with your feet just past shoulder-width apart and slightly tracked out. Squat with your hips back and your legs at a 90-degree angle, then pulse up and down.

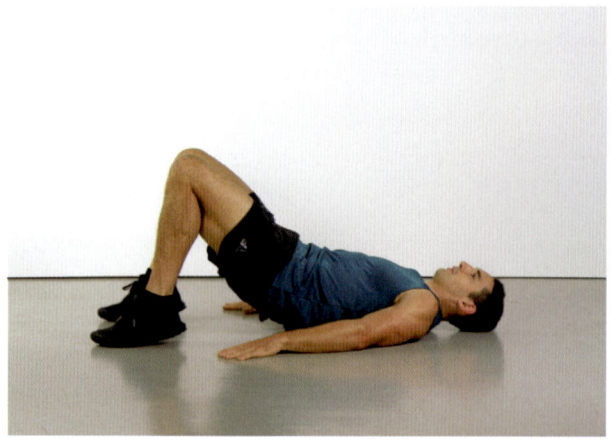

2 Double-leg glute bridge
Lie on your back with your hands on your hips or with your arms straight or beside your body on the ground and your palms facing down. Bring your heels as close as you can to your butt, raising your hips and pressing down on the balls of your feet. Squeeze your butt cheeks (glutes) before lowering yourself down. Don't allow yourself to collapse – stay tight through your core and make sure your butt doesn't hit the ground.

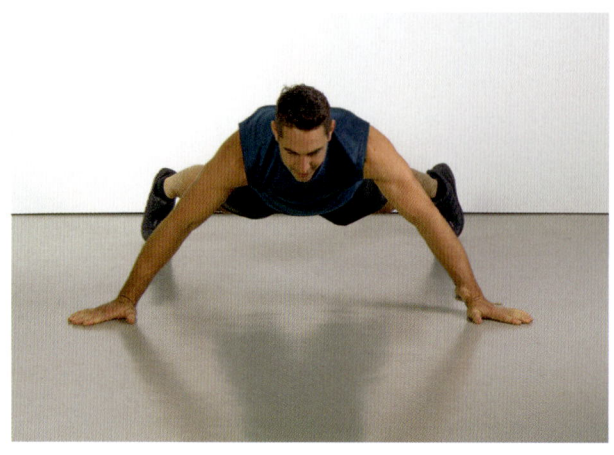

3 Spider-Man holds
Start in a high plank position but with your hands out nice and wide and your legs as wide as your hands. From here, raise your knees and lean forward slightly, engaging your core and squeezing your glutes. You should also feel this movement in your biceps and shoulders.

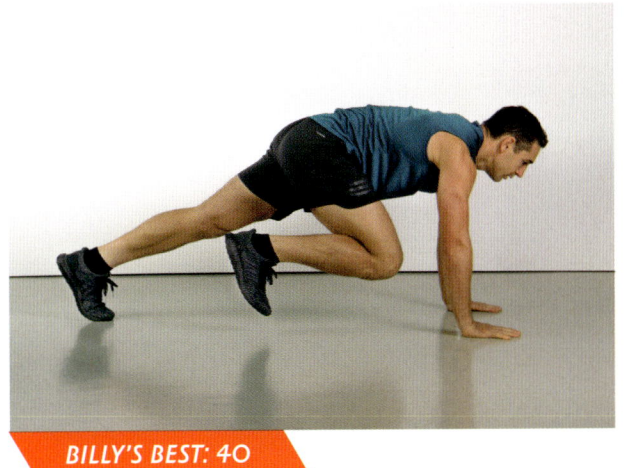

BILLY'S BEST: 40

4 Mountain climbers

Start in a high plank position, with your shoulders over your wrists, your feet together and your core engaged. From here, bring one knee up towards your chest and then return it to the starting position. Repeat on the other side.

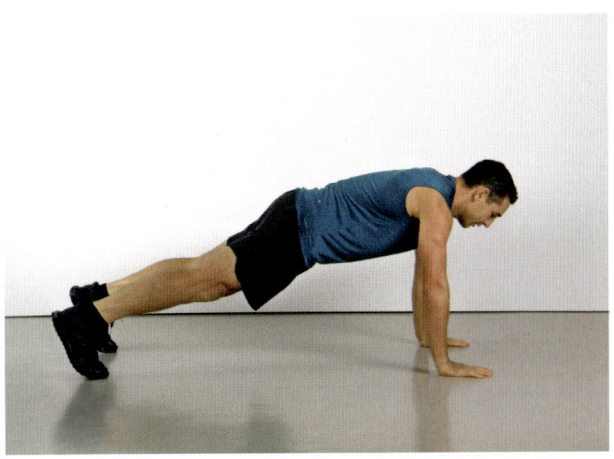

5 Burpees

Stand in a relaxed position with your feet shoulder-width apart. Squat and place your hands firmly on the ground with your feet back. Shoot your legs back so you are in a high plank position, then lower your body so your torso is just touching the ground. Release your hands and then, placing your hands back on the ground, raise your torso and jump your feet back so both hands and both feet are on the ground. Stand back up, then jump up and raise your hands above your head.

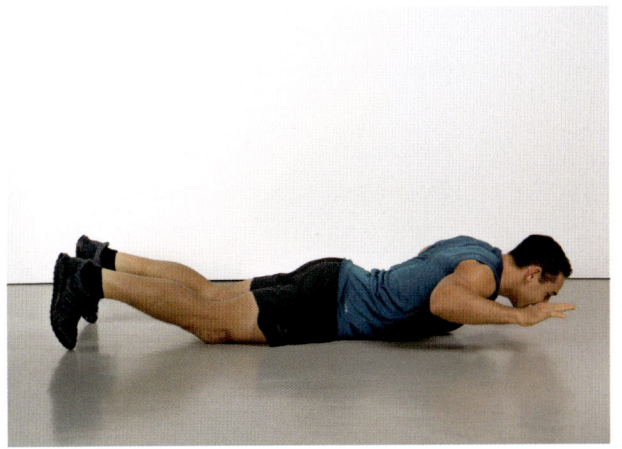

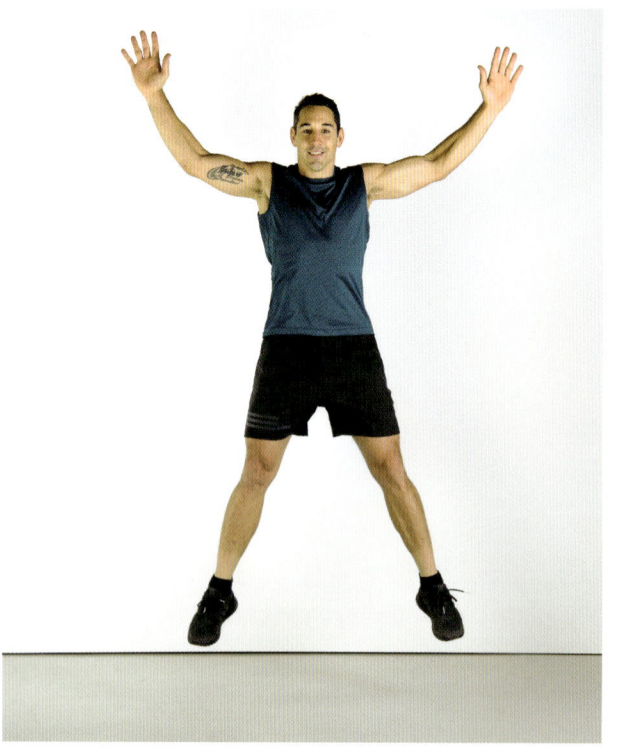

6 Star jumps

Begin in a relaxed stance with your arms close to your body. Jump your feet out wide past shoulder-width and raise both your arms above your head, then land back in the starting position.

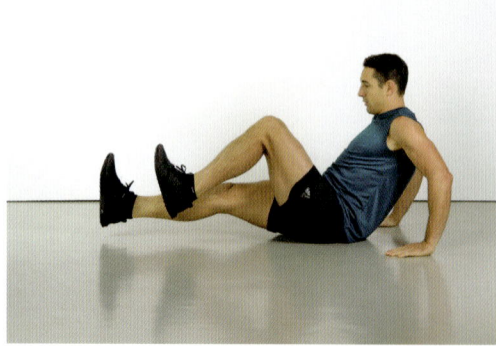

7 Bicycle crunches

Start by sitting on the ground with your hands on the floor by your side and your legs extended in front of you. From here, lean back, engaging your core so your feet are off the ground. Now bring one knee towards your chest, keeping the other leg straight. Return your knee to the earlier position and swap to bring your other knee towards your chest.

Advanced: Take your hands off the ground and bring the opposite elbow to your knee.

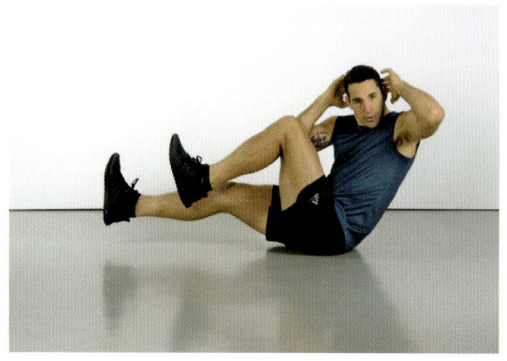

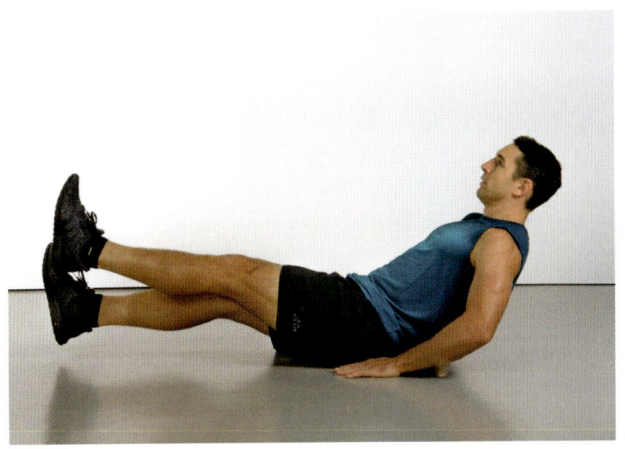

8 Flutter kicks

Starting position is lying on your back with your thumbs tucked under your lower lumbar (base of your back) on either side of your body. Raise your legs and kick them up and down in a small fluttering motion, engaging your core.

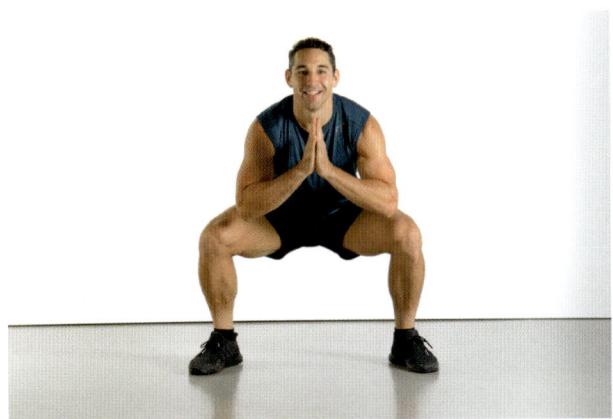

9 Squat kick-outs

Stand with your feet shoulder-width apart and slightly tracked out. Bend at the hips and bring your butt towards the ground so your knees are at a 90-degree angle. Explode back up to standing position, crossing one foot in front of the other and tapping the heel of your front foot in front of the toe of your back foot. Return to the starting position and repeat with your other foot in front.

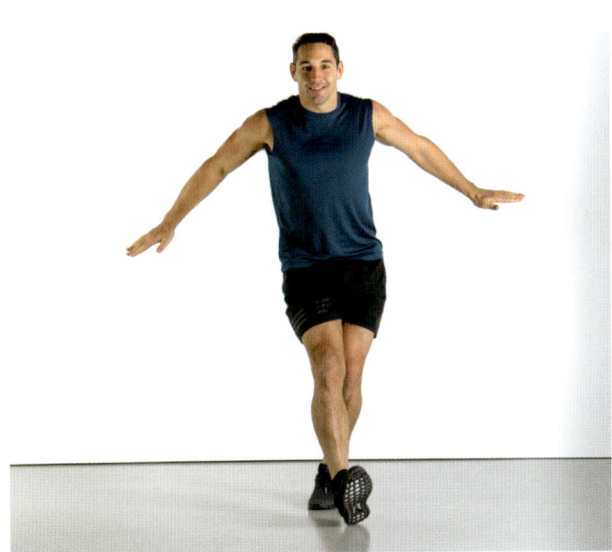

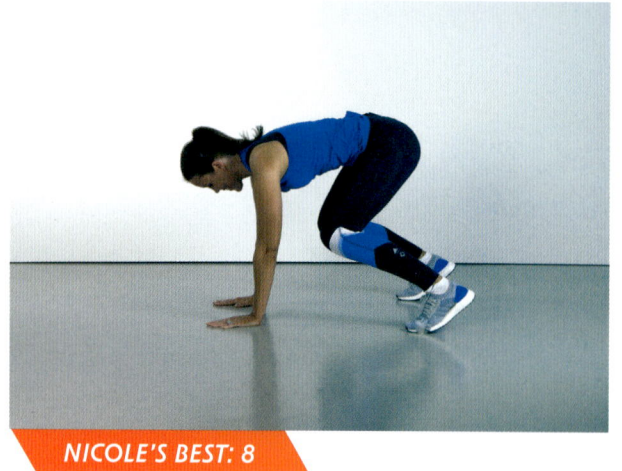

NICOLE'S BEST: 8

10 **Sprawls**

Stand with your feet shoulder-width apart, then squat until both your hands and both your feet are firmly on the ground. From this position transfer your weight into your shoulders and shoot your feet back so that your legs are out wide, then jump your feet back up and stand up into the starting position.

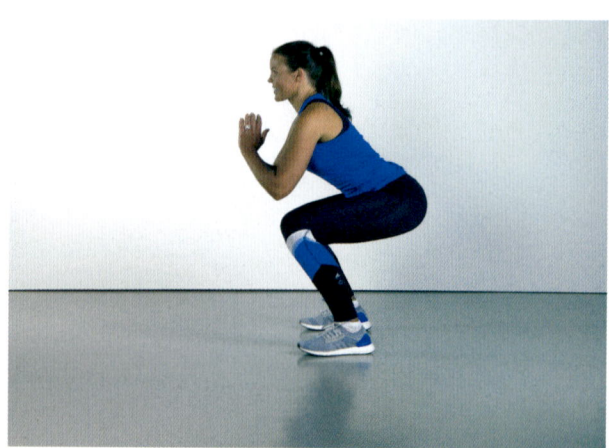

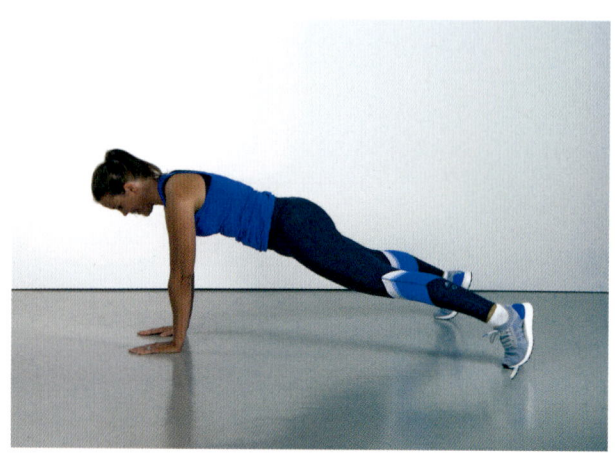

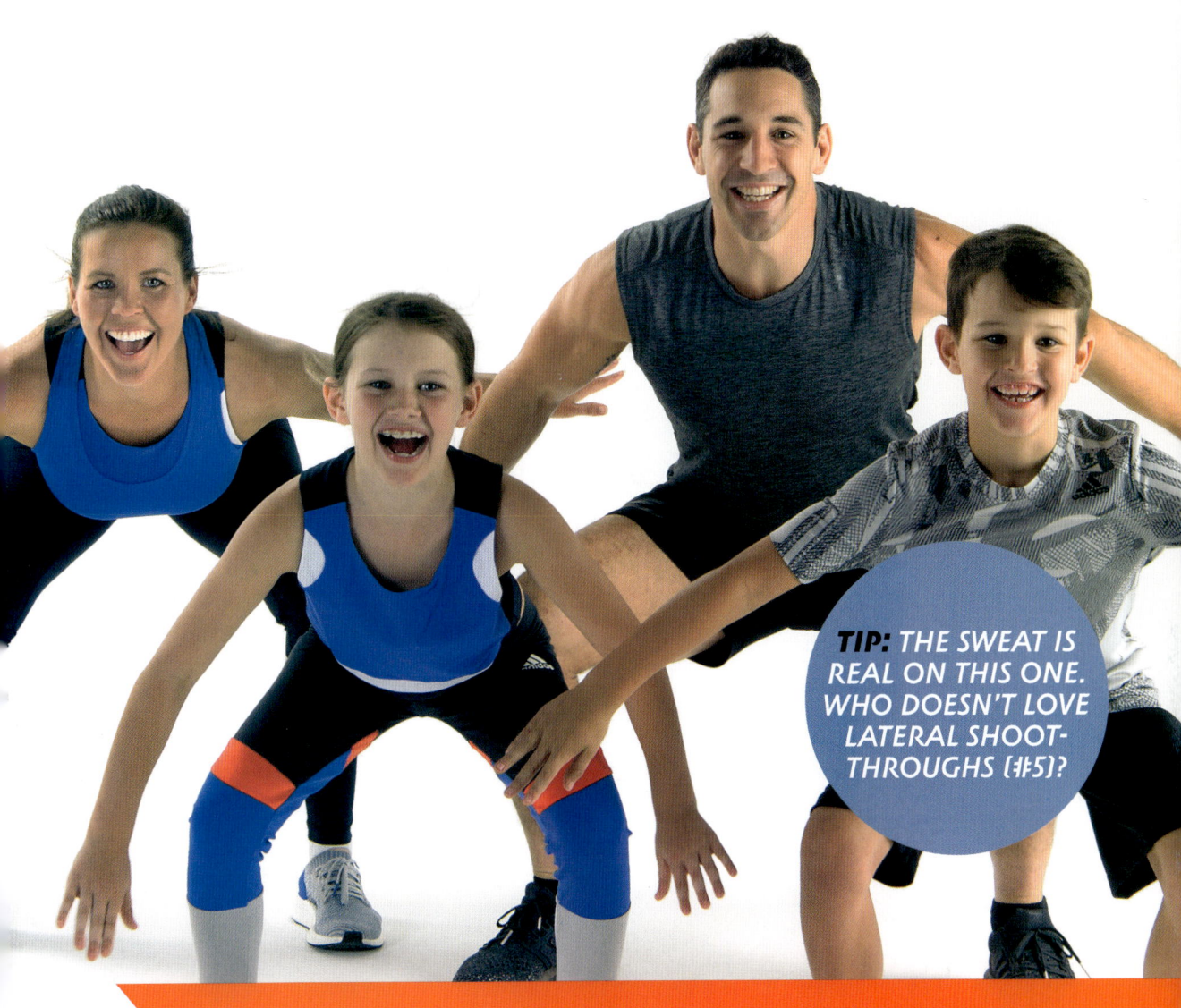

TIP: THE SWEAT IS REAL ON THIS ONE. WHO DOESN'T LOVE LATERAL SHOOT-THROUGHS (#5)?

FRIDAY: MOUNT MAUNGANUI

BPT: ALL-OVER CARDIO

10-MINUTE WORKOUT

20 seconds movement /
10 seconds rest
2 sets of each exercise
(one lap)

20-MINUTE WORKOUT

20 seconds movement /
10 seconds rest
2 sets of each exercise
(two laps)

30-MINUTE WORKOUT

20 seconds movement /
10 seconds rest
2 sets of each exercise
(three laps)

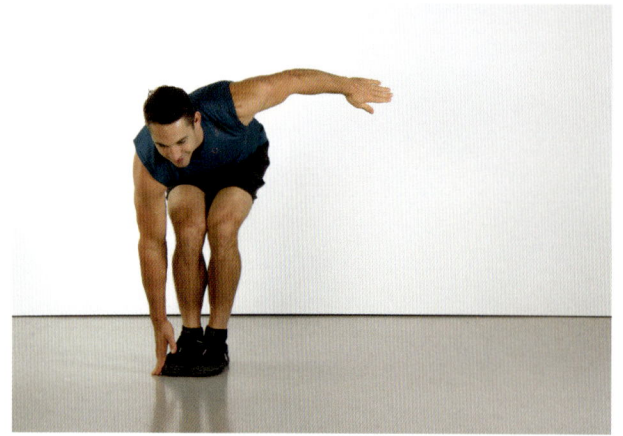

1 Slalom taps

Start with your feet together, then jump to the left to land on both feet, touching your left hand down next to your left foot. Then jump to the right with both feet, touching your right hand to your right foot.

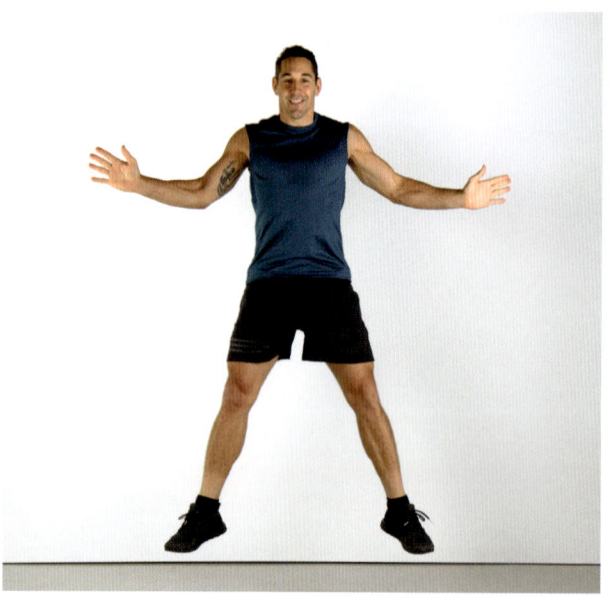

2 Seal jacks

Starting in a relaxed position with your hands touching together in the middle of your chest, jump out so your feet are in a wide stance and your arms split. Bring your feet and hands back together.

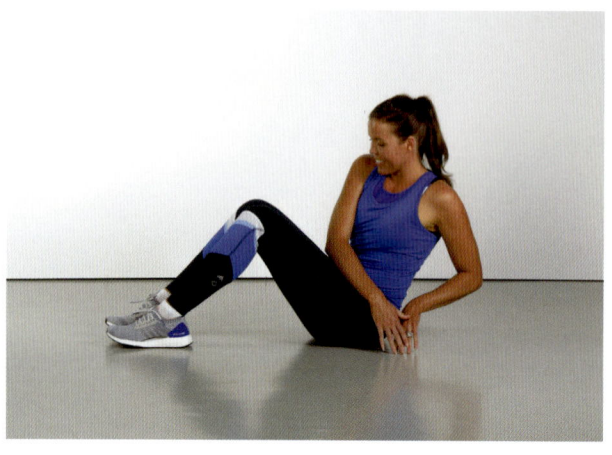

3 Russian twists

Sit on the ground with your knees bent and your feet flat on the ground. Clasping your hands in front of your chest, twist your torso to one side and touch the ground, engaging your core. Then shift your weight and twist your torso to touch the ground on the other side.

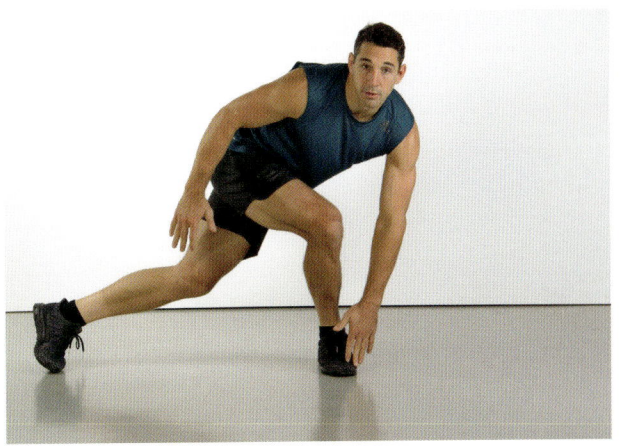

4 Ice skaters

Start with your feet shoulder-width apart. Step half a foot to your left, swing your right leg behind your left leg, and with your right hand touch your left toe. From here, step to your right, swing your left leg behind your right leg, and with your left hand touch your right toe.

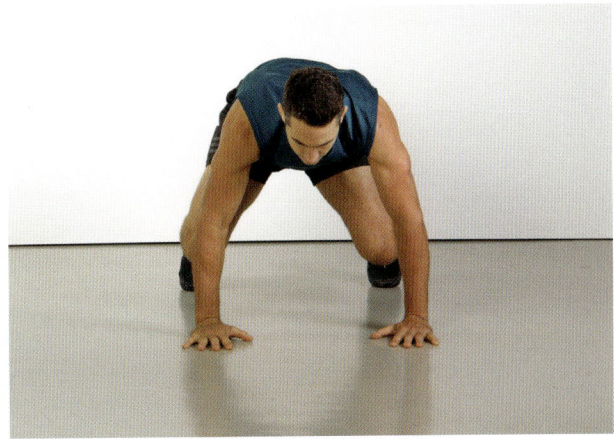

5 Lateral shoot-throughs

Start in high plank position with your hands firmly on the ground and your shoulders above your wrists. Bend your knees at a 90-degree angle and have your toes firmly on the ground and your knees off the ground. This is the starting position. Now turn your left foot so it is flat on the ground. Kick your right foot in front of your left foot and out to the side, so your right leg is now straight and your left foot is firmly on the ground. Now pull your right leg back to the starting position. Repeat on the other side.

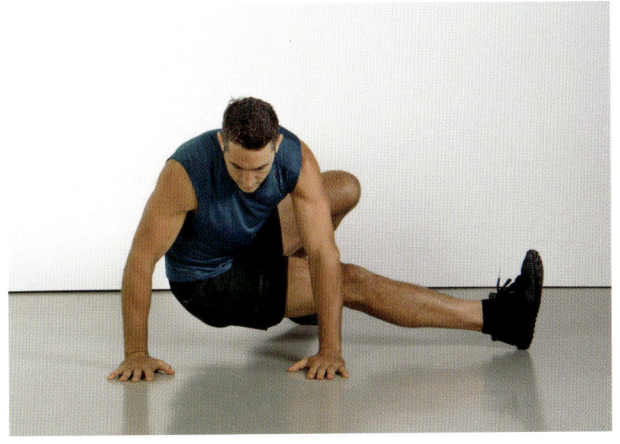

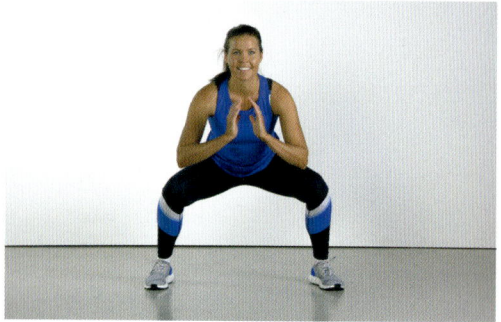

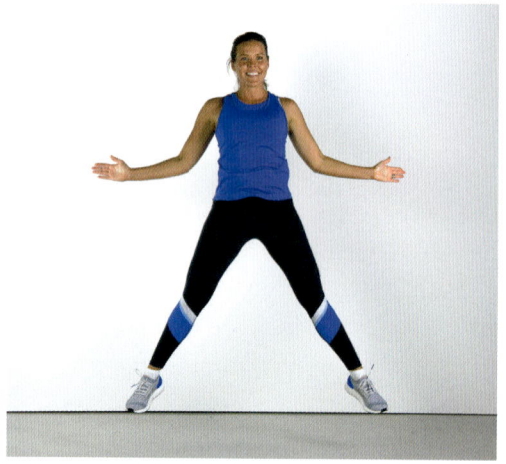

6   In/out jump squats

Stand with your feet just past shoulder-width apart and your hands touching in front of your chest. Squat so your knees are bent and arms are straight and out to the side. Then explode up, bringing your feet together and your arms out to your sides before returning to the starting position.

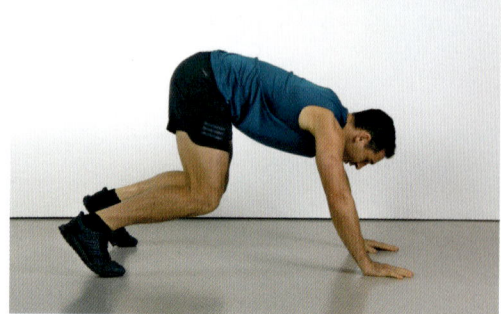

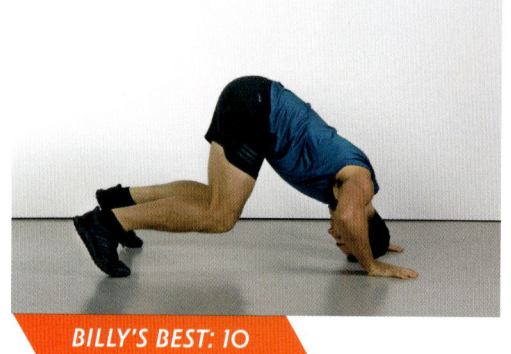

7   A-frame push-ups

Stand with your feet wide apart and slightly tracked out. With your hands shoulder-width apart, and bending at the hips, lean over to touch the ground with your legs straight or bent and your chin slightly tucked. From this starting position, lower yourself down till the top of your head is just off the ground and you're looking through your legs. Your head should be in line with your hands. From here, press back up to the starting position, transferring all the weight into your palms.

BILLY'S BEST: 10

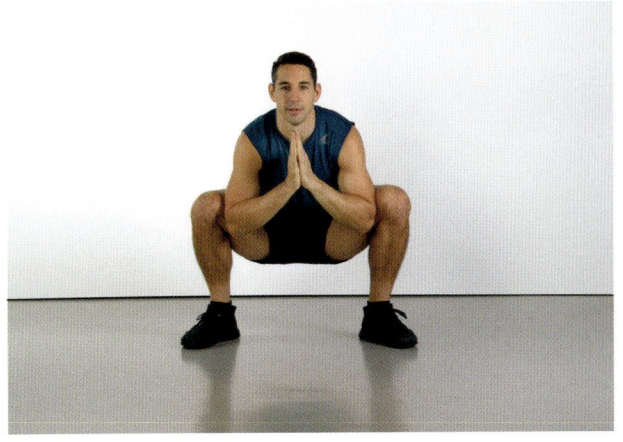

8 Frog squats

Stand with your feet shoulder-width apart and your feet slightly tracked out. Bend down to full squat position with your elbows tucked inside your legs. This is the starting position. From here, raise your hips and then lower them back to the starting position.

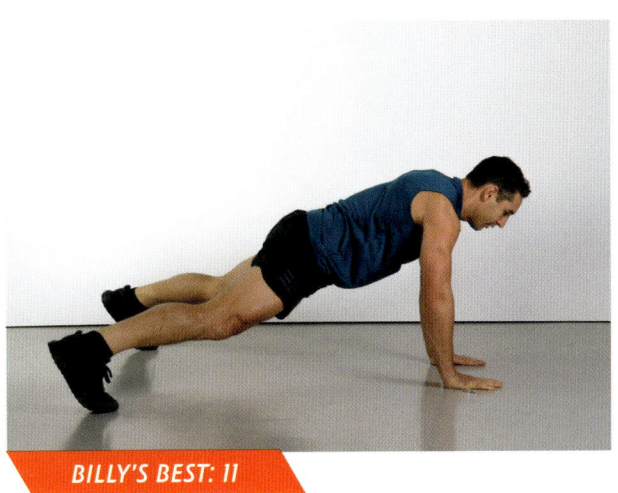

BILLY'S BEST: 11

9 Sprawls

Stand with your feet shoulder-width apart, then squat until both your hands and both your feet are firmly on the ground. From this position transfer your weight into your shoulders and shoot your feet back so that your legs are out wide, then jump your feet back up and stand up into the starting position.

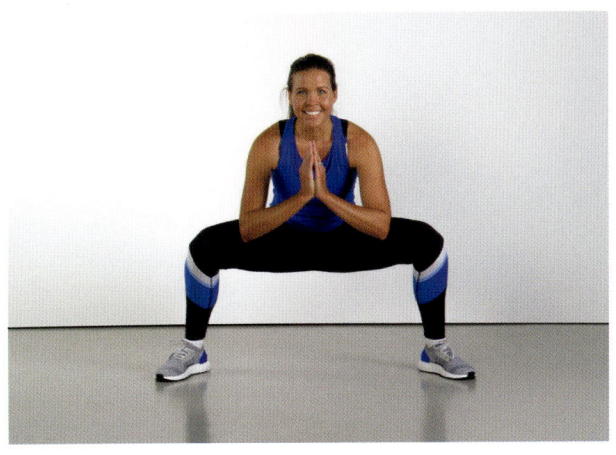

10 Sumo squats

Stand with your feet wide apart and slightly tracked out, and your hands on your hips. Bend at the hips lower your butt towards the ground, bending your knees and keeping your shoulders back and your chest tight. Lower yourself down as far as is comfortable. Return to starting position.

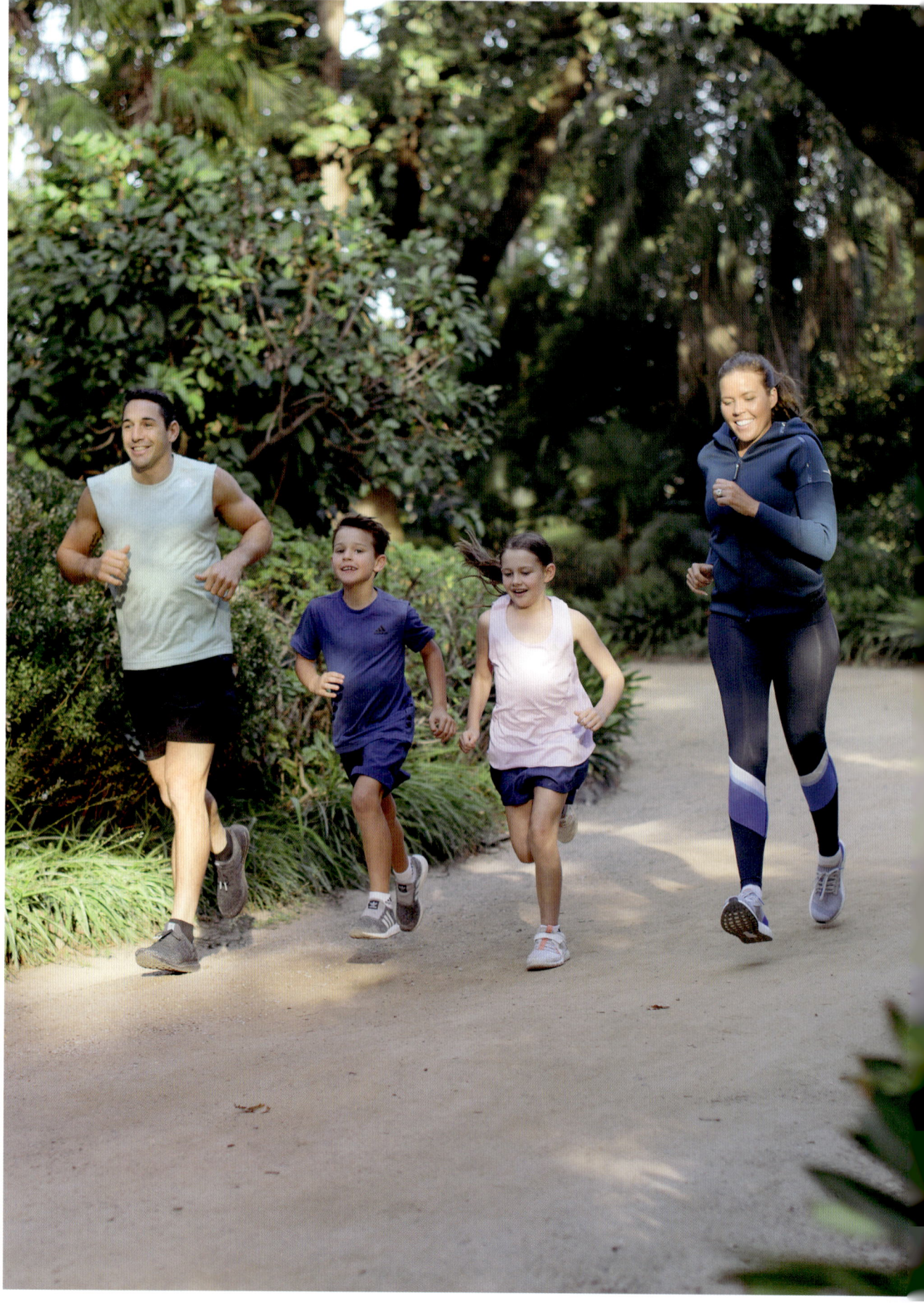

Acknowledgements

I have thoroughly enjoyed bringing this project together. I am passionate about health, fitness and the positive life outcomes they can bring.

Firstly, I must say that I had a lot of support from some very key people to bring this fantastic project to life.

Nicole, my beautiful wife. Thanks for doing the burpees, lunges and many other new exercises with me. It was great to get fitter together and always with a big smile and lots of laughs.

To our kids, Tyla and Jake, we could not be any prouder of you both. Your energy, fun attitude and constant smiles are what it's all about.

To Mike, our superb mentor, coach and trainer for *MOVE*: you inspired us to want to run a bit more, jump a little more and to push ourselves (but to always have fun doing it).

To the film and camera crew, massive shout-outs for your professionalism, patience (at times) and strong commitment to helping us deliver such a great finished book.

Lastly, to my management team, SFX, who have always been there to guide, manage and ensure that what you see before you is the best that it can be.

I hope that you enjoy moving and being healthier with your family and friends.

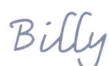